A Concise Guide to The Management of Vitiligo

Rashmi Sarkar • Vignesh Narayan R
Editors

A Concise Guide to The Management of Vitiligo

Springer

Editors
Rashmi Sarkar
Department of Dermatology, Venereology and Leprology
Lady Hardinge Medical College and Hospitals
New Delhi, Delhi, India

Vignesh Narayan R
Department of Dermatology, Venereology and Leprology
New Varalakshmi Hospital
Bangalore, Karnataka, India

ISBN 978-981-95-3856-0 ISBN 978-981-95-3857-7 (eBook)
https://doi.org/10.1007/978-981-95-3857-7

This Springer imprint is published by the registered company Springer Nature Singapore Pte Ltd.
The registered company address is: 152 Beach Road, #21-01/04 Gateway East, Singapore 189721, Singapore

Contents

About the Editors

Rashmi Sarkar is working as the director professor in the Department of Dermatology and Venereology at Lady Hardinge Medical College and Associated SSK and KSC Hospitals, New Delhi, India, affiliated with Delhi University. Previously, she has also worked as a professor at Maulana Azad Medical College, New Delhi, and assistant professor, Government Medical College, Chandigarh, India, and served as an examiner for MD, Diploma, and PhD in Dermatology and DNB. With an H Index of 45 and a research gate score 39.0, she has published over 260 papers in peer-reviewed national and international journals, over 120 chapters in various books, and edited 24 books. She is a global leader in pigmentary disorders.

Vignesh Narayan R has completed his fellowship in Dermatologic Surgery at Bangalore Medical College and Research Institute, Bangalore, India. His areas of interest include pigmentary disorders and dermatologic surgery. He has published many papers in peer-reviewed national and international journals. He had served as the editor-in-chief of the ResiDream Magazine of the Indian Association of Dermatologists, Venereologists, and Leprologists (IADVL) National residents committee and the IADVL YUVA Cell.

Part I
Basic Science

Chapter 1
Introduction to Management of Vitiligo

Vignesh Narayan R and Rashmi Sarkar

Abstract Vitiligo affects approximately 0.5% of the global population, with prevalence peaks in specific regions. Historically misdiagnosed as leprosy, it has carried significant social stigma since ancient times. The earliest reference to vitiligo appears in the Iranian text "Tarkh e Tibble" (2200 BC), and the term was first used by the Roman physician Celsus. Social ostracism associated with vitiligo persists, necessitating patient reassurance about the disease's nature.

Vitiligo's pathophysiology involves the progressive loss of melanocytes, leading to depigmented patches. It is classified into segmental, non-segmental, focal, mixed, and indeterminate types, with segmental vitiligo typically presenting earlier. Theories of vitiligo's aetiology include neurogenic, self-destruction, and autoimmune hypotheses. Differentiating vitiligo from other hypopigmentary disorders is essential for accurate diagnosis.

Wood's lamp examination and biopsy support diagnosis and differentiation. Non-segmental vitiligo often exhibits a pattern of abrupt onset, stability, and rapid evolution, with rare spontaneous repigmentation. Segmental vitiligo, frequently involving hair follicle melanocytes, responds better to surgical treatments.

Management requires a comprehensive approach, addressing medical, psychological, and social aspects. Therapeutic options include aggressive treatments like steroids and JAK inhibitors for rapidly progressing cases, and various surgical techniques for stable disease. Advances in topical therapies and light-based treatments offer hope for improved outcomes.

In summary, vitiligo, an ancient disease now better understood, requires a holistic management approach integrating medical, psychological, and social support to improve patient outcomes and quality of life. Ongoing research promises more personalized and effective treatments for those affected by vitiligo.

V. Narayan R
Department of Dermatology, Venereology and Leprology, New Varalakshmi Hospital, Bangalore, Karnataka, India

R. Sarkar (✉)
Department of Dermatology, Venereology and Leprology, Lady Hardinge Medical College and Hospitals, New Delhi, Delhi, India

R. Sarkar, V. Narayan R (eds.), *A Concise Guide to The Management of Vitiligo*,
https://doi.org/10.1007/978-981-95-3857-7_1

Keywords Introduction · Vitiligo

1.1 Introduction

Vitiligo affects people worldwide, with an overall prevalence of about 0.5%, though certain areas show higher peaks [1]. As Hippocrates noted, "The physician must know what his predecessors have known if he does not deceive both himself and others".

Vitiligo, an ancient disease, has only recently begun to be understood. The earliest reference to vitiligo can be found in an ancient Iranian text, "Tarkh e Tibble", dating back to 2200 BC. Historically, vitiligo was often mistaken for leprosy, leading to significant social stigma. The term "Zaraath" from the Old Testament, which means leprosy, reflects this confusion. The first recorded use of the term "vitiligo" was by the Roman physician Celsus in his book "De Medicina". Derived from the Latin word "vitium", meaning blemish, the term aptly describes the condition [2].

Social stigma has plagued vitiligo patients since ancient times. Historically, individuals with vitiligo were often ostracized, forbidden from ordination, marriage, or entering cities, and were forced to wear tattered clothes and have dishevelled hair. Although these associations have persisted into modern times, patients need reassurance about the true nature of the disease [3].

In the nineteenth century, it was discovered that vitiligo often appears at sites of trauma in affected individuals. Later, it became clear that vitiligo is characterized by the acquired and progressive loss of melanocytes from the skin, resulting in depigmented patches. This understanding led to attempts at classifying the disease based on distribution and proposed aetiology. The three major aetiological theories are the neurogenic theory, the self-destruction theory, and the autoimmune theory. The disease can be broadly classified into segmental, non-segmental, focal, mixed, and indeterminate types. It exhibits a polygenic and multifactorial inheritance pattern, with segmental vitiligo typically having an earlier onset. Clinical observations and genetic associations suggest the existence of various vitiligo phenotypes. Although the classification of the disease into subtypes based on initial area of involvement, extension, and major recognizable patterns is common, there is a lack of scientific evidence to classify them as distinct diseases. Focal vitiligo, for instance, does not clearly fit into segmental or non-segmental categories [4].

It is important to note that not all white patches are vitiligo. Certain conditions, such as inherited or genetically induced hypomelanosis, present at birth, can be mistaken for vitiligo, especially in individuals with lighter skin tones. An example of such a condition is piebaldism. Additionally, hypopigmentation following inflammation must be differentiated from the Koebner phenomenon seen in vitiligo. Other conditions that need differentiation include para-infectious hypopigmentation, such as pityriasis versicolor, which presents with scaling, and indeterminate leprosy, which presents with hypoesthesia. Vitiligo-like depigmentation can also occur following occupational exposure to phenolic derivatives or as a side effect of chemotherapeutic drugs [5].

Wood's lamp examination is useful in identifying areas of depigmentation and early repigmentation after therapy. In darker skin types, a pattern known as multichrome vitiligo, displaying various degrees of depigmentation within a vitiliginous macule, can be observed. Biopsy plays a crucial role in supporting various theories concerning vitiligo development. Pathologists need to be vigilant as the lesions can be easily overlooked. Diagnosis mainly relies on clinical findings rather than histopathology, but histopathological examination is sometimes necessary to differentiate vitiligo from other hypopigmentary disorders like leprosy and mycosis fungoides [6].

Non-segmental vitiligo typically follows a natural course of abrupt onset, periods of stability, and rapid evolution. Spontaneous repigmentation is rare and often results from sunlight exposure. Rare clinical subtypes include inflammatory vitiligo, multichrome vitiligo, vitiligo minor, and blue vitiligo [7].

Classifying segmental vitiligo as a separate entity helps establish its prognosis. It frequently involves hair follicle melanocytes, making it resistant to medical therapies but often responsive to surgical treatments. Patients with universal vitiligo, which affects more than just the skin, are at risk of autoimmune diseases and sunburn. Treatment for these patients often aims at depigmenting small areas of residual pigmentation [8].

An interesting finding in vitiligo patients is the increased incidence of halo nevi. The proposed theory is that the depigmented ring surrounding the nevus is the initial immunological response, which later extends to the surrounding skin. Although distinct pathways have been proposed, they often overlap in certain subsets of patients [9].

Hair follicles serve as reservoirs of melanocytes and are sometimes lost in vitiligo, which can be distressing for patients seeking treatment. Therapeutic techniques include hair follicle and melanocyte transplantation. In some cases, vitiligo patients may experience loss of non-skin melanocytes, such as those in the iris, anterior chamber, and choroid. Subtle abnormalities in hearing and brainstem auditory responses may be seen in patients with otic melanocytic involvement. In diseases like Vogt-Koyanagi-Harada syndrome, there is a loss of leptomeningeal melanocytes [10].

Although vitiligo is considered an autoimmune disease, the association with other autoimmune disorders varies widely based on patient ethnicity. Some associations may simply represent the coexistence of two disorders. Thyroid disorders are common in Caucasian and Indian populations, while alopecia areata is more prevalent in Chinese populations [11].

Vitiligo affects both children and adults, with differences in prevalence and presentation. Children tend to have a higher prevalence of segmental type, halo nevi, family history of vitiligo, and associated autoimmune diseases. The lack of long-term follow-up studies makes childhood vitiligo a grey area, but early diagnosis often correlates with better treatment outcomes. Similarly, late-onset vitiligo occurs in patients over 50 years old, with non-segmental phenotypes being more common.

The increasing human lifespan has led to renewed interest in this condition. Possible causes include the senescence of melanocytes and the immune system [12].

Thorough assessment and evaluation of patients with vitiligo are crucial during the initial consultation. This involves assessing the extent of the disease in terms of body surface area involved and the activity of depigmentation. Several tools are available for this purpose, including the Vitiligo Extent Tensity Index (VETI), Vitiligo Area Scoring Index (VASI), and Vitiligo Disease Activity (VIDA) scores. Additionally, subjective tools that evaluate the impact on quality of life are essential in guiding treatment interventions and providing appropriate support [13].

Patients with vitiligo often face significant social challenges. Society tends to treat individuals with vitiligo differently, subjecting them to stares, whispered comments, social isolation, and antagonism. This can lead to feelings of embarrassment, discomfort, and anxiety about the disease. These issues are particularly pronounced in patients with lesions in visible areas such as the face, or sensitive areas like the genitals. The socio-economic and educational impacts are also considerable, as patients may need to take time off for therapy. Childhood trauma associated with vitiligo can have lasting effects on activities and self-esteem [14].

Effective management of vitiligo involves a holistic approach, considering not just the affected patches but the patient as a whole. Key factors include the patient's skin colour, tanning ability, disease duration, and activity. In patients with non-segmental vitiligo experiencing a phase of rapid progression, aggressive therapies such as mini-pulse steroid therapy and Janus kinase (JAK) inhibitors may be used. These can be combined with therapies promoting repigmentation, such as ultraviolet (UV)-based treatments. However, light-based therapies pose challenges, including the need for frequent visits and the necessity to tailor the dose for different treatment sites while shielding areas with a lower minimal erythema dose [15].

Topical therapies can be effective for localized disease and are often combined with light-based treatments. They typically result in a more diffuse pattern of repigmentation compared to the perifollicular type seen with light-based therapies. Agents like topical calcineurin inhibitors are advantageous as they can be used on non-light-exposed sites and promote repigmentation without causing immunosuppression. Emerging treatment options include prostaglandin analogues, band-pass filters, and topical JAK inhibitors [16].

Surgical techniques for repigmentation are suitable for patients with stable vitiligo, particularly those with the stable subtype. Treatment options range from micropigmentation, which provides immediate results, to cell and tissue grafting techniques. The choice of technique depends on the disease location, type, patient age, and the availability of facilities and expertise [17].

Vitiligo, though an ancient disease, is now being more thoroughly understood thanks to advancements in dermatological research. Historically misdiagnosed and socially stigmatized, vitiligo presents not only a medical challenge but also significant psychosocial impacts on patients. The disease affects approximately 0.5% of the global population and can manifest in various forms, including segmental, non-segmental, and mixed types. Recent discoveries about the disease's aetiology, including its autoimmune components and genetic predispositions, have paved the way for more effective classification and management strategies.

Comprehensive patient assessment, involving tools like the VETF, VASI, and VIDA scores, alongside considerations of quality of life, is crucial for effective management. Advances in therapeutic options, from topical and light-based therapies to emerging pharmacological treatments and surgical interventions, provide hope for improved outcomes. The integration of medical, psychological, and social support is essential in addressing the holistic needs of patients with vitiligo. As research continues to unveil the intricacies of this condition, the future holds promise for more personalized and effective treatments, ultimately enhancing the quality of life for those affected by vitiligo.

Acknowledgement None

Conflicts of Interest None

Source of Funding None

Ethics Statement N/a

References

1. Gandhi K, Ezzedine K, Anastassopoulos KP, Patel R, Sikirica V, Daniel SR, et al. Prevalence of vitiligo among adults in the United States. JAMA Dermatol. 2022;158(1):43–50.
2. Joge RR, Kathane PU, Joshi SH. Vitiligo: a narrative review. Cureus. 2022;14(9):e29307.
3. Millington GW, Levell NJ. Vitiligo: the historical curse of depigmentation. Int J Dermatol. 2007;46(9):990–5.
4. Faraj S, Kemp EH, Gawkrodger DJ. Patho-immunological mechanisms of vitiligo: the role of the innate and adaptive immunities and environmental stress factors. Clin Exp Immunol. 2022;207(1):27–43.
5. Delgado P, Crumpton K. A practical guide to vitiligo differential diagnoses in primary care. Nurse Pract. 2021;46(11):29–36.
6. Mazzei Weiss ME. Vitiligo: to biopsy or not to biopsy? Cutis. 2020;105(4):189–90.
7. Bae JM, Jung YS, Jung HM, Park JH, Hann SK. Classification of facial vitiligo: a cluster analysis of 473 patients. Pigment Cell Melanoma Res. 2018;31(5):585–91.
8. AlGhamdi KM, Kumar A. Depigmentation therapies for normal skin in vitiligo universalis. J Eur Acad Dermatol Venereol. 2011;25(7):749–57.
9. Ezzedine K, Diallo A, Léauté-Labrèze C, Seneschal J, Mossalayi D, AlGhamdi K, et al. Halo nevi association in nonsegmental vitiligo affects age at onset and depigmentation pattern. Arch Dermatol. 2012;148(4):497–502.
10. Lotti T, D'Erme AM. Vitiligo as a systemic disease. Clin Dermatol. 2014;32(3):430–4.
11. Sawicki J, Siddha S, Rosen C. Vitiligo and associated autoimmune disease: retrospective review of 300 patients. J Cutan Med Surg. 2012;16(4):261–6.
12. Dogra S, Parsad D, Handa S, Kanwar AJ. Late onset vitiligo: a study of 182 patients. Int J Dermatol. 2005;44(3):193–6.
13. Feily A. Vitiligo extent tensity index (VETI) score: a new definition, assessment and treatment evaluation criteria in vitiligo. Dermatol Pract Concept. 2014;4(4):81–4.

14. Bidaki R, Majidi N, Moghadam Ahmadi A, Bakhshi H, Sadr Mohammadi R, Mostafavi SA, et al. Vitiligo and social acceptance. Clin Cosmet Investig Dermatol. 2018;11:383–6.
15. Hamzavi IH, Lim HW, Syed ZU. Ultraviolet-based therapy for vitiligo: what's new? Indian J Dermatol Venereol Leprol. 2012;78(1):42–8.
16. Rodrigues M, Ezzedine K, Hamzavi I, Pandya AG, Harris JE. Current and emerging treatments for vitiligo. J Am Acad Dermatol. 2017;77(1):17–29.
17. Thakur V, Narayan RV, Parsad D. Transplantation procedures in vitiligo: what's new. Dermatol Rev. 2022;3(5):276–83.

Chapter 2
Melanocyte and Melanogenesis

Anuradha Bishnoi, K. B. Meghana, and Davinder Parsad

Abstract Melanocytes are pigment-producing cells derived from neural crest cells and are responsible for the color of skin. They also have an important role in protection from UV rays. There are multiple steps involved in the synthesis of melanin pigment. Any congenital or acquired defects in the pathway and enzymes involved in the pathway cause pigmentary disorders. The rate of synthesis of melanin, size, and distribution of melanosomes are all involved in the pathogenesis of pigmentary disorders. This chapter explores the development, function, and regulatory mechanisms of melanocytes, as well as the pathogenesis of melanocyte-related disorders.

Keywords Melanocyte · Melanogenesis · Pigment · Tyrosinase · α-MSH · Eumelanin · Pheomelanin

2.1 Introduction

Melanocytes are specialized cells with a dendritic morphology that produce melanin pigment which is responsible for the color of the skin. They migrate to the basal layer of the epidermis and hair follicles, playing a crucial role in determining skin and hair color during fetal development. Additionally, the melanin protects the skin from UV damage and possesses immune functions crucial for maintaining skin health. The regulation of pigmentation involves a complex interplay of intrinsic signals within melanocytes and external factors. The ability of melanocytes to regenerate facilitates variable restoration of skin and hair pigmentation following different types of insults. This chapter explores the biology of melanocytes, tracing their origin and lifecycle and examining their roles in skin pigmentation through processes such as melanogenesis. It further delves into the regulation of melanin synthesis and the implications of melanocyte behavior in various disease conditions.

A. Bishnoi (✉) · K. B. Meghana · D. Parsad
Department of Dermatology, Venereology and Leprology, Postgraduate Institute of Medical Education and Research, Chandigarh, India

R. Sarkar, V. Narayan R (eds.), *A Concise Guide to The Management of Vitiligo*,
https://doi.org/10.1007/978-981-95-3857-7_2

2.2 Origin and Life Cycle of Melanocytes

Melanocytes are embryonically derived from neural crest cells. Neural crest cells start as multipotent cells but progressively adopt lineage-specific roles during development. These cells are categorized into four distinct regional populations: cranial, vagal, trunk, and sacral. Melanocytes primarily derive from cranial and trunk neural crest cells [1]. In humans, cranial neural crest cells give rise to melanocytes found in the head region, while those in the rest of the body originate mainly from trunk neural crest cells. Apart from melanocytes, cranial neural crest cells also form the skeletal framework, muscles, and dermis of the head [2]. Based on embryonic migratory theory, trunk neural crest cells segregate into two groups: dorsally and ventrally migrating cells. Conventionally, dorsolaterally migrating cells are considered the primary origin of melanocytes, whereas ventrally migrating cells contribute to the development of the peripheral nervous system and adrenal medulla [3].

Melanoblasts are the melanocyte-specific progenitor cells that originate from the neural crest cells and develop into melanocytes through several stages of growth, division, and maturation. After their specification, melanoblasts continue to proliferate and migrate to their ultimate locations in the epidermis and hair follicles, a step vital for their correct distribution within the skin. Subsequently, they differentiate and begin to produce melanin pigment. While migrating through the dermis towards the epidermis and hair follicles, melanoblasts gradually activate a series of genes involved in melanin production, many of which are regulated by the transcription factor MITF. Maturation of melanocytes is a critical process where melanoblasts evolve into fully functional melanocytes. A key aspect of this maturation/differentiation is the activation of tyrosinase, an enzyme essential for melanin synthesis [1].

This process typically occurs between 6 and 8 weeks of embryonic development, with the majority localizing to the epidermis by 12–13 weeks [4]. Commonly identified *molecular markers* for melanocyte precursors include the tyrosine kinase receptor KIT (c-kit), transcription factors such as MITF, SOX10, Pax 3, and the melanogenic enzyme tyrosinase-related protein (TYRP-2). Key *growth factors* that regulate melanocyte development from neural crest cells include endothelins, stem cell factor (SCF) as the ligand for c-kit, Wnt proteins, and neuregulin-1 [5]. The early differentiation process of melanocytes is governed by the Wnt/β-catenin pathway [6]. A key transcription factor known as Mi, initially discovered in the microphthalmia (mi) mutant, exhibits a relatively specific role in promoting melanocyte differentiation. Mi corresponds to the MITF transcription factor, which plays a crucial role in regulating various genes specific to melanocytes [7].

Throughout an individual's life, melanocytes can undergo cycles of activation and dormancy, influenced by genetic factors, hormonal changes, and environmental exposure, which affect melanin production and distribution, thus impacting skin coloration and response to sunlight. Melanocytes generally exhibit low proliferative activity under normal physiological conditions in adult skin. They are long-lived cells that maintain their population mainly through longevity rather than active proliferation. However, under certain conditions, such as exposure to ultraviolet (UV) light, inflammatory processes, or hormonal changes, melanocytes can be stimulated to proliferate. Additionally, pathological conditions like vitiligo or melanoma can also affect the proliferation rates and behavior of melanocytes.

2.3 Epidermal Melanin Unit

Melanocytes are present in the basal layer of the epidermis. "Epidermal melanin unit" as described by Fitzpatrick and Breathnach in 1963, consists of melanocytes together with surrounding epidermal cells [8]. The ratio of melanocytes to keratinocytes is 1: 10 in the epidermal basal layer, which is consistent throughout life. Three dimensionally, a single melanocyte supplies melanosomes to approximately 36 keratinocytes [9].

Approximately 1200 melanocytes are present per square millimeter of skin, regardless of an individual's racial background [10]. Adhesion molecules like E-cadherin, P-cadherin, and desmogleins facilitate binding between melanocyte and keratinocytes. These connections between the dendritic processes of mature melanocytes and keratinocytes are essential for stabilizing the melanocytes and transferring melanin into keratinocytes, which determines skin color and contributes to photoprotection [11]. Melanin granules are present above the nucleus of keratinocytes and are shed along with the epidermal cells. Defective E-cadherin expression has been postulated to lead to melanocytorrhagy in vitiligo.

The epidermal melanin units are consistent across different human races but vary in the organization of melanocytic dendrites and the intensity of melanogenesis. Studies have shown that darker skin has higher tyrosinase activity, leading to increased melanin production compared to lighter skin, with differences in pigmentation also attributed to the catalytic efficiency of tyrosinase and other proteins such as tyrosinase-related protein-1 and dopachrome tautomerase involved in the process of melanin synthesis also called melanogenesis [12, 13].

2.4 Hair Follicle Melanocytes

Melanocytes are situated in the proximal *bulb* of each hair follicle [14]. The bodies of bulbar melanocytes are present at the apex of the dermal papilla, with their dendrites extending between cortical and medullary keratinocytes [15]. The ratio of melanocytes to keratinocytes in this region is 1:5, denser than in the epidermis [16]. Follicular pigmentation results from complex interactions among follicular melanocytes, matrix keratinocytes, and dermal papilla fibroblasts, collectively known as the *hair melanin unit*.

Similar to the epidermis where melanosome phagocytosis from melanocytes to keratinocytes is mediated by the PAR2 receptor on keratinocytes, melanin granules are transported to keratinocytes within the growing hair shaft. However, differences arise in the degradation and quality of melanosomes [16]. Hair follicle melanocytes have shorter lifespans and undergo apoptosis at the end of the hair cycle, which lasts over 3–8 years. Melanogenesis occurs exclusively during the anagen phase of the hair growth cycle; pigment synthesis ceases during the catagen phase and is absent in the telogen phase [14]. During the catagen phase, fully differentiated bulbar melanocytes undergo apoptosis, while new melanocytes originate from melanoblasts located in the hair *bulge* [15].

2.5 Melanogenesis

The process of melanin synthesis is known as melanogenesis. Melanin exhibits various beneficial properties for the body, including absorption and scattering of UV light, scavenging of free radicals, involvement in oxidation-reduction reactions, and storage of ions. Two distinct forms of melanin, pheomelanin and eumelanin, are produced, each following a different synthesis pathway and yielding a different color. The specific type of melanin synthesized depends on the substrates available and the activity of enzymes involved in melanogenesis [17].

Tyrosinase (TYR) catalyzes the hydroxylation of tyrosine to L-3,4-dihydroxyphenylalanine (DOPA), which rapidly oxidizes to DOPAquinone [18]. In the presence of cysteine, DOPAquinone reacts to form 3- or 5-cysteinyl DOPAs, which are further oxidized and polymerize to produce yellow-red soluble melanin, known as pheomelanin. In the absence of thiols such as "cysteine, glutathione, or thioredoxin," DOPAchrome is formed leading finally to the production of brown-black eumelanin [19]. When the carboxylic acid in the DOPAchrome is spontaneously lost, 5,6-dihydroxyindole (DHI) is produced. DHI-melanin is insoluble and dark brown to black eumelanin. On the other hand, DOPAchrome will produce DHI-2-carboxylic acid (DHICA) if DOPAchrome tautomerase (TYRP2/DCT) is present. Further conversions are catalyzed by tyrosinase and TYRP1 to produce DHICA-melanin, which is lighter brown eumelanin [19] (Figure 2.1).

Overall pigmentation and color of the skin in an individual is partially determined by the ratio of the various forms of melanin present in human skin [20]. Pheomelanin is found in both light and dark skin types. Skin color is determined by the ratio of eumelanin to total melanin [21]. Eumelanin offers superior photoprotection compared to pheomelanin because it is more resistant to degradation and has a greater ability to neutralize reactive oxygen species (ROS). Because of this, lighter skin has a 30–40-fold increased chance of developing skin cancer compared to darker skin [19]. Products of melanogenesis, especially the intermediate molecules in this process, like quinones and hydrogen peroxide, are inherently cytotoxic. To mitigate this, melanocytes localize melanogenesis within melanosomes and elevate the production of anti-apoptotic proteins such as Bcl-2 [22].

Melanogenesis takes place in melanosomes, lysosomes like structures in melanocytes. There are four stages of development of melanosomes [23] (Fig. 2.2):

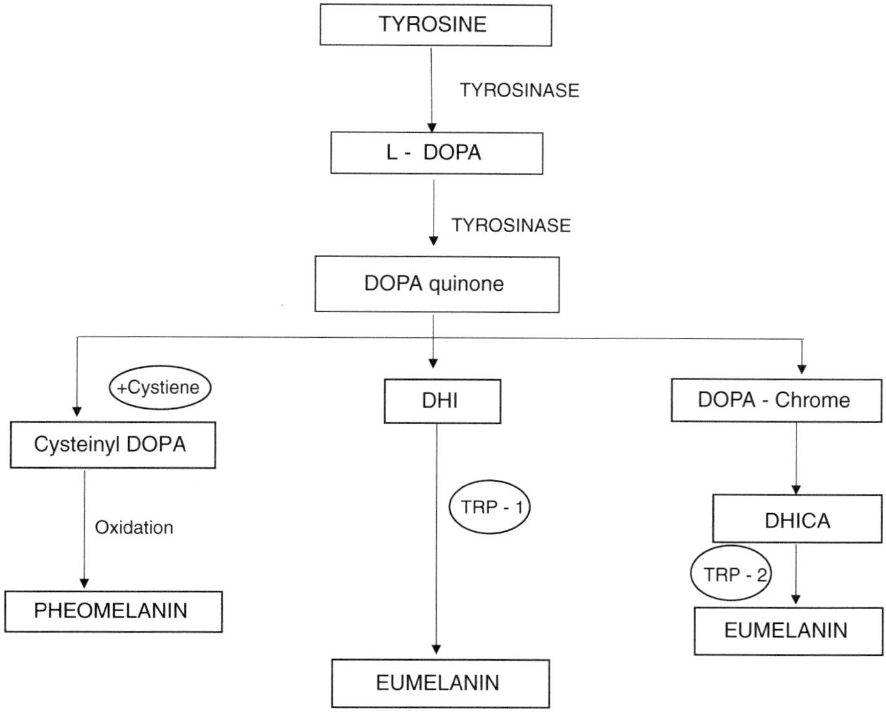

Fig. 2.1 Melanin synthesis pathway. DHI (5,6-dihydroxyindole); TRP-1 (tyrosinase-related protein 1); L-DOPA (L-dihydroxyphenylalanine); tyrosinase-related protein 2 (TRP-2), also known as dopachrome tautomerase; DHICA 5,6-dihydroxyindole-2-carboxylic acid

- Phase 1: Small dots or vesicles in amorphous matrix.
- Phase 2: Fibril matrix structures have developed, and tyrosinase is present, although melanin synthesis has not started.
- Phase 3: Beginning of melanin production and pigment deposition on fibrils.
- Phase 4: Whole melanosome is filled with pigment. Tyrosinase activity is lost.

Individuals with lighter skin tones have melanosomes predominantly in stages I and III within their melanocytes, whereas melanosomes in keratinocytes are generally in stage III. In lighter-skinned individuals, melanosome degradation is faster, and there are typically fewer than 20 melanosomes per cell. Conversely, individuals with darker skin tones typically possess melanosomes predominantly in stage IV. Melanosomes within keratinocytes also tend to be in stage IV and exhibit slower mobility. The average number of melanosomes per cell is generally over 200 [24]. Studies have identified various genes, such as MC1R, TYR, OCA2, and SLC24A5, that influence human skin pigmentation and contribute to normal physiological variation in skin color. Variants in the MC1R gene are linked to lighter skin, red hair, and freckles in populations of European ancestry. MC1R influences the balance between eumelanin and pheomelanin [25, 26].

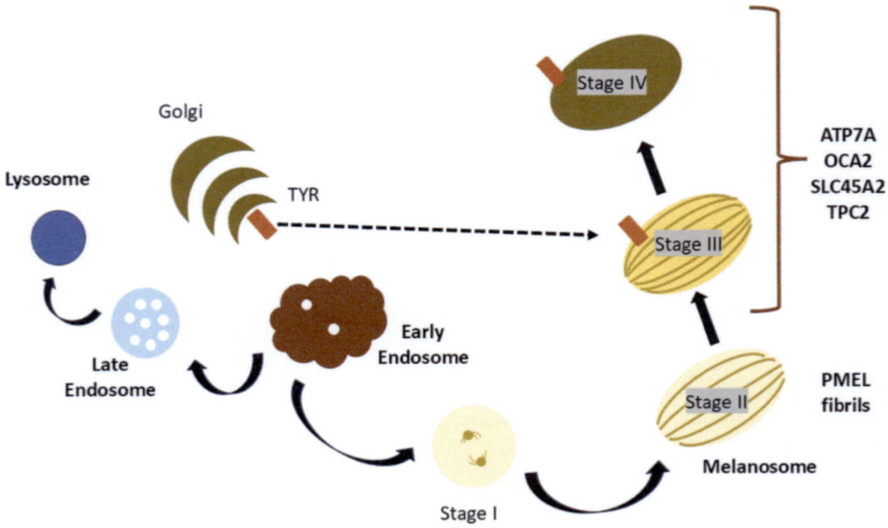

Fig. 2.2 Melanosome development

2.5.1 Transfer of Melanosomes

There are three proposed theoretical mechanisms to explain melanosome transfer [27]:

1. Direct inoculation of melanosomes into keratinocytes via nanotubular membrane filopodia.
2. Phagocytosis pathway where melanocytes release melanosomes that are subsequently engulfed by keratinocytes.
3. Partial cytophagocytosis involves the transfer of melanosomes to keratinocytes through the tips of melanocyte dendrites containing melanosomes in close proximity to keratinocytes.
4. Ando et al.'s model of melanosome transfer [28]:

   - Membrane-bound pigment globules (PG) containing multiple melanosomes and a few mitochondria are generated within the filopodia of melanocyte dendrites.
   - These PGs are released from various regions of the dendrites into the extracellular space.
   - Subsequently, microvilli on keratinocytes capture these PGs in a protease-activated receptor-2 (PAR-2) pathway-dependent manner.
   - The membrane-surrounded PGs undergo degradation, releasing individual melanosomes into the cytosol of keratinocytes, where they migrate to the perinuclear area.

Defects in these pathways may lead to pigment dilution disorders such as Hermansky–Pudlak Syndrome (HPS) and Chediak–Higashi Syndrome (CHS).

Hermansky–Pudlak Syndrome (HPS) is a group of autosomal recessive disorders characterized by hypopigmentation and platelet storage disease, caused by defects in intracellular protein trafficking systems affecting melanosomes and platelet granules. Chediak–Higashi Syndrome (CHS), also marked by hypopigmentation, includes severe immunological defects, lymphoproliferative disorder, and neuropathies, with large lysosomes and cytoplasmic granules as key diagnostic features, resulting from mutations in the CH1 gene. Griscelli syndrome is linked to defects in Rab27a, myosin Va, or melanophilin proteins, disrupting melanosome transport and uptake, leading to melanosome accumulation in melanocytes [29].

2.6 Regulation of Melanin Synthesis

The production of melanin in an individual is influenced by various factors, including enzyme activity levels, transport mechanisms, and the relative proportions of proteins involved in melanogenesis. Key proteins regulating the transition between eumelanin and pheomelanin include "α-MSH, agouti signaling protein (ASIP), endothelin-1, basic fibroblast growth factor (bFGF)," along with external factors such as UVR.

Melanocortin receptors (MC-Rs) are integral membrane proteins consisting of seven transmembrane domains and are coupled with G-proteins. There are five subtypes known as "MC1-R, MC2-R, MC3-R, MC4-R, and MC5-R." [30] These receptors are encoded by genes located on chromosome 16 and play a central role in regulating pigmentation. MC-Rs are expressed in various cell types including melanocytes, melanoma cells, monocytes, endothelial cells, and keratinocytes. MC-R agonists include melanocyte-stimulating hormone (α-MSH) and adrenocorticotropic hormone (ACTH), both of which are derived from the cleavage of proopiomelanocortin (POMC). POMC is broken down by carboxypeptidase-1 into ACTH and β-lipotrophin, and by carboxypeptidase-2 into β-endorphin and ACTH. ACTH is further cleaved into ACTH 1–17 and α-MSH.

Activation of MC1R leads to the activation of adenylyl cyclase, which initiates the production of cyclic AMP (cAMP) [31]. This process results in the phosphorylation of CREB (cAMP responsive-element-binding protein) family of transcription factors. CREB, in turn, promotes the transcription of various genes, including MITF (microphthalmia-associated transcription factor), a critical regulator of pigment enzymes and differentiation factors [32].

Alpha-melanocyte-stimulating hormone (α-MSH) activates intracellular protein kinase C (PKC) and regulates tyrosinase, a key enzyme in melanin biosynthesis. PKC, a serine/threonine kinase, participates in various cellular processes such as growth factor signaling, cellular transformation, and differentiation. This enzyme resides in the cytoplasm and gets activated by inositol triphosphate-diacylglycerol (IP3-DAG). The expression of different forms of PKC (PKC-α, β, ε, Δ, and ξ) induces alterations in melanocyte activity. PKC-β upon activation helps in phosphorylation of tyrosinase [33]. Catecholamines enhance melanogenesis by activating the cAMP/PKA pathway through stimulation of β2 adrenergic receptors. Additionally, the α1 adrenergic receptor can trigger the IP3/DAG pathway, which raises intracellular levels of PKC-β and activates tyrosinase, further influencing melanin production [34].

Growth factors like SCF, GM-CSF, and hepatocyte growth factor (HGF) activate signaling pathways mediated by their respective receptors: c-KIT, GM-CSFR, and HGFR leading to autophosphorylation and activation of MAP kinase. This process phosphorylates MITF and upregulates the expression of melanogenesis-related enzymes. [35] The WNT signaling pathway activates the MITF-M promoter, thereby enhancing MITF expression to regulate melanogenesis further [36] (Fig. 2.3).

Melanocytes produce POMC peptides, prostaglandins, cytokines, leukotrienes and nitric oxide, influencing keratinocytes through autocrine or paracrine signaling, playing roles in immune and inflammatory responses. Keratinocytes also respond to UVR by releasing factors that affect melanocytes, either stimulating or inhibiting melanogenesis [37]. The primary melanogenic effect of α-MSH is an increase in the eumelanin-to-phaeomelanin ratio, which explains the skin-darkening effect observed in humans. α-MSH's influence on melanogenesis is mediated through tyrosinase by enhancing both its expression and activation. Higher levels of tyrosinase are essential for eumelanogenesis compared to phaeomelanogenesis [38].

2.6.1 Melanocyte Response to Ultraviolet Radiation (UVR)

Acquired pigmentation is a visible effect of UVR exposure variably perceived as "sunburn" or "sun-tan." Sun sensitivity refers to the skin's response to UVR, characterized by erythema (inflammation) and changes in pigmentation. Immediate tanning, appears 5–10 min post-exposure to UVR, is mainly due to UVA, and goes away minutes or days later. It is caused by the oxidation of pre-existing melanin followed by the redistribution of melanosomes within the epidermis. Delayed tanning, appears 3–4 days after exposure to UVR, goes away within weeks, is due to UVA and mainly UVB radiation, and is caused by a rise in epidermal melanin content, especially eumelanin, which provides photoprotection. UVR stimulates melanocyte proliferation and recruitment, enhances dendrite formation, and promotes the transfer of melanosomes to a supranuclear position in keratinocytes for DNA protection. Simultaneously, UVR elevates the expression of POMC peptides in keratinocytes and boosts the production of melanogenic enzymes and MC1-R in melanocytes. Even at low UVR doses, DNA damage can occur before visible skin alterations appear [39]. UVR, particularly UVB, causes breaks in thymidine-forming cyclobutene dimer formation [40]. DNA damage can itself then act as a trigger in enhancing pigment production.

The inability to tan is attributed to several genetic characteristics that provide insights into the UV-induced pigmentation response. Variants of MC1R, which

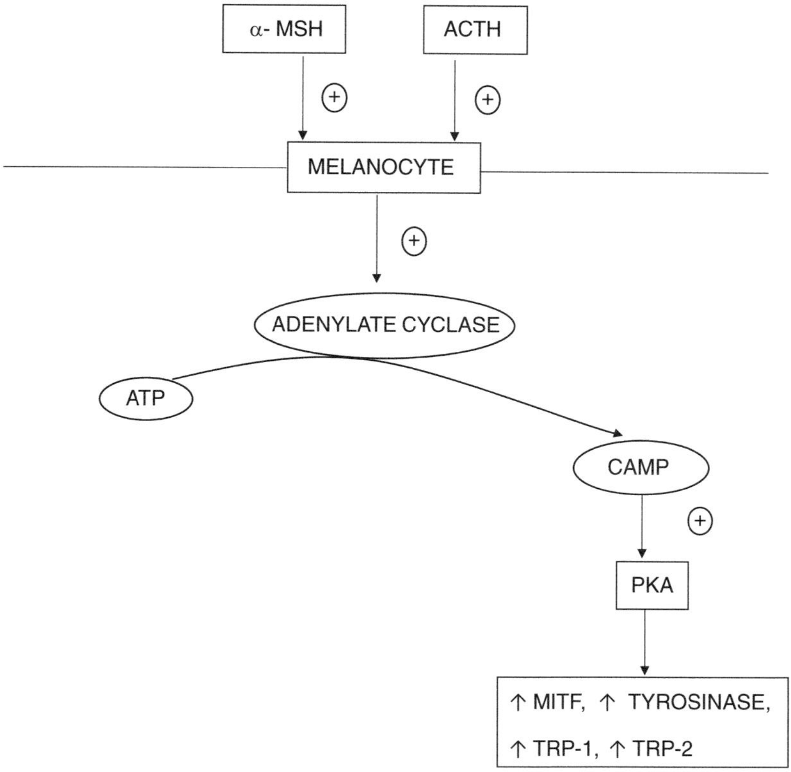

Fig. 2.3 α-MSH and melanocyte pathway

result in a poorly functional receptor due to reduced ligand binding or diminished activation of adenylyl cyclase, are associated with a relative inability to tan (individuals with red hair). Such individuals tend to develop freckles but do not produce a uniform, protective pigment. They also experience heightened susceptibility to sunburn, although the precise mechanisms triggering this response remain unclear [41]. Ephelides/freckles are small, red to light brown spots that appear in childhood, darken in summer, and often fade with age. They are most common on the face, arms, neck, and chest in fair-skinned individuals. In contrast, lentigines are larger, darker spots that typically appear after age 50 on sun-exposed areas. Ephelides have larger, more pigmented melanocytes with extended dendrites and large melanosomes, while SLs show thicker epidermis, elongated rete ridges, and hyperpigmented keratinocytes. Unlike ephelides, melanocytes in lentigines have normal-sized melanosomes but show more mitochondria and a disrupted dermal-epidermal junction. Although both share increased melanin production, their distinct cellular features suggest they arise from different mechanisms.

Although the presumed mechanism is melanin providing straightforward shielding, our understanding of this process remains incomplete. Variants of MC1R have been linked to heightened risks of melanoma and non-melanoma skin cancers independently of skin pigment, such as in individuals with red hair phenotype [42]. Pheomelanin, a type of pigment associated with blond and red hair, may act as a photosensitizer capable of generating reactive oxygen species upon UV exposure. This property has been linked to increased rates of TUNEL-positive (apoptotic) cells after UV exposure, suggesting that higher production of pheomelanin might contribute to melanoma risk. However, the exact mechanisms underlying this process are not fully understood, and it remains unclear whether pheomelanin is solely a marker of melanoma risk or directly involved in carcinogenesis [43].

2.7 Dermal Melanocytosis and Dermal Pigmentation

During embryonic development, sometimes the migration of melanocytes gets arrested at the epidermal-dermal junction, without reaching basal epidermis. These lesions present at birth characterized by slate gray to bluish color patches in the affected sites due to Tyndall effect. Mongolian spot presents at birth as gray to faint blue patch measuring up to few centimeters, most commonly located in the lumbosacral region. Nevus of Ota presents mostly as unilateral blue to light brown specks of pigmentation distributed along ophthalmic and m axillary division of trigeminal nerve with involvement of conjunctiva. Naevus of Ito is relatively rare and involves the acromioclavicular region and upper chest. Histopathologically, they are characterized by the presence of elongated dendritic melanocytes in the dermis and absence of melanophages [44].

Acquired dermal melanocytosis presents mostly in adult women with bilateral pigmentation similar to nevus of Ota, but the conjunctiva is spared, also known as Hori's nevus. It is also reported rarely in other areas of the face especially the nose, which should be differentiated from post-inflammatory pigmentation seen in chikungunya fever, known as "chik sign." On histopathological examination, post-inflammatory hyperpigmentation contains only dermal melanin and melanophages, with no presence of dermal melanocytes [45].

2.8 Melanocytes and Vitiligo

Vitiligo is the most common acquired pigmentary disorder characterized by depigmented patches. It occurs due to selective loss of melanocytes in the lesional skin. There are many theories for the pathogenesis of the disease. These include autoimmune responses, genetics, oxidative stress, melanocyte detachment mechanisms, and the generation of inflammatory mediators. Both innate and acquired immunity have a role in its pathogenesis. Among these the autoimmunity theory is the most widely accepted one [46]. The innate immune cells such as inflammatory dendritic cells and natural killer cells are activated in the skin of vitiligo patients. These cells may migrate to lymph nodes and present melanocyte antigens to T cells, thus activating adaptive immune responses. Innate cells can directly attack melanocytes by releasing cytokines that attract and activate autoreactive T cells [38]. Antibodies to cytoplasmic and surface melanocytic antigens have been identified in the sera of vitiligo patients. These antibodies may hypothetically cause the destruction of melanocytes through antibody-dependent cellular cytotoxicity and complement-mediated lysis. However, cytotoxic CD8+ T cells, which specifically target melanocytes, are chiefly responsible for the destruction of melanocytes in vitiligo. Melanocytes in vitiligo patients are more susceptible to oxidative damage, and the process of melanogenesis by itself produces a pro-oxidant environment in the skin. Exposure to external factors can also generate oxidative byproducts. Monobenzone, a depigmenting agent used in the treatment of widespread vitiligo, acts by inducing oxidative stress in the melanocytes [47].

The main aim in treatment of vitiligo is to halt the progression of disease by targeting immune system and in aiding repigmentation of the lesions by stimulating melanocytes. Various modalities of treatment are available for the treatment ranging from topical steroids, topical calcineurin inhibitors to systemic steroids and immunomodulators. Topical corticosteroids function through local immunomodulation by binding to the glucocorticoid receptor, which leads to the suppression of gene expression for numerous cytokines such as IL-1, IL-2, IL-3, IL-4, IL-5, IL-6, IL-8, IL-10. IL-13, TNF-α, and interferon-γ, thereby inhibiting the activation of cytotoxic T lymphocytes. Similarly topical calcineurin inhibitors and topical JAK inhibitors act on different pathways ultimately leading to suppression of cytotoxic T lymphocytes. Systemic corticosteroids and other oral immunosuppressants are used in the management of rapidly progressing active vitiligo.

Recently afamelanotide, a synthetic analogue of α–melanocyte-stimulating hormone (α-MSH), (whose circulating levels and in lesional skin were found to be low in vitiligo patients) has been mostly studied as adjuvant therapy mainly with phototherapy in clinical trials. α-MSH functions through the melanocortin-1 receptor, which is typically absent in early-stage melanoblasts. The combined use of NB–UVB phototherapy and afamelanotide facilitated enhanced differentiation of melanoblasts and increased expression of the melanocortin-1 receptor.

Phototherapy is the most efficacious and safest treatment option for generalized vitiligo, and also has systemic immunomodulatory actions. Phototherapy influences various cell types, including immune cells (cytotoxic and regulatory T cells), keratinocytes, melanocytes, and fibroblasts, affecting both stabilization and repigmentation. NBUVB treatment has been shown to reduce the frequencies of circulating CD4+ and CD8+ central memory T cells, indicating a possible immunosuppressive effect. Additionally, it downregulates chemokines CXCL9 and CXCL10, which are important in directing memory T cells to vitiligo lesions. It was also found that phototherapy increases the expression of E-cadherin and matrix metalloproteinase 2 (MMP 2) in stable vitiligo lesions which might help in repigmentation [48].

For stable vitiligo, surgery is the preferred option that helps in definite repigmentation by transplanting melanocytes from normal skin to vitiligo patches either using tissue grafting or cellular grafting. The proposed mechanism of repigmentation post-grafting is migration of melanocytes from the graft to the basal layer in the recipient area and recolonization of the epidermis with active and functional melanocytes. Multiple factors influence the outcome of repigmentation like stability of the disease, type of graft, location of the lesion and postoperative care.

2.9 Congenital Disorders of Pigmentation

Albinism is a congenital pigmentation disorder, characterized by complete absence of melanin in the skin, hair, and eyes from birth. It occurs due to the absence of tyrosinase enzyme activity. In addition to the visible lack of pigment, the condition causes significant eye abnormalities, such as a reddish appearance of the iris and retina, severe photophobia, and impaired vision due to nystagmus and amblyopia. Ocular albinism may manifest solely in the eyes, while pigmentation remains normal elsewhere. Patients with oculocutaneous albinism (OCA) are also more prone to sunburn and overall sensitivity to sunlight, which can restrict outdoor activities if they are unable to use sun-protective clothing or sunscreen. They also have more risk of developing squamous cell carcinoma, basal cell carcinoma, melanoma, and, less frequently, Merkel cell carcinoma [49]. Other disorders, such as Hermansky–Pudlak syndrome, Chediak–Higashi syndrome, and others, as discussed before are caused by mutations in genes involved in intracellular trafficking and organelle transport including melanosomes (Table 2.1).

On the other hand, reticulate pigmentary disorders present with hyperpigmented and/or hypopigmented macules of varying sizes. Dowling-Degos disease is caused due to mutation in KRT5, POFUT1, POGLUT1 genes that are responsible for the transport of melanin. Dyschromatosis universalis hereditaria is caused by the mutation in the gene ABCB6. Here the number of melanocytes is normal, but there is defect in melanosome synthesis and maturation. Reticulate acropigmentation of Kitamura occurs due to mutation in ADAM 10 gene, essential for activating NOTCH1, which may influence the distribution or transport of melanosomes within keratinocytes [50].

A flowchart of various factors influencing melanogenesis is given in Fig. 2.4.

Table 2.1 Congenital hypopigmented disorders and defective pathways

Defect in pathway	Disorders	Genes
Defect in embryological development and migration of melanocytes	*Piebaldism*	KIT
	Waardenburg syndrome	PAX3 MITF EDNRB, EDN3 SOX10
Defect in melanogenesis	*Oculocutaneous albinism*	TYR TYRP1 OA1, MATP
Defect in biogenesis of melanosomes	*Hermansky–Pudlak syndrome*	HPS1, HPS3, HPS4, HPS5, HPS6 DTNBP1 AP3B1
	Chediak–Higashi syndrome	LYST
Defect of melanosomes transport	*Griscelli–Prunieras syndrome*	MYO5A RAB27A MLPH

EDN3 endothelin 3, *EDNRB* endothelin receptor type B, *MITF* microphthalmia-associated transcription factor, *MYO5A* myosin VA, *MLPH* melanophilin, *LYST* lysosomal trafficking regulator, *DTNBP1* dystrobrevin-binding protein 1, *AP3B1* adaptor protein complex 3 beta 1 subunit, *TYR* tyrosinase, *TYRP1* tyrosinase-related protein 1, *OA1* ocular albinism type 1, *MATP* membrane-associated transporter protein

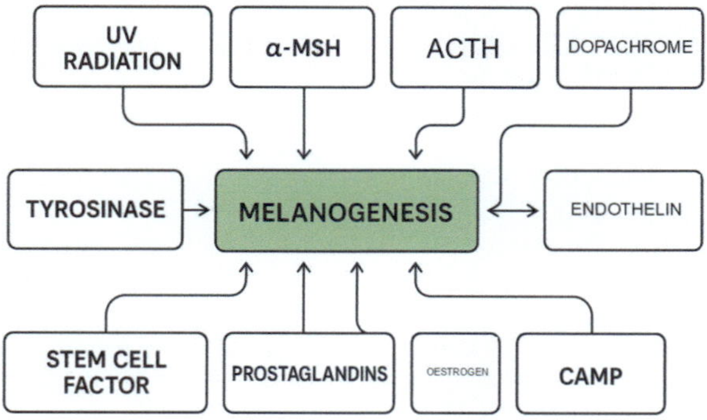

Fig. 2.4 Flowchart of factors influencing melanogenesis

2.10 Conclusion

Melanocyte biology and the process of melanogenesis are important as they are implicated in many congenital and acquired disorders of hypopigmentation and hyperpigmentation. The knowledge helps in better understanding of the pathogenesis of various pigmentary diseases and also in research for targeted therapies.

References

1. Ernfors P. Cellular origin and developmental mechanisms during the formation of skin melanocytes. Exp Cell Res. 2010;316(8):1397–407.
2. Betters E, Liu Y, Kjaeldgaard A, et al. Analysis of early humanneural crest development. Dev Biol. 2010;344:578–92.
3. Le Douarin NM, Creuzet S, Couly G, et al. Neural crest cell plasticity and its limits. Development. 2004;131:4637–50.
4. Cramer SF, Fesyuk A. On the development of neurocutaneous units-implications for the histogenesis of congenital, acquired, and dysplastic nevi. Am J Dermatopathol. 2012;34:60–81.
5. Hirobe T. How are proliferation and differentiation of melanocytes regulated? Pigment Cell Melanoma Res. 2011;24:462–78.
6. Dunn JD, Brady M, Ochsebauer-Jambor C, et al. WNT1 and WNT3a promote expansion of melanocytes through distinct modes of action. Pigment Cell Res. 2005;18:167–80.
7. Baxter LL, Pavan WJ. Pmel17 expression is Mitf-dependent and reveals cra nial melanoblasts migration during murine development. Gene Expr Patterns. 2003;3:703–7.
8. Fitzpatrick TB, Breathnach AS. Das epidermale Melamim-Einheit System. Dermatol Wochenschr. 1963;147:481–9.
9. Haass NK, Herlyn M. Normal human melanocyte homeostasis as a paradigm for understanding melanoma. J Invest Dermatol Symp Proc. 2005;10:153–63.
10. Miot LD, Miot HA, Silva MG, et al. Physiopathology of melasma. An Bras Dermatol. 2009;84:623–35.
11. Haass NK, Smalley KS, Li L, et al. Adhesion, migration and communications in melanocytes and melanoma. Pigment Cell Res. 2005;18:150–9.
12. Fuller BB, Spaulding DT, Smith DR. Regulation of the catalytic activity of preexisting tyrosinase in black and Caucasian human melanocyte cell cultures. Exp Cell Res. 2001;262:197–208.
13. Maeda K, Yokokawa Y, Hatao M, Naganuma M, Tomita Y. Comparison of the melanogenesis in human black and light brown melanocytes. J Dermatol Sci. 1997;14:19–206.
14. Tobin DJ. The cell biology of human hair follicle pigmentation. Pigment Cell Melanoma Res. 2011;24:75–88.
15. Commo S, Bernard BA. Melanocyte subpopulation turnover during the human hair cycle: an immunohistochemical study. Pigment Cell Res. 2000;13:253–9.
16. Slominski A, Wortsman J, Plonka PM, et al. Hair follicle pigmentation. J Invest Dermatol. 2005;124:13–21.
17. Riley PA. Melanin. Int J Biochem Cell Biol. 1997;29:1235–9.
18. Fitzpatrick TB, Miyamoto M, Ishikawa K. The evolution of concepts of melanin biology. Arch Dermatol. 1967;96:305–23.
19. Hearing VJ. Determination of melanin synthetic pathway. J Invest Dermatol. 2011;131:8–11.
20. Slominski A, Tobin DJ, Shibahara S, et al. Melanin pigmentation in mammalian skin and its hormonal regulation. Physiol Rev. 2004;84:1155–228.
21. Ito S, Wakamatsu K. Diversity of human hair pigmentation as studied by chemical analysis of eumelanin and pheomelanin. J Eur Acad Dermatol Venereol. 2011;25:1369–80.
22. Sulaimon SS, Kitchell BE. The biology of melanocytes. Vet Dermatol. 2003;14:57–65.
23. Cichorek M, Wachulska M, Stasiewicz A, Tymińska A. Skin melanocytes: biology and development. Adv Dermatol Allergol. 2013;1:30–41.
24. Schallreuter KU. Advances in melanocyte basic science research. Dermatol Clin. 2007;25(3):283–91.
25. Makova K, Norton H. Worldwide polymorphism at the MC1R locus and normal pigmentation variation in humans. Peptides. 2005;26:1901–8.
26. Saternus R, Pilz S, Gräber S, et al. A closer look at evolution: variants (SNPs) of genes involved in skin pigmentation, including EXOC2, TYR, TYRP1 and DCT, are associated with 25(OH) D serum concentration. Endocrinology. 2015;156:39–47.

27. Ando H, Niki Y, Ito M, Akiyama K, Matsui MS, Yarosh DB, et al. Melanosomes are transferred from melanocytes to keratinocytes through the processes of packaging, release, uptake, and dispersion. J Invest Dermatol. 2012;132(4):1222–9.
28. Ando H, Niki Y, Yoshida M, et al. Involvement of pigment globules containing multiple melanososmes in the transfer of melanosomes from melanocytes to keratinocytes. Cellular Logistics. 2011;1:12–20.
29. Hershkovitz D, Sprecher E Monogenic pigmentary skin disorders: genetics and pathophysiology. Israel Med Assoc J. 2008;10:713–7.
30. Tsatmali M, Ancans J, Thody AJ. Melanocyte function and its control by melanocortin peptides. J Histochem Cytochem. 2002;50(2):125–33.
31. Mountjoy KG, Robbins LS, Mortrud MT, Cone RD. The cloning of a family of genes that encode the melanocortin receptors. Science. 1992;257(5074):1248–51.
32. Levy C, Khaled M, Fisher DE. MITF: master regulator of melanocyte development and melanoma oncogene. Trends Mol Med. 2006;12(9):406–14.
33. Yaar M, Park H-Y. Melanocytes: a window into the nervous system. J Invest Dermatol. 2012;132:835–45.
34. Grando SA, Pittelkow MR, Schallreuter KU. Adrenergic and cholinergic control in the biology of epidermis: physiological and clinical significance. J Invest Dermatol. 2006;126(9):1948.
35. Bonaventure J, Domingues MJ, Larue L. Cellular and molecular mechanisms controlling the migration of melanocytes and melanoma cells. Pigment Cell Melanoma Res. 2013;26:316–25.
36. Dorsky RI, Raible DW, Moon RT. Direct regulation of nacre, a zebrafish MITF homolog required for pigment cell formation, by the Wnt pathway. Genes Dev. 2000;14:158–62.
37. Videira IF, Moura DF, Magina S. Mechanisms regulating melanogenesis. An Bras Dermatol. 2013;88(1):76–83.
38. Thody AJ, Graham A. Does alpha-MSH have a role in regulating skin pigmentation in humans? Pigment Cell Res. 1998;11(5):265–74.
39. Heenen M, Giacomoni PU, Golstein P. Individual variations in the correlation between erythemal threshold, UV-induced DNA damage and sun-burn cell formation. J Photochem Photobiol B. 2001;63:84–7.
40. Eller MS, Ostrom K, Gilchrest BA. DNA damage enhances melanogenesis. Proc Natl Acad Sci USA. 1996;93:1087–92.
41. Kamb A. Sun protection factor p53. Nature. 1994;372:730–1.
42. Kennedy C, et al. Melanocortin 1 receptor (MC1R) gene variants are associated with an increased risk for cutaneous melanoma which is largely independent of skin type and hair color. J Invest Dermatol. 2001;117:294–300.
43. Takeuchi S, et al. Melanin acts as a potent UVB photosensitizer to cause an atypical mode of cell death in murine skin. Proc Natl Acad Sci USA. 2004;101:15076–81.
44. Franceschini D, Dinulos JG. Dermal melanocytosis and associated disorders. Curr Opin Pediatr. 2015;27(4):480–5.
45. Chuah SY, Hammami Ghorbel H, Lacour JP, Passeron T. Acquired dermal melanocytosis of the nose. J Eur Acad Dermatol Venereol. 2015;29(4):827–9.
46. Bergqvist C, Ezzedine K. Vitiligo: a focus on pathogenesis and its therapeutic implications. J Dermatol. 2021;48(3):252–70.
47. Chen J, Li S, Li C. Mechanisms of melanocyte death in vitiligo. Med Res Rev. 2021;41(2):1138–66.
48. Bishnoi A, Parsad D. Phototherapy for vitiligo: a narrative review on the clinical and molecular aspects, and recent literature. Photodermatol Photoimmunol Photomed. 2024;40(3):e12968.
49. Okulicz JF, Shah RS, Schwartz RA, Janniger CK. Oculocutaneous albinism. J Eur Acad Dermatol Venereol. 2003;17(3):251–6.
50. Zhang J, Li M, Yao Z. Updated review of genetic reticulate pigmentary disorders. Br J Dermatol. 2017;177(4):945–59.

Chapter 3
Genetics and Epidemiology of Vitiligo

Alessia Paganelli, Rohit Gupta, and Mauro Picardo

Abstract Epidemiologically, vitiligo affects approximately 0.5–2% of the global population, with no significant sex or ethnic predisposition, though certain environmental triggers may influence onset. Genetic studies have identified multiple susceptibility loci associated with immune regulation, melanocyte function, and oxidative stress pathways, suggesting a polygenic inheritance. Recent genome-wide association studies (GWAS) highlight key genes such as TYR, NLRP1, and HLA as contributors to disease risk. Understanding the interaction between genetic predisposition and environmental factors is crucial for developing new targeted effective therapies. The aim of the present chapter is to explore the epidemiology and genetics of vitiligo.

Keywords Vitiligo · Genetics · Epigenetic · GWAS · Mendelian randomization · Auto-immunity

3.1 General Epidemiology of Vitiligo

Recent estimates indicate a global prevalence of vitiligo of approximately 0.5–2% [1–3]. However, important regional variations have been documented so far and give reason for the high prevalence range variability emerging from epidemiological studies, ranging from less than 0.1% to greater than 8% worldwide [4]. A meta-analysis from Zhang and co-authors pointed out significant differences

A. Paganelli
Istituto Dermopatico Immacolata, IDI IRCCS, Rome, Italy

R. Gupta
National Institute of Immunology, New Delhi, India

M. Picardo (✉)
Istituto Dermopatico Immacolata, IDI IRCCS, Rome, Italy

National Institute of Immunology, New Delhi, India

R. Sarkar, V. Narayan R (eds.), *A Concise Guide to The Management of Vitiligo*,
https://doi.org/10.1007/978-981-95-3857-7_3

also based on the type of study, with higher disease prevalence rates registered in hospital-based studies compared to population- or community-based studies [2].

The mean age of onset ranges from 20 to 30 years of age, with both children and elderly possibly being affected. However, approximately half of all patients develop the disease before the age of 20 [4]. Onset at an advanced age should raise concerns about associated diseases, such as autoimmune thyroiditis, diabetes mellitus, or alopecia areata. Interestingly, earlier disease onset has been documented in familial forms of the disease [5].

Several authors reported a slight predilection for the female sex, biased by the higher chances of female patient requiring medical attention for cosmetic issues [2, 4]. However, sex distribution is still debated with most reports suggesting equal frequency of the disease in males and females [6–8].

3.2 The Genetic Bases of Vitiligo

Based on large-scale epidemiological studies, vitiligo has been demonstrated mostly to occur sporadically; however, up to 20% of patients have at least one affected relative [9].

Familial aggregation of vitiligo displays a non-Mendelian pattern. Several authors hypothesized polygenic, multifactorial inheritance, with an estimated vitiligo heritability of approximately 50% [10–12]. Not surprisingly, familial cases are characterized by earlier onset of the disease, with decreased risk of developing vitiligo with increasing genetic distance from affected subjects [13]. These features strongly support the hypothesis of a polygenic disorder and genetic segregation analyses indicating vitiligo is a complex trait, with multiple contributory genetic loci [12, 14].

Notably, vitiligo is strongly associated with other immune-mediated disorders. Recently this association has been demonstrated to have a genetic basis. Approximately 10–20% of vitiligo patients, in fact, develop other concomitant autoinflammatory and/or autoimmune diseases including, among others, thyroid disease, type 1 diabetes, lupus erythematosus, Addison's disease, alopecia areata [5, 9, 15]. Of note, most of the renowned genetic susceptibility loci for such comorbidities have also been demonstrated to play a role in the occurrence of vitiligo. Moreover, vitiligo is also part of genetically determined clinical syndromes such as APECED (autoimmune polyendocrinopathy, candidiasis, ectodermal dystrophy, also known as APS1, autoimmune polyendocrine syndrome type 1; OMIM #240300) [16]. Taken together, these data highlight the presence of a strong genetic background in the setting of vitiligo, therefore paving the way for genetic studies in this field.

For an overview of the most important genetic modifications associated with vitiligo see Table 3.1.

Three main technical approaches have been used to identify loci of genetic susceptibility for vitiligo: the *candidate gene* approach, the *genome-wide* approach,

Table 3.1 List of the most relevant genes in vitiligo pathogenesis and their involvement in physiology and/or disease

Gene	Physiological and/or pathological process
AIRE	APECED/APS1 (*autoimmune poliEndocripothy, candidiasis, ectodermal dystrophy/autoimmune polyendocrine syndrome type 1*
HLA	Antigen presentation
PTPN22	Negative regulator of T cell activation
CTLA4	T cell co-stimulation
NLRP1	Inflammasome activation, IL1 secretion
TYR, OCA2, MC1R	Melanocyte differentiation and melanogenesis
IL4	Th2-driven response, atopic dermatitis
PCSK9	Cholesterol homeostasis

and the *genes' expression* approach. Genome-wide association studies (GWAS) have been found to be the most reliable method and are currently considered the "gold standard" for disease gene identification.

The *candidate gene* approach is aggravated by a high rate of false-positive results but few of the many published candidate gene associations have also been confirmed by GWAS. Among these, several genes involved in the immune response such as *HLA*, *PTPN22*, and *CTLA4*. However, genetic association of PTPN22 and CTLA4 is yet to be confirmed in non-European populations [17–19]. Of note, genetic associations of vitiligo with HLA class I and II alleles were particularly strong in patients with relatives affected by other immune-mediated disorders, which are often associated themselves with genetic variation in the MHC class I or class II gene regions [20, 21].

Genome-wide linkage studies enabled the identification of a locus on chromosome 17p13, called SLEV1, associated with vitiligo and other autoimmune diseases [22]. Fine mapping in vitiligo families ultimately identified the underlying gene as NLRP1 (previously termed NALP1) [23]. Next-generation DNA sequencing showed that the most represented high-risk NLRP1 haplotype is associated with enhanced activation of the IL-1β pathway [24].

Approximately 50 chromosomal loci have been identified so far as possibly associated with vitiligo through GWAS. Specific pathogenic gene variants have also been determined in part of such cases, therefore filling gaps of knowledge in vitiligo pathogenesis for the first time. For example, genes involved in immune regulation and cellular apoptosis have been identified through GWAS as possibly involved in vitiligo pathogenesis. Susceptibility in genes encoding proteins crucial for melanocyte function has also been demonstrated in both vitiligo and melanoma, involving exactly the same genetic variants but with opposite alleles [17]. These include—among others—TYR, OCA2, and MC1R, encoding tyrosinase, a melanocyte melanogenic protein and melanocortin 1 receptor, respectively. Interestingly, TYR, OCA2, and MC1R are also thought to act as vitiligo autoantigens. On the one hand vitiligo may represent an epiphenomenon of immune surveillance against melanoma [25], which is in line with the lower risk for vitiligo-affected subjects of developing melanoma [26]. This theory is also supported by the better outcomes of melanoma immunotherapy of patients developing vitiligo, in terms of overall survival [27].

3.3 Mendelian Randomization Studies in Vitiligo

Mendelian randomization (MR) studies are epidemiological studies that exploit naturally occurring genetic variations as instrumental variables to determine the causal relationship between a risk factor (such as a biomarker, behaviour, or environmental exposure) and a disease outcome. The rationale for this kind of study resides in the strict association between specific genetic variables and the exposures of interest. By examining the relationship between these genetic variants and the disease outcome, MR helps provide more robust evidence for causal inference compared to traditional observational studies.

For example, Li and collaborators explored the hypothesis of a causal association between psoriasis and vitiligo based on the observation of both the morbid conditions in a single patient [28]. However, MR studies did not support a causal relationship, but only suggested a possible association between psoriasis and vitiligo based on shared mechanisms of immune dysfunction.

Another MR-based research revealed that genetically determined increased IL4 levels could determine a higher risk of developing vitiligo [29]. The availability of effective therapeutic options for blocking IL-4 (already widely prescribed for atopic dermatitis) paves the way for their use for the treatment of vitiligo.

Other studies found vitiligo risk to be associated with increased counts in specific leucocyte subclasses, including basophils, monocytes, eosinophils and neutrophils [30].

Further evidence of the importance of a MR-based approach in the setting of vitiligo is provided by a recent study aimed at exploring the impact of genetically proxied lipid-lowering agents on the risk of vitiligo and potentially associated mediators [31]. Lipid-lowering MR indicated a potential role of PCSK9 (proprotein convertase subtilisin/kexin type 9) inhibitors in reducing the risk of developing vitiligo. Multivariable MR suggested that well-known lipid profiles do not mediate the relationship between PCSK9 and vitiligo, while two-step MR analyses identified five potential protein mediators (CCN5, CXCL12, FCRL1, LGMN, and FGF2). As a consequence, PCSK9 inhibitors could represent a therapeutic option for the prevention and the treatment of vitiligo.

3.4 Epigenetic Modifications in Vitiligo

3.4.1 MicroRNAs

MicroRNAs (miRNAs) are single-stranded RNAs that modulate gene expression affecting the stability and, as a consequence, the translation of mRNAs post-transcriptionally [32]. In the last decades, miRNAs have been recognized as an important component of epigenetic regulation, with strong implications in the therapeutic setting [33]. With regards to miRNA origin, long, polyadenylated primary precursors undergo sequential cleavage by different RNases (Drosha, Dicer) and then bind Argonaute to form the RNA-induced silencing complex (RISC), which targets mRNA for regulation.[[34] Subsequently, base pairing to the 3′ untranslated region (3′UTR) of target mRNA leads to repression of gene expression.

Interestingly, Dicer expression has been demonstrated to be under direct transcriptional regulation by MITF (microphthalmia-associated transcription factor) in melanocytes [35]. Several miRNAs have been described as directly regulating MITF expression, including miR-218, miR-137, and miR-429 [36–38]. MITF is a key regulator of melanogenesis and skin pigmentation and all the aforementioned miRNAs were shown to interfere with these processes. Recently, Kim et al. demonstrated miR-675 to be released extracellularly from keratinocytes and delivered to neighbouring melanocytes, affecting MITF expression [39]. Other studies in murine models showed UV exposure to significantly downregulate miR-145 levels, which, in turn, determined increased expression of genes involved in melanocyte differentiation and melanogenesis, such as MITF, Tyr, Trp1, Sox 9 [40].

Not less importantly, miRNAs are crucial also for immune tolerance maintenance: murine models with deletions of Dicer in CD4+CD25+Foxp3+ regulatory T (Treg) cells and invariant natural killer T (iNKT) cells unveiled the critical role of miRNAs in Tregs and iNKT function.

Notably, numerical and/or functional defects in Tregs and iNKTs are associated with the development of autoimmune disorders [41, 42].

The involvement of miRNAs in both melanogenesis and immune tolerance strongly suggests a critical role for miRNAs in vitiligo pathogenesis. The analysis of serum miRNA expression profiles of patients affected by vitiligo compared to healthy controls enabled the identification of a panel of three miRNAs (miR-16, miR-19b, and miR-720) as potential disease biomarkers [43, 44]. Other studies led to the identification of miRNAs differentially expressed in vitiligo patients both from PBMCs and skin biopsies [45, 46]. Similarly, specific miRNAs were differentially expressed in murine models of vitiligo compared to control mice [47].

Several authors tried to better characterize the contribution of genetic variations in miRNAs in the setting of vitiligo. Specific miR-196a-2 alleles, for example, have been found to be protective against vitiligo, through downregulation of TYRP1 gene expression in melanocytes and, consequently, prevention of oxidative stress-induced apoptosis [48]. On the contrary, upregulation of miR-25 (targeting MITF) is associated with increased ROS production and is possibly involved in vitiligo development [49].

3.4.2 DNA Methylation

Notably, methylation of CpG islands in gene promoter regions determines silencing of gene expression through interference with transcription activators and/or recruitment of chromatin repressor complexes [50]. More recently, non-CpG DNA methylation in both the intragenic and intergenic sites is also important for regulation of differential gene expression [51].

Interestingly, increased DNA methylation levels have been reported in vitiligo patients compared to healthy controls, consistent with similar observations in other organ-specific autoimmune diseases (e.g. type 1 diabetes mellitus) [52]. More in detail, reduced IL10 expression in vitiligo patient PBMCs has been associated with DNA hyper methylation within the IL-10 gene. However, further research into gene-specific DNA methylation patterns is necessary to clarify the role of DNA methylation dysregulation in the development of vitiligo.

3.4.3 Histone Modifications

Histone post-translational modifications, including acetylation, methylation, ubiquitination, and phosphorylation, are another major source of epigenetic alteration, influencing chromatin accessibility to transcription factors at gene promoters and enhancers, therefore modulating related gene expression. Evidence for altered histone acetylation/deacetylation has already been demonstrated for several immune-mediated disorders, such as type 1 diabetes and rheumatoid arthritis [53, 54]. This is at least partially explained by impaired regulation of specific genes involved in the immune response, including HLA molecules, toll-like receptors, cytokines, and transcription factors [55]. Nucleosome alterations have also been documented to impact melanocyte differentiation and senescence [56]. However, specific histone or nucleosome modification patterns associated with the development of vitiligo have yet to be clarified.

3.5 Conclusion

The genetics and epigenetics of vitiligo provide critical insights into its complex pathogenesis, highlighting the interplay between genetic susceptibility, immune dysregulation, and environmental factors. Key susceptibility loci, including TYR, HLA, and NLRP1, emphasize the involvement of melanocyte function and immune pathways in the development of the disease. Additionally, epigenetic mechanisms, such as DNA methylation, histone modifications, and non-coding RNAs, have been identified as pivotal regulators of gene expression, potentially mediating the effects of environmental triggers on genetic predisposition. These findings not only advance the understanding of vitiligo's aetiology but also inform the development of novel therapeutic strategies, including precision medicine approaches targeting specific genetic and epigenetic pathways. Continued research that integrates genetic, epigenetic, and environmental data is essential to further refine treatment modalities and improve outcomes for individuals with vitiligo.

References

1. Picardo M, Dell'Anna ML, Ezzedine K, Hamzavi I, Harris JE, Parsad D, et al. Vitiligo. Nat Rev Dis Primers. 2015;1(1):15011.
2. Zhang Y, Cai Y, Shi M, Jiang S, Cui S, Wu Y, et al. The prevalence of vitiligo: a meta-analysis. PLoS One. 2016;11(9):e0163806.
3. Harris JE, Ezzedine K, Bibeau K, Jones H, Na L, Pandya A. 17755 global survey investigating the prevalence of vitiligo and vitiligo signs among adults in Europe, Japan, and the United States. J Am Acad Dermatol. 2020;83(6):AB198.
4. Alikhan A, Felsten LM, Daly M, Petronic-Rosic V. Vitiligo: a comprehensive overview. J Am Acad Dermatol. 2011;65(3):473–91.
5. Laberge G, Mailloux CM, Gowan K, Holland P, Bennett DC, Fain PR, et al. Early disease onset and increased risk of other autoimmune diseases in familial generalized vitiligo. Pigment Cell Res. 2005;18(4):300–5.
6. Handa S, Kaur I. Vitiligo: clinical findings in 1436 patients. J Dermatol. 1999;26(10):653–7.
7. Khoury M, Dabit T, Siniora H, Fashho J, Toubasi AA. The prevalence of vitiligo and its associated risk factors in the middle east and Africa: a systematic review and meta-analysis. Health Sciences Review. 2024;12:100187.
8. Vedamurthy M, Kumar M, Boda S. Exploring the spectrum of vitiligo: clinical and demographic perspectives—a cross-sectional study. CSDM. 2024;4:40.
9. Alkhateeb A, Fain PR, Thody A, Bennett DC, Spritz RA. Epidemiology of vitiligo and associated autoimmune diseases in Caucasian probands and their families. Pigment Cell Res. 2003;16(3):208–14.
10. Hafez M, Sharaf L, Abd el-Nabi SM. The genetics of vitiligo. Acta Derm Venereol. 1983;63(3):249–51.
11. Das SK, Majumder PP, Majumdar TK, Haldar B. Studies on vitiligo. II. Familial aggregation and genetics. Genet Epidemiol. 1985;2(3):255–62.
12. Sun X, Xu A, Wei X, Ouyang J, Lu L, Chen M, et al. Genetic epidemiology of vitiligo: a study of 815 probands and their families from South China. Int J Dermatol 2006;45(10):1176–1181.
13. Majumder PP, Nordlund JJ, Nath SK. Pattern of familial aggregation of vitiligo. Arch Dermatol. 1993;129(8):994–8.
14. Nath SK, Majumder PP, Nordlund JJ. Genetic epidemiology of vitiligo: multilocus recessivity cross-validated. Am J Hum Genet. 1994 Nov;55(5):981–90.
15. Schallreuter KU, Lemke R, Brandt O, Schwartz R, Westhofen M, Montz R, et al. Vitiligo and other diseases: coexistence or true association? Hamburg study on 321 patients. Dermatology. 1994;188(4):269–75.
16. Bjørklund G, Pivin M, Hangan T, Yurkovskaya O, Pivina L. Autoimmune polyendocrine syndrome type 1: clinical manifestations, pathogenetic features, and management approach. Autoimmun Rev. 2022;21(8):103135.

17. Jin Y, Andersen G, Yorgov D, Ferrara TM, Ben S, Brownson KM, et al. Genome-wide association studies of autoimmune vitiligo identify 23 new risk loci and highlight key pathways and regulatory variants. Nat Genet. 2016;48(11):1418–24.
18. Birlea SA, LaBerge GS, Procopciuc LM, Fain PR, Spritz RA. *CTLA4* and generalized vitiligo: two genetic association studies and a meta-analysis of published data. Pigment Cell Melanoma Res. 2009;22(2):230–4.
19. Laberge GS, Birlea SA, Fain PR, Spritz RA. The PTPN22-1858C>T (R620W) functional polymorphism is associated with generalized vitiligo in the Romanian population. Pigment Cell Melanoma Res. 2008;21(2):206–8.
20. Foley LM, Lowe NJ, Misheloff E, Tiwari JL. Association of HLA-DR4 with vitiligo. J Am Acad Dermatol. 1983;8(1):39–40.
21. Liu JB, Li M, Chen H, Zhong SQ, Yang S, Du WD, et al. Association of vitiligo with HLA-A2: a meta-analysis. J Eur Acad Dermatol Venereol. 2007;21(2):205–13.
22. Nath SK, Kelly JA, Namjou B, Lam T, Bruner GR, Scofield RH, et al. Evidence for a susceptibility gene, SLEV1, on chromosome 17p13 in families with vitiligo-related systemic lupus erythematosus. Am J Hum Genet. 2001;69(6):1401–6.
23. Jin Y, Mailloux CM, Gowan K, Riccardi SL, LaBerge G, Bennett DC, et al. NALP1 in vitiligo-associated multiple autoimmune disease. N Engl J Med. 2007;356(12):1216–25.
24. Levandowski CB, Mailloux CM, Ferrara TM, Gowan K, Ben S, Jin Y, et al. NLRP1 haplotypes associated with vitiligo and autoimmunity increase interleukin-1β processing via the NLRP1 inflammasome. Proc Natl Acad Sci USA. 2013;110(8):2952–6.
25. Das PK, van den Wijngaard RM, Wankowicz-Kalinska A, Le Poole IC. A symbiotic concept of autoimmunity and tumour immunity: lessons from vitiligo. Trends Immunol. 2001;22(3):130–6.
26. Paradisi A, Tabolli S, Didona B, Sobrino L, Russo N, Abeni D. Markedly reduced incidence of melanoma and nonmelanoma skin cancer in a nonconcurrent cohort of 10,040 patients with vitiligo. J Am Acad Dermatol. 2014;71(6):1110–6.
27. Carbone ML, Capone A, Guercio M, Reddel S, Silvestris DA, Lulli D, et al. Insight into immune profile associated with vitiligo onset and anti-tumoral response in melanoma patients receiving anti-PD-1 immunotherapy. Front Immunol. 2023;14:1197630.
28. Li J, Shen Q, Wang Y, Guo C, Ma Y, Zhang Y. The relationship between psoriasis and vitiligo: from a comprehensive study. Skin Res Technol. 2024;30(7):e13868.
29. Liu C, Liu X, Xin H, Li X. A Mendelian randomization study on the causal effects of circulating cytokines on the risk of vitiligo. Front Med. 2024;11:1375339.
30. Xin Y, Yuan T, Wang J. Circulating immune cells and vitiligo: a bidirectional two-sample Mendelian randomization study. Front Immunol. 2024;15:1391186.
31. Kang TJ, Lee SY, Yoon S, Kim EG, Kim JO, Kim JS, et al. PCSK9 inhibitors and the risk of vitiligo: a Mendelian randomization study. J Invest Dermatol 2024 Aug;S0022202X24019857.
32. Kozomara A, Griffiths-Jones S. miRBase: annotating high confidence microRNAs using deep sequencing data. Nucleic Acids Res. 2014;42(Database issue):D68–73.
33. Fabian MR, Sonenberg N, Filipowicz W. Regulation of mRNA translation and stability by microRNAs. Annu Rev Biochem. 2010;79:351–79.
34. Pasquinelli AE. MicroRNAs and their targets: recognition, regulation and an emerging reciprocal relationship. Nat Rev Genet. 2012;13(4):271–82.
35. Levy C, Khaled M, Robinson KC, Veguilla RA, Chen PH, Yokoyama S, et al. Lineage-specific transcriptional regulation of DICER by MITF in melanocytes. Cell. 2010;141(6):994–1005.
36. Dong C, Wang H, Xue L, Dong Y, Yang L, Fan R, et al. Coat color determination by miR-137 mediated down-regulation of microphthalmia-associated transcription factor in a mouse model. RNA. 2012 Sep;18(9):1679–86.
37. Yan B, Liu B, Zhu CD, Li KL, Yue LJ, Zhao JL, et al. microRNA regulation of skin pigmentation in fish. J Cell Sci. 2013;126(Pt 15):3401–8.

38. Guo J, Zhang J-F, Wang W-M, Florence W-KC, Lu Y-F, Ng C-F, et al. MicroRNA-218 inhibits melanogenesis by directly suppressing microphthalmia-associated transcription factor expression. RNA Biol. 2014;11(6):732–41.
39. Kim NH, Choi SH, Kim CH, Lee CH, Lee TR, Lee AY. Reduced MiR-675 in exosome in H19 RNA-related melanogenesis via MITF as a direct target. J Invest Dermatol. 2014 Apr;134(4):1075–82.
40. Dynoodt P, Mestdagh P, Van Peer G, Vandesompele J, Goossens K, Peelman LJ, et al. Identification of miR-145 as a key regulator of the pigmentary process. J Invest Dermatol. 2013 Jan;133(1):201–9.
41. Berzins SP, Smyth MJ, Baxter AG. Presumed guilty: natural killer T cell defects and human disease. Nat Rev Immunol. 2011 Feb;11(2):131–42.
42. Tang Q, Bluestone JA. The Foxp3+ regulatory T cell: a jack of all trades, master of regulation. Nat Immunol. 2008 Mar;9(3):239–44.
43. Shi YL, Weiland M, Li J, Hamzavi I, Henderson M, Huggins RH, et al. MicroRNA expression profiling identifies potential serum biomarkers for non-segmental vitiligo. Pigment Cell Melanoma Res. 2013 May;26(3):418–21.
44. Jiang S, Li C, Olive V, Lykken E, Feng F, Sevilla J, et al. Molecular dissection of the miR-17-92 cluster's critical dual roles in promoting Th1 responses and preventing inducible Treg differentiation. Blood. 2011;118(20):5487–97.
45. Wang Y, Wang K, Liang J, Yang H, Dang N, Yang X, et al. Differential expression analysis of miRNA in peripheral blood mononuclear cells of patients with non-segmental vitiligo. J Dermatol. 2015;42(2):193–7.
46. Mansuri MS, Singh M, Dwivedi M, Laddha NC, Marfatia YS, Begum R. MicroRNA profiling reveals differentially expressed microRNA signatures from the skin of patients with nonsegmental vitiligo. Br J Dermatol. 2014;171(5):1263–7.
47. Shi YL, Weiland M, Lim HW, Mi QS, Zhou L. Serum miRNA expression profiles change in autoimmune vitiligo in mice. Exp Dermatol. 2014;23(2):140–2.
48. Huang Y, Yi X, Jian Z, Wei C, Li S, Cai C, et al. A single-nucleotide polymorphism of miR-196a-2 and vitiligo: an association study and functional analysis in a Han Chinese population. Pigment Cell Melanoma Res. 2013;26(3):338–47.
49. Shi Q, Zhang W, Guo S, Jian Z, Li S, Li K, et al. Oxidative stress-induced overexpression of miR-25: the mechanism underlying the degeneration of melanocytes in vitiligo. Cell Death Differ. 2016;23(3):496–508.
50. Costello JF, Plass C. Methylation matters. J Med Genet. 2001;38(5):285–303.
51. Maunakea AK, Nagarajan RP, Bilenky M, Ballinger TJ, D'Souza C, Fouse SD, et al. Conserved role of intragenic DNA methylation in regulating alternative promoters. Nature. 2010;466(7303):253–7.
52. Zhao M, Gao F, Wu X, Tang J, Lu Q. Abnormal DNA methylation in peripheral blood mononuclear cells from patients with vitiligo. Br J Dermatol. 2010 Oct;163(4):736–42.
53. Miao F, Smith DD, Zhang L, Min A, Feng W, Natarajan R. Lymphocytes from patients with type 1 diabetes display a distinct profile of chromatin histone H3 lysine 9 dimethylation: an epigenetic study in diabetes. Diabetes. 2008 Dec;57(12):3189–98.
54. Trenkmann M, Brock M, Gay RE, Kolling C, Speich R, Michel BA, et al. Expression and function of EZH2 in synovial fibroblasts: epigenetic repression of the Wnt inhibitor SFRP1 in rheumatoid arthritis. Ann Rheum Dis. 2011;70(8):1482–8.
55. Miao F, Chen Z, Zhang L, Liu Z, Wu X, Yuan YC, et al. Profiles of epigenetic histone post-translational modifications at type 1 diabetes susceptible genes. J Biol Chem. 2012;287(20):16335–45.
56. Koludrovic D, Laurette P, Strub T, Keime C, Le Coz M, Coassolo S, et al. Chromatin-Remodelling complex NURF is essential for differentiation of adult melanocyte stem cells. PLoS Genet. 2015 Oct;11(10):e1005555.

Chapter 4
Pathogenesis and Histopathology of Vitiligo

Niharika Dhattarwal, Geeti Khullar, and Amit Kumar Yadav

Abstract Pathogenesis of vitiligo is complex and involves interplay between inherent susceptibility of melanocytes to stress, external and internal factors leading to oxidative stress and immune dysfunction. Various theories have been proposed with scientific evidence supporting each one of them. Role of genetics and inherited genetic susceptibility loci in the pathogenesis has been proven. Neural theory implicates neuromediators and catecholamines, while biochemical theory blames melanogenesis byproducts and other biochemicals in damaging melanocytes. According to the oxidative stress theory, which is one of the widely accepted theories, it is the internal imbalance between reactive oxygen species and antioxidants, along with mitochondrial dysfunction which leads to melanocyte death. As per melanocytorrhagy theory, deficiency of cell adhesion molecules leads to detachment of melanocytes from basal layers and their loss. Whereas intrinsic death theory proposes activation of apoptotic cascade due to internal defects in melanocytes as the melanocyte death mechanism. Immune theory describes the role of both adaptive and innate immunity and activation of immune system to be ultimately responsible for disease progression and continuation. Stem cell theory hypothesizes decreased capacity of stem cells to regenerate lost melanocytes to be the basis of depigmentation. A flowchart summarizing and interconnecting all the possible pathways of pathogenesis has also been depicted. The role of histopathology in the diagnosis of vitiligo is not yet fully established. The diagnosis is made primarily on clinical grounds. Biopsy is usually done in difficult cases to rule out the differential diagnoses.

N. Dhattarwal
Department of Dermatology, Deen Dayal Upadhyaya Hospital, New Delhi, Delhi, India

G. Khullar (✉)
Department of Dermatology, Lady Hardinge Medical College and Associated Hospitals, New Delhi, Delhi, India

A. K. Yadav
Department of Pathology, Vardhman Mahavir Medical College and Safdarjung Hospital, New Delhi, Delhi, India

R. Sarkar, V. Narayan R (eds.), *A Concise Guide to The Management of Vitiligo*,
https://doi.org/10.1007/978-981-95-3857-7_4

Keywords Genetics · Neuromediators · Oxidative stress · Melanocytorrhagy · Apoptosis · Immune system · Innate immunity · CD8 cells · Treg cells · Memory T cells · Stem cells

4.1 Introduction

Vitiligo is a common pigmentary disorder resulting from a reduction in melanin production and the number of melanocytes. The underlying pathogenesis is complex and multifactorial. Although many theories have been proposed and studied extensively over the years, the precise mechanism is still not fully elucidated. This chapter will discuss all these implicated factors in detail for better understanding of vitiligo pathogenesis and subsequent successful treatment. An integrated flowchart of all pathomechanisms is shown in Fig. 4.1.

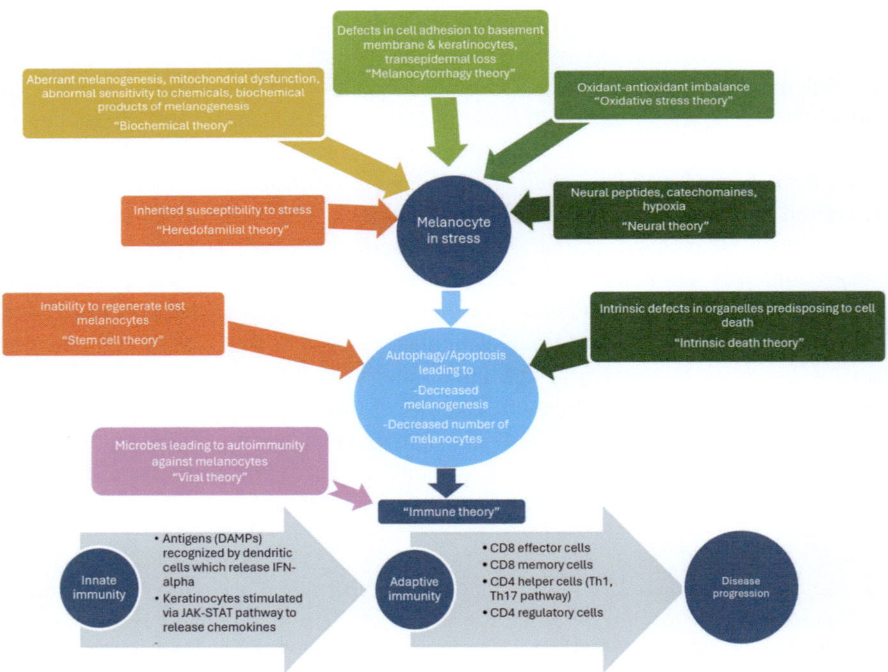

Fig. 4.1 A flowchart integrating and describing overview of proposed pathogenic theories of vitiligo

4.2 Theories of Vitiligo

4.2.1 *Heredofamilial Theory*

Vitiligo cases can be classified as "simplex" when there is no family history of vitiligo or "multiplex" when there is an affected first-degree relative. The percentage of "multiplex" patients varies across studies among different populations and ethnic groups. But large-scale epidemiological surveys have shown that the vast majority of cases (91%) are "simplex" [1, 2]. Pattern of inheritance is non-Mendelian polygenic, which means that multiple genes interact additively to influence the phenotypic trait [3].

Over time, multiple technologies have been used to elucidate the genetic basis of vitiligo including heritability studies, candidate gene association studies, genetic linkage studies and genome-wide association studies (GWAS). Fifty-four vitiligo susceptibility loci have been identified till now, each contributing to overall vitiligo heritability. Of these loci, 50 were detected by GWAS which is the gold standard and preferred study. Although the majority of these loci were identified from cases of European ancestry, they are shared across populations suggesting similarity in genetics [4, 5]. On identification of corresponding genes and genetic variants of these loci, 85% were found to encode proteins involved in immune regulation, apoptosis and melanogenesis [6]. Many of these genes are shared by other autoimmune diseases that are epidemiologically associated with vitiligo like Addison's disease, pernicious anaemia, autoimmune thyroid disease, type 1 diabetes and idiopathic thrombocytopenic purpura, supporting their role in pathogenesis [5]. Epidemiological studies also suggest a bimodal distribution of age-of-onset similar to these diseases, further suggesting shared genetic predisposition [7].

4.2.2 *Neural Theory*

This theory originated due to characteristic dermatomal distribution in some cases (known as segmental vitiligo) and development of vitiligo following nerve injury or neuropathy [8, 9]. Histopathological studies have shown ultrastructural changes in nerve fibres and Schwann cells in lesional skin [10]. Levels of neuromediators like neuropeptide Y (NPY), calcitonin gene-related peptide (CGRP), vasoactive intestinal polypeptide (VIP), polyclonal general neuronal marker (PGP) and substance P have also been found increased in lesions on vitiligo [8, 11, 12]. It is postulated that release of these neurochemicals from peripheral nerve endings can affect melanocytes and modulate immune responses.

Stress is another factor that is linked with etiopathogenesis of vitiligo. Almost one-third of patients stated that significant emotional upset preceded the onset of disease [10]. Patients with vitiligo also exhibit alexithymia, insecure attachment and poor social support [13]. Physical or psychological stress especially in patients with increased susceptibility to stress increases the levels of catecholamines. Neuropeptides like NPY are found to be co-localized and released along with norepinephrine leading to neuromodulatory effects on melanocytes. Catecholamines can be directly cytotoxic to melanocytes as well. Vascular effects of catecholamines lead to hypoxia and production of free radicals [14].[r]

4.2.3 Biochemical Theory

According to this theory, normal biochemical metabolites of melanogenesis like quinones can become autotoxic if insufficiently contained within the melanosomal organelle [15]. Some authors have suggested the involvement of cellular pathway of pteridines. 5,6,7,8-tetrahydrobiopterin (6BH4) is an essential cofactor for phenylalanine hydroxylase, the enzyme catalysing formation of tyrosine from phenylalanine. There is defective recycling of 6BH4 which leads to increased 6BH4 levels. These are toxic at high concentrations and drive the metabolic pathway forward leading to accumulation of byproducts 7RI-L-erythro 5,6,7,8 tetrahydrobiopterin (7BH4) and H2O2. 7BH4 can inhibit phenylalanine hydroxylase and thus affect melanogenesis [10, 16, 17]. 7BH4 was found in suction blister material from the skin of vitiligo patients [10].

Chemical leukoderma refers to contact depigmentation occurring due to chemicals like monobenzyl ether of hydroquinone (used in rubber industry), monomethyl ether of hydroquinone, pyrocatechol, hydroquinone (used in bleaching creams), *p*-tertiary butylphenol (used as adhesive), paraphenylenediamine (used in hair dyes) and azo dyes (red dye used to colour the feet and hands of women). The exact mechanism by which these chemicals act is not known. Phenolic compounds react with tyrosinase and cause oxidative damage to the melanocyte. 4-tertiary butyl phenol can induce apoptosis in melanocytes. Azo dyes can also cause apoptosis by binding to DNA and also inhibit melanogenesis by competitive inhibition of tyrosinase [9, 18].

Reduced antioxidant defences play an important role in the toxic effects of these chemicals as they do not cause depigmentation in all individuals [15].

4.2.4 Oxidative Stress Theory

According to this theory, it is the oxidative stress inside melanocytes which is responsible for disrupting cell homeostasis by altering the structural and functional integrity of DNA, lipids and proteins ultimately leading to cell death. Mitochondrial dysregulation has also been implicated in oxidative stress-induced melanocyte destruction in vitiligo [19]. Reactive oxygen species (ROS) disrupt mitochondrial dynamics which further increases ROS production, creating a vicious cycle and destroying melanocytes [20]. The role of transient receptor potential cation channel

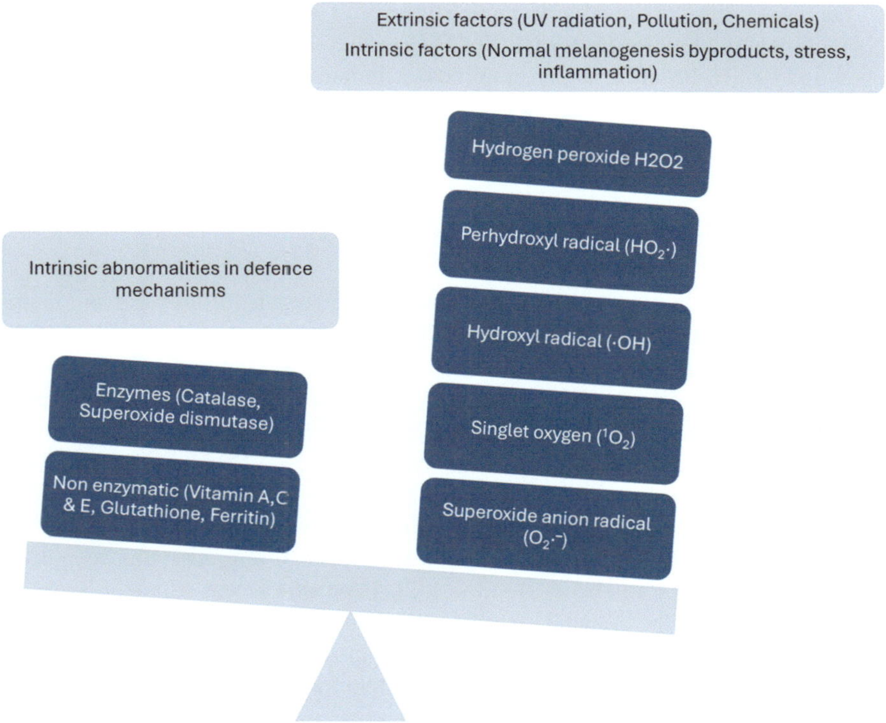

Fig. 4.2 Factors leading to imbalance between oxidants and antioxidants inside melanocytes

subfamily M member 2 (TRPM2) and nicotinamide adenine dinucleotide (NAD+)-dependent deacetylase sirtuin-3 (SIRT3) has been postulated [21]. TRPM2, increases mitochondrial calcium influx and SIRT3 leads to mitochondrial fission, both leading to impaired electron transport chain and stimulation of apoptotic cascade in melanocytes.

ROS also affect cell functions (melanogenesis) and in vitro tests have shown reduced melanogenesis following exposure to H2O2 [22]. Possible mechanisms include the release of high mobility group box 1 (HMGB1) protein which down-regulates melanin synthesis-related proteins [19].

Oxidative stress results from various intrinsic and extrinsic factors which create an imbalance between reactive oxygen species and its scavengers (Fig. 4.2). Patients with vitiligo have increased sensitivity to oxidative stress probably due to impaired antioxidant defence mechanisms. Patients with vitiligo had significantly lower levels of catalase, superoxide dismutase, glutathione peroxidase and glutathione S-transferase and increased levels of hydrogen peroxide (H_2O_2) [23–25]. A systematic review and meta-analysis concluded that these enzymatic alterations and lipid peroxidation were reported in other inflammatory diseases such as psoriasis and lichen planus, suggesting that these are not disease-specific [26].

Oxidative stress is linked to immune stimulation as it promotes the secretion of chemokines (notably IL-15, CXCL16, CXCL9, IL −17 and IL-1b) from keratinocytes and T cell infiltration, which amplifies the inflammation and immune responses against melanocytes [20, 27, 28].

4.2.5 Melanocytorrhagy Theory

According to this theory, there is detachment of melanocytes from basement membrane and neighbouring keratinocytes leading to transepidermal loss. It is possibly related to altered expression of cell adhesion molecules (CAM) like integrins and cadherins in melanocytes [29]. Studies have shown reduced E-cadherin in melanocytes from normal skin of patients with vitiligo [30]. Decreased expression of beta1 integrin, laminin and vascular cell adhesion molecules (VCAM-1) has also been noted [31]. These detached, morphologically altered melanocytes then migrate to the upper layers of epidermis predisposing them to transepidermal loss and apoptosis (known as "anoikis"). The retraction of dendrites and migration has been demonstrated in response to chemical stress [32]. Poor attachment of melanocytes to type IV collagen of the basement membrane in vitiligo patients has also been documented [33]. Although the exact mechanism of apoptosis has not been established, there is loss of fibronectin adhesion-mediated apoptosis suppression in these melanocytes and more exposure to UV radiation in upper epidermis. Perturbed intercellular relationship with neighbouring keratinocytes affects melanosome transfer which induces further oxidative stress through the transfer of immature melanosomes.

Mechanical stress can further decrease levels of E-cadherin; this can explain the development of vitiligo by Koebner phenomenon. Inflammatory mediators like interferon (IFN)-γ and tumour necrosis factor (TNF)α can also lead to loss of E-cadherin suggesting a link with immune dysregulation [31].

4.2.6 Intrinsic Death Theory

According to this theory, melanocytes in vitiligo have intrinsic defects which make them more susceptible to undergo apoptosis [34, 35]. Abnormal rough endoplasmic reticulum, deficiency of growth factors and decreased c-kit receptor expression have been demonstrated in lesional skin [8]. Apoptosis is activated either by an extracellular signal (Fas/FasL and TNF-α/TNFR1) activating the death receptor (extrinsic pathway) or when BCL-2-family proteins cause the permeabilization of the mitochondrial outer membrane (intrinsic pathway). Lower ratios of Bcl-2 (anti-apoptotic)/Bax (pro-apoptotic) have been detected in perilesional melanocytes as compared to the control [36]. TRPM2 was overexpressed in lesional melanocytes of vitiligo, which is a calcium channel sensitive to oxidative stress and leads to abnormal mitochondrial calcium accumulation and apoptosis [37]. Polymorphisms of the FAS gene and elevated level of Fas were implicated by some authors while others suggest involvement of TNF-α/TNFR pathway [38, 39]. All these studies suggest susceptibility to the induction of apoptosis. Apoptosis is considered the main mechanism for loss of melanocytes as supported by histological and laboratory data, although other mechanisms also exist [29].

Many studies have shown that autophagy might play a role in vitiligo, which is not cell "death" per se but a highly conserved cytoprotective catabolic process undertaken to deal with pathophysiological stresses [40]. Autophagy deficiency could affect a melanocyte's ability to defend against oxidative stress. A study has shown that polymorphism of an autophagy-promoting gene may contribute to increased susceptibility to vitiligo [41]. Autophagy deficiency could facilitate oxidative stress-induced apoptosis and autophagy may even lead to IL-17-mediated cell death known as "autophagic cell death" [35].

Some researchers have demonstrated necrotic cells in non-lesional vitiliginous skin suggesting that melanocytes can also undergo necrosis. However, current evidence suggests that this happens in few scenarios only like exposure to high concentrations of H2O2 and mono-benzyl ether of hydroquinone [42, 43].

4.2.7 Immune Theory

According to this theory, autoreactive immune cells are involved in attacking and killing melanocytes. Histochemical and immunohistochemical data confirms infiltration of a large number of T lymphocytes in vitiligo lesions and there is response to immunosuppressive treatment, both supporting this theory.

4.2.7.1 Innate Immunity

Melanocytes secrete exosomes when under stress which are recognized by dendritic cells, macrophages and NK (natural killer) cells inducing their maturation into antigen-presenting cells. ROS and products inside exosomes like melanocyte-specific antigens, miRNAs, heat shock proteins (especially HSP-70) and other proteins (calreticulin and high-mobility group protein B1 [HMGB1]) act as damage-associated molecular patterns (DAMPs) [44, 45]. Aberrant activation of dendritic cells and granzyme-B-expressing activated NK cells in vitiligo has been seen [46, 47]. In vitro studies have demonstrated the expression of HSP70 Lox-1 receptors on the surface of dendritic cells in vitiligo [48]. After activation, dendritic cells locally synthesize cytokines IFN-α and induce T-cell activation and recruitment via type 1 IFN pathway. NLR family pyrin domain containing 3 (NLRP3) is a multiprotein complex which may be activated by DAMPs and initiate the processing and release of pro-inflammatory cytokines IL-1β and IL-18. Recently, perilesional keratinocytes from vitiligo skin have been shown to exhibit increased expressions of NLRP3 and downstream cytokine IL-1β [49]. IL1-β from keratinocytes stimulates expression of chemokines and their receptors which are critical in promoting infiltration of cytotoxic CD8+ lymphocytes in the vitiligo areas. It can also strengthen the function of CD8+ and CD4+ T cells and stimulates polarization of T cells towards Th17 pathway which is involved in the pathogenesis [9, 44].

4.2.7.2 Adaptive Immunity

CD8 Cells

Dendritic cells result in activation and recruitment of melanocyte-specific cytotoxic T lymphocytes (CD8+) of the adaptive immune system. Vitiligo patients have elevated numbers of CD8+ T cells in their peripheral blood compared to healthy individuals. CD8+ T cells are demonstrated from the lesional borders, with their numbers often correlating with disease severity [50]. Some researchers have also shown that in some circumstances, stressed melanocytes can directly activate melanocyte-specific CD8+ T cells [51]. CD8+ T cells produce cytokines such as IFN-γ and TNF. The binding of IFN-γ to its receptor on keratinocytes activates the Janus kinase/signal transducers and activators of transcription (JAK/STAT) signalling the pathway to release chemokines. Notable chemokines include CXCL9, CXCL10 and CXCL11, all acting via CXCR3 receptor. CXCL9, CXCL10 and CXCL11 were the most highly expressed genes in a transcriptional profile of lesional skin of vitiligo patients [52]. CXCL9 promotes further recruitment of CD8+ T cells and CXCL10 is required for localization within the epidermis where melanocytes reside and effector function i.e. inducing apoptosis. CXCL9 and CXCL10 expression strongly correlates with disease activity supporting them as potential biomarkers of disease progression [53]. Animal studies have confirmed that IFN-γ, the IFN-γ receptor, STAT1, CXCL10 and CXCR3 are critical for the development of hypopigmentation in vitiligo [45].

Memory T cells (Trm) are long-lived T cells that persist within tissues and quickly convert to a large number of effector T cells upon re-exposure to the initial pathogenic process. One study found that stable and active vitiligo perilesional skin was highly infiltrated with a population of CD8 Trm cells with control normal human skin [54]. Trm are implicated in disease maintenance and disease flares. The expression of certain cell surface molecules is essential for the functioning of Trm. CD103 and CD96 expression is crucial for their retention, development and survival [55]. CD49, CD122 and IL15 are important for induction of cytotoxic response [56, 57]. Activated CD8+ CD49a + Trm cells were found to be involved in the stimulation of IFN-γ, granzyme B and perforin via IL-15 induction [56].

CD4 Cells

CD4+ helper T cells are mainly responsible for the activation of other immune cells. Th1 and Th17 pathways are thought to be involved in vitiligo development [44, 58, 59]. Decreased Th1/Tc1, Th17/Tc17, and Th1/Th17-Tc1/Tc17 cells were seen in the circulation of vitiligo patients [60]. Increased concentration of IL-2 (a Th1 pathway cytokine) has been noted in lesions [61]. The role of the Th17 pathway has been debated by some researchers as evidenced by a few studies on IL-17 levels and poor response to secukinumab [44, 62].

CD4+ T-regulatory cells (Tregs) maintain peripheral tolerance to their own tissues by suppressing the activity of T-effector cells. Diseases like vitiligo where there is immune dysregulation often either lack Treg or have decreased function of Treg. In the animal model of vitiligo, repigmentation was accompanied by an elevated infiltration of Tregs into the skin, possibly resulting in the prevention of immune responses against melanocytes [63]. Some authors have reported an increase in vitiligo severity when Treg cells were depleted [64].

B Cells

The role of autoantibodies has also been suggested. Proposed mechanisms of generation of these anti-melanocyte antibodies include:

- Primary immune dysregulation and loss of tolerance to pigment cell antigens or
- Primary melanocyte destruction and secondary generation of antibodies against released antigens

IgG and IgA antibodies against tyrosinase and other proteins (L-dopachrome tautomerase, tyrosinase-related protein-1 and 2 [TRP-1 & 2] and human melanocyte-specific protein PMEL17) of the melanogenic pathway have been found at significantly elevated levels in the sera of vitiligo patients. These have been found correlating with extent and activity of vitiligo as well [44, 65, 66].

4.2.8 Stem Cell Theory

According to this theory, it is the inability of melanocyte stem cells to replace the lost melanocytes which is responsible for depigmentation. Whether the renewal capacity of melanocyte stem cells is primarily hampered or the produced melanocytes are destroyed at a rate faster than the producing capacity is unclear and requires more research [30]. However, this theory is debatable as evidence supports that melanocyte stem cells are present in the lesional epidermis of patients with vitiligo, even after 25 years and these stem cells can be used to achieve repigmentation [67, 68].

4.2.9 Viral Theory

This theory has been proposed to identify the role of infections like H. *pylori*, HIV, herpes etc. in vitiligo. Although the exact pathomechanism is not fully established, these microbes may lead to abnormal activation of immune system. Consequently the cytokines and effector cells affect not only the microbes but also melanocytes, highlighting the importance of immune system in vitiligo [15].

4.3 Histopathology of Vitiligo

In order to understand the histopathology of vitiligo it is essential to first understand the concept of epidermal melanin unit [69]. Melanocytes are neural crest derivatives and they reach their final destination of the basal layer of epidermis and hair follicles via a process of migration. In the normal skin in the basal layer of the epidermis, for every five basal keratinocytes, there is one melanocyte [70]. Functionally, these melanocytes provide melanosomes to approximately 36 neighbouring keratinocytes. Keratinocytes produce factors that are important for proliferation, differentiation, functioning and survival of melanocytes.

4.3.1 Melanocytes

The fundamental histopathological finding in vitiligo is loss of functional melanocytes in the basal layer of the epidermis (Fig. 4.3). This loss of melanin can also be demonstrated by using special stains like Fontana-Masson (Fig. 4.4a, b). While earlier research reported complete loss of melanin and absence of melanocytes from the lesional skin, it was later documented that vitiligo lesions may not be fully devoid of melanocytes [71, 72]. Tobin et al. demonstrated melanocytes from in vitro samples of lesional and normal skin, independent of disease duration and treatment [73]. Bartosik et al. detected non-negligible amounts of melanin in basal keratinocytes in one to 3 year old vitiligo lesions, suggesting the possibility of ongoing melanogenesis [74]. In a study of 100 cases of vitiligo, 16% showed the presence of melanin with Fontana-Masson staining [75]. The exact significance of these remaining melanocytes is still unclear. Whether it is a part of early pathogenic inflammatory process where these melanocytes are in the process of destruction or these actually represent

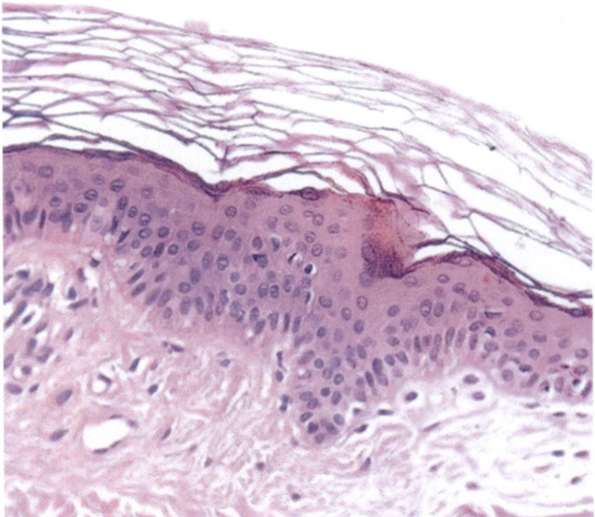

Fig. 4.3 Absence of melanocytes in basal layer of the epidermis in vitiligo (H&E, X400)

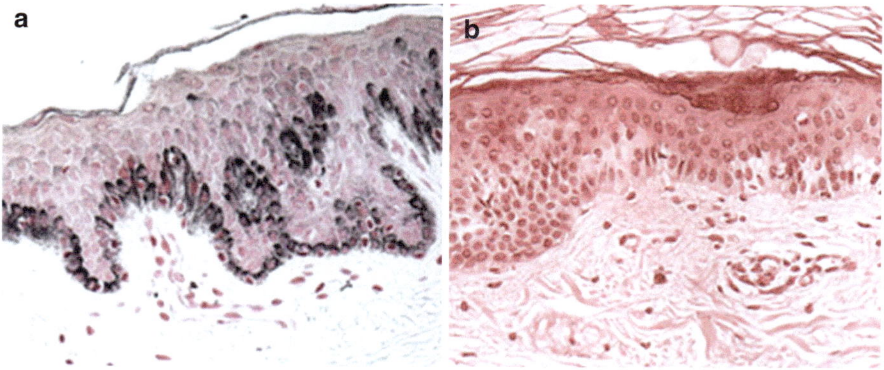

Fig. 4.4 (**a**) Fontana-Masson showing presence of melanin pigment and melanocytes in the epidermis (X400). (**b**) Fontana-Masson showing absence of melanin pigment and melanocytes in the epidermis (x400)

a functional percentage of melanocytes capable of contributing to repigmentation, needs further evaluation. Till then, it is mainly the melanoblasts of outer follicular root sheath which are considered the main source of repigmentation in vitiligo.

4.3.2 Epidermal Changes

Melanin is the first line of defence against ultraviolet radiation. Because vitiliginous skin lacks melanocytes, epidermis may compensate for the absence of pigmentation by undergoing epidermal hyperplasia. Several studies have documented the presence of hyperkeratosis or acanthosis in vitiligo skin [76–78]. In a study of 206 patients (412 sections), significant differences in the thickness of epidermis between vitiligo skin and adjacent normal-appearing skin were noted [79]. These changes were more pronounced in sun-exposed areas than sun-protected areas, suggesting that they indeed occur as a compensatory photoprotective response to UV exposure. Some researchers even use dermabrasion as a therapeutic modality, where they remove the hyperkeratotic skin to increase the penetration of topical agents and narrowband ultraviolet B [80, 81].

Increased number of Langerhans cells in the epidermis has also been reported in some studies, suggesting a possible role in the pathogenesis of vitiligo [75, 76, 82].

4.3.3 Inflammatory Changes

Dermal inflammation is the second most consistent histopathological finding seen in around 48% of cases of vitiligo apart from decreased basal pigmentation [9, 76]. Mostly a superficial lymphocytic infiltrate and occasionally a lichenoid interface dermatitis are seen [83]. In a histopathologic study of 25 patients, both epidermal and dermal inflammatory changes were noted. These changes were more prominent in perilesional skin with perivascular and periadnexal distribution compared to vitiliginous or uninvolved skin [9, 75, 84]. Some researchers also found that the inflammatory changes are more avidly seen in unstable vitiligo and can be correlated with disease activity [85]. Five histopathological variables were evaluated by the researchers: spongiosis, epidermal lymphocytes, basal cell vacuolation, dermal lymphocytes and melanophages (Fig. 4.5a–e). The histopathological criteria for

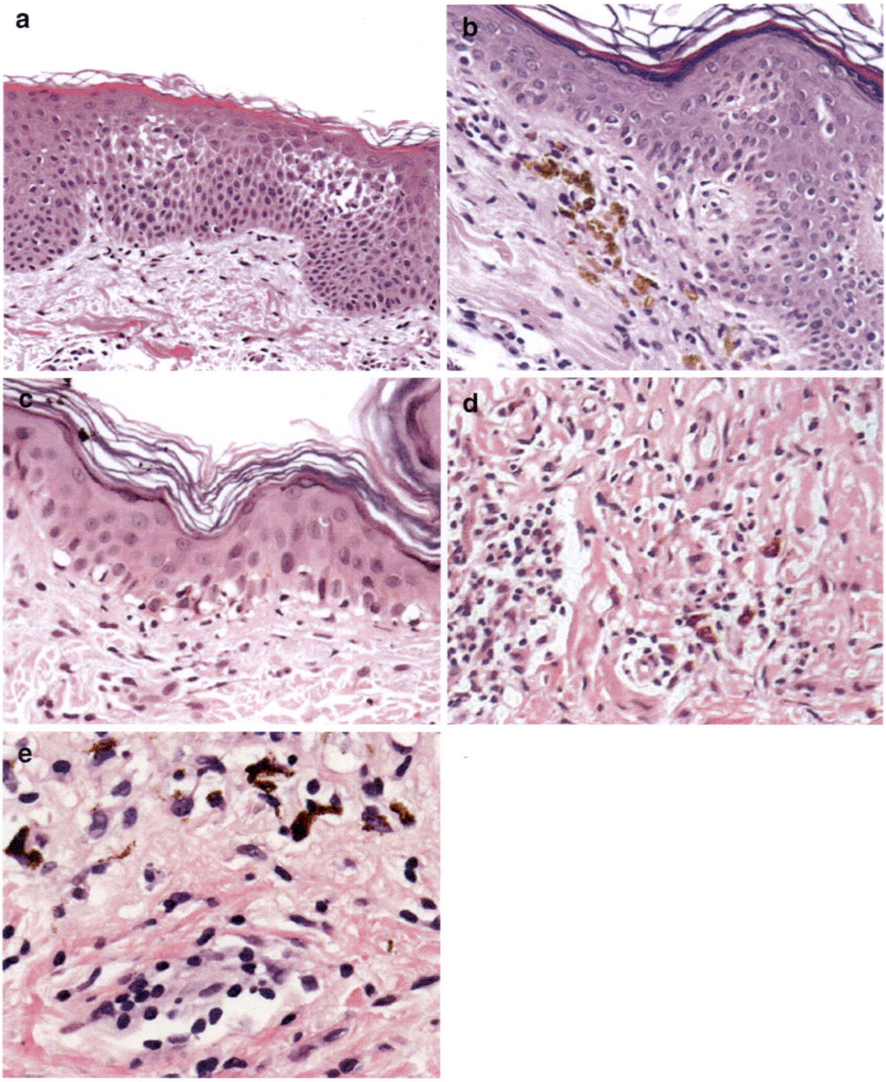

Fig. 4.5 (**a**) Spongiosis (H&E, x400). (**b**) Intraepidermal lymphocytes (H&E, x400). (**c**) Basal cell vacuolation (H&E, x400). (**d**) Dermal lymphocytosis (H&E, x200). (**e**) Dermal melanophages (H&E, x400)

Table 4.1 Histomorphological criteria for spongiosis, epidermal lymphocytes, basal vacuolation and melanophages

S. no.	Histological feature	Criteria
1.	Spongiosis	Presence of at least one focus showing intercellular oedema in the epidermis
2.	Epidermal lymphocytes	Presence of at least one lymphocyte in the epidermis
3.	Basal cell vacuolation	Presence of at least one focus showing basal cell degeneration in the form of vacuolation
4.	Melanophages	Presence of at least one focus in the superficial reticular dermis showing melanophages

Table 4.2 Vitiligo histological scoring system

S. no.	Histological feature	Observation	Score
1.	Spongiosis	Present/absent	1/0
2.	Epidermal lymphocytes	Present/absent	1/0
3.	Basal vacuolation	Present/absent	1/0
4.	Dermal lymphocytes >100	Present/absent	1/0
5.	Melanophages	Present/absent	1/0

Table 4.3 Recommended diagnostic categories based on the score

S. no.	Total score	Diagnosis
1.	5	Unstable vitiligo
2.	4	Unstable vitiligo
3.	3	Favours unstable, clinical corelation required
4.	2	Favours stable, clinical corelation required
5.	0–1	Strongly favours stable vitiligo, clinical correlation essential

these variables are shown in Table 4.1 and a proposed scoring system based on these criteria is shown in Table 4.2. The diagnostic recommendations based on the score obtained are shown in Table 4.3 [85].

4.3.4 Degenerative Changes

Degeneration of basal and suprabasal keratinocytes in the form of vacuolar alterations has also been noted. According to an analysis of 74 cases of vitiligo, these alterations were more marked in long-term disease [83]. Both affected and normal adjacent skin as well as cutaneous nerves and adnexal structures can have foci of vacuolar alterations [9, 83]. Basal cell vacuolization is one of the variables considered by Yadav et al. for histopathological scoring as mentioned above.

4.3.5 Special Stains

Stains that can be used in histopathological analysis of vitiligo include Fontana-Masson stain specific for melanin, dihydroxyphenyl alanine technique for demonstration of tyrosinase, DOPA, HMB-45, Mel-5 and NKI/beteb [83, 86, 87].

4.3.6 Electron Microscopy

Melanocytes from perilesional area of active vitiligo showed retractable dendrites with reduced melanosomes as compared to normal long, thin dendrites and a moderate number of melanosomes in control skin [88]. Abnormalities like cytoplasm vacuolization, rough endoplasmic reticulum dilatation, DNA marginalization in the nucleus, loss of dendrites and detachment have been seen in melanocytes. Keratinocytes show swelling of membrane-bound organelles, formation of vacuoles and cytoplasm condensation [8].

4.3.7 Immunohistochemistry

The major application of immunohistochemistry in vitiligo has been to identify melanocytes. Various markers that have been used for melanocytes include Melan-A, S-100, TP1, dopachrome tautomerase (DCT) and melanogenesis-associated transcription factor (MITF). CD8+ cytotoxic T lymphocytes are the predominant cells identified in the infiltrate. CD103+ resident memory T cells and CD4+ T helper cells have also been found by certain authors [89]. FOXP3+ T regulatory cells (Tregs) have been reported to be under-expressed [90]. CD1a has shown a markedly increased number of Langerhans cells in the epidermis.

Melanocyte stem cells that reside in the outer root sheath of the hair follicle and are responsible for repigmentation, can be demonstrated using immunohistochemical markers against TRP1 and TRP 2.

4.4 Conclusion

There are many interrelated pathomechanisms underlying onset and progression of vitiligo. Intrinsic susceptibility of melanocytes due to genetics, altered structure of organelles, aberrant melanogenesis or adhesion defects in the presence of external stressors like trauma, chemicals, infections, rise of catecholamines and neuromediators gives rise to oxidative stress inside melanocytes. This results in defective melanogenesis, autophagy and apoptosis. Resultant release of antigens stimulates innate as well as adaptive immune response, which is responsible for initiating a cascade of continual melanocyte destruction and disease progression. A multimodal treatment is thus warranted to address the “stressors” of melanocytes and immunosuppressants to control the immune dysregulation.

The fundamental histopathological finding in vitiligo is loss of functional melanocytes in the basal layer of the epidermis. Histopathology can be done in selected cases to rule out close differential diagnosis like nevus depigmentosus and post inflammatory hypopigmentation. Inflammatory changes especially in perilesional skin like spongiosis, epidermal and dermal lymphocytic infiltration may serve as markers for disease activity and severity. Scoring these histopathological parameters can bring more objectivity and consistency in reporting the biopsies.

References

1. Alkhateeb A, Fain PR, Thody A, Bennett DC, Spritz RA. Epidemiology of vitiligo and associated autoimmune diseases in Caucasian probands and their families. Pigment Cell Res. 2003;16:208–14.
2. Roberts GHL, Paul S, Yorgov D, Santorico SA, Spritz RA. Family clustering of autoimmune vitiligo results principally from polygenic inheritance of common risk alleles. Am J Hum Genet. 2019;105:364–72.
3. Roberts GHL, Santorico SA, Spritz RA. The genetic architecture of vitiligo. Pigment Cell Melanoma Res. 2020;33(1):8–15.
4. Spritz RA, Andersen GH. Genetics of vitiligo. Dermatol Clin. 2017;35:245–55.
5. Roberts GHL, Spritz RA. Genetics of vitiligo. eLS. Wiley; 2018.
6. Roberts GHL, Santorico SA, Spritz RA. Deep genotype imputation captures virtually all heritability of autoimmune vitiligo. Hum Mol Genet. 2020;29(5):859–63.
7. Jin Y, Roberts GHL, Ferrara TM, Ben S, van Geel N, Wolkerstorfer A, et al. Early-onset autoimmune vitiligo associated with an enhancer variant haplotype that upregulates class II HLA expression. Nat Comms. 2019;10:391.
8. Mohammed GF, Gomaa AH, Al-Dhubaibi MS. Highlights in pathogenesis of vitiligo. World J Clin Cases. 2015;3(3):221–30.
9. Marchioro HZ, Silva de Castro CC, Fava VM, Sakiyama PH, Dellatorre G, Miot HA. Update on the pathogenesis of vitiligo. An Bras Dermatol. 2022;97(4):478–90.
10. Malhotra N, Dytoc M. The pathogenesis of vitiligo. J Cutan Med Surg. 2013;17(3):153–72.
11. Lazarova R, Hristakieva E, Lazarov N, Shani J. Vitiligo-related neuropeptides in nerve fibers of the skin. Arch Physiol Biochem. 2000;108:262–7.
12. Falabella R, Barona MI, Echeverri IC, Alzate A. Substance P mayplay a part during depigmentation in vitiligo. A pilot study. J Eur Acad Dermatol Venereol. 2003;17:355–6.
13. Picardi A, Pasquini P, Cattaruzza MS, Gaetano P, Melchi CF, Baliva G, et al. Stressful life events, social support, attachment security and alexithymia in vitiligo. A case-control study. Psychother Psychosom. 2003;72(3):150–8.
14. Al Abadie MS. The neuronal theory in the pathogenesis of vitiligo: past and present. J Dermatol Dermatitis. 2021;6(3):1–6.
15. Kundu RV, Mhlaba JM, Rangel SM, Le Poole IC. The convergence theory for vitiligo: a reappraisal. Exp Dermatol. 2019;28(6):647–55.
16. Schallreuter KU, Beazley WD. Wood JM biochemical theory of vitiligo: a role of pteridines in pigmentation. In: Hann SK, Nordlund JJ, editors. Vitiligo. Oxford: Blackwell Science; 2000. p. 151–9.

17. Allam M, Riad H. Concise review of recent studies in vitiligo. Qatar Med J. 2013;2013(2):1–19.
18. Bajaj AK, Saraswat A, Srivastav PK. Chemical leucoderma: Indian scenario, prognosis, and treatment. Indian J Dermatol. 2010;55(3):250–4.
19. Yi X, Guo W, Shi Q, Yang Y, Zhang W, Chen X, et al. SIRT3-dependent mitochondrial dynamics Remodeling contributes to oxidative stress-induced melanocyte degeneration in vitiligo. Theranostics. 2019;9(6):1614–33.
20. Białczyk A, Wełniak A, Kamińska B, Czajkowski R. Oxidative stress and potential antioxidant therapies in vitiligo: a narrative review. Mol Diagn Ther. 2023;27(6):723–39.
21. Kaushik H, Kumar V, Parsad D. Mitochondria-melanocyte cellular interactions: an emerging mechanism of vitiligo pathogenesis. J Eur Acad Dermatol Venereol. 2023;37(11):2196–207.
22. Jimenez-Cervantes C, Martinez-Esparza M, Perez C, Daum N, Solano F, Garcia-Borron JC. Inhibition of melanogenesis in response to oxidative stress: transient downregulation of melanocyte differentiation markers and possible involvement of microphthalmia transcription factor. J Cell Sci. 2001;114:2335–44.
23. Mulayim MK, Kurutas EB, Nazik H, Ozturk P. Assessment of oxidative/nitrosative stress and raftlin in vitiligo. Indian J Dermatol. 2022;67:624.
24. Mathachan SR, Khurana A, Gautam RK, Kulhari A, Sharma L, Sardana K. Does oxidative stress correlate with disease activity and severity in vitiligo? An analytical study. J Cosmet Dermatol. 2021;20:352–9.
25. Said ER, Nagui NAER, Rashed LA, Mostafa WZ. Oxidative stress and the cholinergic system in non-segmental vitiligo: effect of narrow band ultraviolet b. Photodermatol Photoimmunol Photomed. 2021;37:306–12.
26. Speeckaert R, Dugardin J, Lambert J, Lapeere H, Verghaehe E, Speeckaert MM, et al. Critical appraisal of the oxidative stress pathway in vitiligo: a systematic review and meta-analysis. J Eur Acad Dermatol Venereol. 2018;32:1089–98.
27. Li S, Zhu G, Yang Y, Jian Z, Guo S, Dai W, et al. Oxidative stress drives CD8þ T-cell skin trafficking in patients with vitiligo through CXCL16 upregulation by activating the unfolded protein response in keratinocytes. J Allergy Clin Immunol. 2017;140:177e89.e9.
28. He S, Xu J, Wu J. The promising role of chemokines in vitiligo: from oxidative stress to the autoimmune response. Oxidative Med Cell Longev. 2022;2022:8796735.
29. Kumar R, Parsad D. Melanocytorrhagy and apoptosis in vitiligo: connecting jigsaw pieces. Indian J Dermatol Venereol Leprol. 2012;78(1):19–23.
30. Delmas V, Larue L. Molecular and cellular basis of depigmentation in vitiligo patients. Exp Dermatol. 2019;28(6):662–6.
31. Srivastava N, Gupta S, Parsad D. Melanocyte adhesion and apoptosis in vitiligo: linking puzzle blocks. Curr Mol Med. 2023;23(8):709–11.
32. Schallreuter KU, Wood JM, Lemke KR, Levenig C. Treatment of vitiligo with a topical application of pseudocatalase and calcium in combination with short-term UVB exposure: a case study on 33 patients. Dermatology. 1995;190:223–9.
33. Kumar R, Parsad D, Kanwar AJ. Role of apoptosis and melanocytorrhagy: a comparative study of melanocytes adhesion in stable and unstable vitiligo. Br J Dermatol. 2011;164:187–91.
34. Gong Q, Li X, Sun J, Ding G, Zhou M, Zhao W, et al. The effects of calcipotriol on the dendritic morphology of human melanocytes under oxidative stress and a possible mechanism: is it a mitochondrial protector? J Dermatol Sci. 2015;77(2):117–24.
35. Wu X, Yang Y, Xiang L, Zhang C. The fate of melanocyte: mechanisms of cell death in vitiligo. Pigment Cell Melanoma Res. 2021;34(2):256–67.
36. Kumar R, Parsad D, Kanwar AJ, Kanwar A, Kaul D. Altered levels of LXR-α: crucial implications in the pathogenesis of vitiligo. Exp Dermatol. 2012;21(11):853–8.
37. Kang P, Zhang W, Chen X, Yi X, Song P, Chang Y, et al. TRPM2 mediates mitochondria-dependent apoptosis of melanocytes under oxidative stress. Free Radic Biol Med. 2018;126:259–68.
38. Jimbo H, Nagai H, Fujiwara S, Shimoura N, Nishigori C. Fas-FasL interaction in cytotoxic T cell-mediated vitiligo: the role of lesional expression of tumor necrosis factor-α and interferon-γ in Fas-mediated melanocyte apoptosis. Exp Dermatol. 2019;29(1):61–70.

39. Sastry KS, Naeem H, Mokrab Y, Chouchane AI. RNA-seq reveals dysregulation of novel melanocyte genes upon oxidative stress: implications in vitiligo pathogenesis. Oxidative Med Cell Longev. 2019;2019:2841814.
40. Yu H, Cen J, Lin X, He J, Wang Y, Cheng H. Expressions of autophagy-related proteins in perilesional melanocytes of vitiligo in vitro. Zhejiang Med J. 2019;41(24):2592–5.
41. Jeong TJ, Shin MK, Uhm YK, Kim HJ, Chung JH, Lee MH. Association of UVRAG polymorphisms with susceptibility to non-segmental vitiligo in a Korean sample. Exp Dermatol. 2010;19(8):e323–5.
42. Zhang Y, Liu L, Jin L, Yi X, Dang E, Yang Y, et al. Oxidative stress-induced calreticulin expression and translocation: new insights into the destruction of melanocytes. J Invest Dermatol. 2014;134(1):183–91.
43. Hariharan V, Klarquist J, Reust MJ, Koshoffer A, McKee MD, Boissy RE, et al. Monobenzyl ether of hydroquinone and 4-tertiary butyl phenol activate markedly different physiological responses in melanocytes: relevance to skin depigmentation. J Invest Dermatol. 2010;130(1):211–20.
44. Faraj S, Kemp EH, Gawkrodger DJ. Patho-immunological mechanisms of vitiligo: the role of the innate and adaptive immunities and environmental stress factors. Clin Exp Immunol. 2022;207(1):27–43.
45. Bergqvist C, Ezzedine K. Vitiligo: a review. Dermatology. 2020;236(6):571–92.
46. Yu R, Broady R, Huang Y, et al. Transcriptome analysis reveals markers of aberrantly activated innate immunity in vitiligo lesional and non-lesional skin. PLoS One. 2012;7:e51040.
47. Mosenson JA, Zloza A, Nieland JD, et al. Mutant HSP70 reverses autoimmune depigmentation in vitiligo. Sci Transl Med. 2013;5:174ra28.
48. Jacquemin C, Rambert J, Guillet S, Thiolat D, Boukhedouni N, Doutre M-S, et al. Heat shock protein 70 potentiates interferon alpha production by plasmacytoid dendritic cells: relevance for cutaneous lupus and vitiligo pathogenesis. Br J Dermatol. 2017;177:1367–75.
49. Li S, Kang P, Zhang W, et al. Activated NLR family pyrin domain containing 3 (NLRP3) inflammasome in keratinocytes promotes cutaneous T-cell response in patients with vitiligo. J Allergy Clin Immunol. 2020;145:632–45.
50. Strassner JP, Rashighi M, Ahmed Refat M, Richmond JM, Harris JE. Suction blistering the lesional skin of vitiligo patients reveals useful biomarkers of disease activity. J Am Acad Dermatol. 2017;76:847–855.e5.
51. van den Boorn JG, Picavet DI, van Swieten PF, et al. Skin depigmenting agent monobenzone induces potent T-cell autoimmunity toward pigmented cells by tyrosinase haptenation and melanosome autophagy. J Invest Dermatol. 2011;131:1240–51.
52. Rashighi M, Agarwal P, Richmond JM, Harris TH, Dresser K, Su MW, et al. CXCL10 is critical for the progression and maintenance of depigmentation in a mouse model of vitiligo. Sci Transl Med. 2014;6(223):223ra23
53. Wang XX, Wang QQ, Wu JQ, Jiang M, Chen L, Zhang CF, et al. Increased expression of CXCR3 and its ligands in patients with vitiligo and CXCL10 as a potential clinical marker for vitiligo. Br J Dermatol. 2016;174(6):1318–26.
54. Boniface K, Jacquemin C, Darrigade AS, et al. Vitiligo skin is imprinted with resident memory CD8 T cells expressing CXCR3. J Invest Dermatol. 2018;138:355–64.
55. Mackay LK, Rahimpour A, Ma JZ, et al. The developmental pathway for CD103(+)CD8+ tissue-resident memory T cells of skin. Nat Immunol. 2013;14:1294–301.
56. Cheuk S, Schlums H, Gallais Sérézal I, et al. CD49a expression defines tissue-resident CD8+ T cells poised for cytotoxic function in human skin. Immunity. 2017;46:287–300.
57. Richmond JM, Strassner JP, Zapata L, et al. Antibody blockade of IL-15 signaling has the potential to durably reverse vitiligo. Sci Transl Med. 2018;10:eaam7710.
58. Frączek A, Owczarczyk-Saczonek A, Placek W. The role of T_{RM} cells in the pathogenesis of vitiligo-a review of the current state-of-the-art. Int J Mol Sci. 2020;21(10):3552.
59. Matos TR. Is targeting circulating T blood cells a therapeutic option for vitiligo? Br J Dermatol. 2020;183:803.

60. Martins C, Darrigade AS, Jacquemin C, et al. Phenotype and function of circulating memory T cells in human vitiligo. Br J Dermatol. 2020;183:899–908.
61. Das D, Akhtar S, Kurra S, Gupta S, Sharma A. Emerging role of immune cell network in autoimmune skin disorders: an update on pemphigus, vitiligo and psoriasis. Cytokine Growth Factor Rev. 2019;45:35–44.
62. Giordano D, Magri F, Persechino F, et al. Vitiligo with progressive repigmentation during secukinumab treatment in a patient with Psoriatic Arthritis: a case report. Case Rep Dermatol. 2021;13:209–15.
63. Eby JM, Kang HK, Klarquist J, et al. Immune responses in a mouse model of vitiligo with spontaneous epidermal de- and repigmentation. Pigment Cell Melanoma Res. 2014;27:1075–85.
64. Chatterjee S, Eby JM, Al-Khami AA, et al. A quantitative increase in regulatory T cells controls development of vitiligo. J Invest Dermatol. 2014;134:1285–94.
65. Rocha IM, Oliveira LJ, De Castro LC, et al. Recognition of melanoma cell antigens with antibodies present in sera from patients with vitiligo. Int J Dermatol. 2000;39:840–3.
66. Kemp EH, Waterman EA, Gawkrodger DJ, Watson PF, Weetman AP. Autoantibodies to tyrosinase-related protein-1 detected in the sera of vitiligo patients using a quantitative radiobinding assay. Br J Dermatol. 1998;139:798–805.
67. Vinay K, Dogra S. Stem cells in vitiligo: current position and prospects. Pigment Int. 2014;1(1):8–12.
68. Birlea SA, Costin GE, Roop DR, Norris DA. Trends in regenerative medicine: repigmentation in vitiligo through melanocyte stem cell mobilization. Med Res Rev. 2017;37(4):907–35.
69. Haass NK, Herlyn M. Normal human melanocyte homeostasis as a paradigm for understanding melanoma. J Investig Dermatol Symp Proc. 2005;10:153–63.
70. Lee AY, Kim NH, Choi WI, Youm YH. Less keratinocyte-derived factors related to more keratinocyte apoptosis in depigmented than normally pigmented suction blistered epidermis may cause passive melanocyte death in vitiligo. J Invest Dermatol. 2005;124:976–83.
71. Le Poole IC, Das PK. Microscopic changes in vitiligo. Clin Dermatol. 1997;15:863–73.
72. Le Poole IC, van den Wijngaard RM, Westerhof W, Dutrieux RP, Das PK. Presence or absence of melanocytes in vitiligo lesions: an immunohistochemical investigation. J Invest Dermatol. 1993;100:816–22.
73. Tobin DJ, Swanson NN, Pittelkow MR, et al. Melanocytes are not absent in lesional skin of long duration vitiligo. J Pathol. 2000;191:407–16.
74. Bartosik J, Wulf HC, Kobayasi T. Melanin and melanosome complexes in long standing stable vitiligo—an ultrastructural study. Eur J Dermatol. 1998;8:95–9.
75. Kim YC, Kim YJ, Kang HY, Sohn S, Lee ES. Histopathologic features in vitiligo. Am J Dermatopathol. 2008;30:112–6.
76. Montes LF, Abulafia J, Wilborn WH, et al. Value of histopathology in vitiligo. Int J Dermatol. 2003;42:57–61.
77. El-Khateeb EA, Ragab NF, Mohamed SA. Epidermal photoprotection: comparative study of narrowband ultraviolet B minimal erythema doses with and without stratum corneum stripping in normal and vitiligo skin. Clin Exp Dermatol. 2011;36:393–8.
78. Stylianos V, Eleftherios I, Nikolaos K, et al. Correlating epidermal thickness and basement membrane length to angiogenesis in the centre and the periphery of vitiligo lesion. Indian J Dermatol Venereol Leprol. 2012;78:368–71.
79. Jung SE, Kang HY, Lee ES, Kim YC. Changes of epidermal thickness in vitiligo. Am J Dermatopathol. 2015;37(4):289–92.
80. Awad SS. Dermabrasion may repigment vitiligo through stimulation of melanocyte precursors and elimination of hyperkeratosis. J Cosmet Dermatol. 2012;11:318–22.
81. Bayoumi W, Fontas E, Sillard L, et al. Effect of a preceding laser dermabrasion on the outcome of combined therapy with narrowband ultraviolet B and potent topical steroids for treating nonsegmental vitiligo in resistant localizations. Br J Dermatol. 2012;166:208–11.
82. Faria AR, Tarlé RG, Dellatorre G, Mira MT, Castro CC. Vitiligo – Part 2 – classification, histopathology and treatment. An Bras Dermatol. 2014;89(5):784–90.

83. Sharquie KE, Mehenna SH, Naji AA, Al-Azzawi H. Inflammatory changes in vitiligo: stage I and II depigmentation. Am J Dermatopathol. 2004;26(2):108–12.
84. Yadav AK, Singh P, Khunger N. Clinicopathologic analysis of stable and unstable vitiligo: a study of 66 cases. Am J Dermpathol. 2016;38:608–13.
85. Pauncio AL, Vignale R. Ultrastructural studies in stable vitiligo. Am J Dermatopathol. 2003;2:16–20.
86. Yaghoobi R, Omidian M, Bagherani N. Vitiligo: a review of the published work. J Dermatol. 2011;38:419–31.
87. Alikhan A, Felsten LM, Daly M, Petronic-Rosic V. Vitiligo: a comprehensive overview part I. Introduction, epidemiology, quality of life, diagnosis, differential diagnosis, associations, histopathology, etiology, and work-up. J Am Acad Dermatol. 2011;65:473–91.
88. Xiong XX, Ding GZ, Zhao WE, Li X, Ling YT, Li S, et al. Differences in the melanosome distribution within the epidermal melanin units and its association with the impairing back-ground of leukoderma in vitiligo and halo nevi: a retrospective study. Arch Dermatol Res. 2017;309:323–33.
89. Frączek A, Owczarczyk-Saczonek A, Placek W. The role of TRM cells in the pathogenesis of vitiligo-a review of the current state-of-the-art. Int J Mol Sci. 2020;21:3552.
90. Kidir M, Karabulut AA, Ercin ME, Atasoy P. Regulatory T-cell cytokines in patients with nonsegmental vitiligo. Int J Dermatol. 2017;56:581–8.

Chapter 5
Mechanism of Repigmentation in Vitiligo

Anuradha Bishnoi, K. B. Meghana, and Davinder Parsad

Abstract Repigmentation and its maintenance have always been important from the viewpoint of patients with vitiligo and treating physicians, and now have been classified as the core outcome domains. Various treatment approaches, including medical and surgical methods, aim to stimulate melanocyte activity and regeneration. This chapter explores the mechanisms involved in repigmentation, clinical patterns observed, and repigmentation responses to different modalities of treatment used in vitiligo.

Keywords Repigmentation · Melanocytes · NBUVB · Stability · JAK inhibitors · Patterns of repigmentation

5.1 Introduction

Melanocytes are generally long-lived cells, but they are not strictly permanent. They are typically stable in their location within the basal layer of the epidermis, where they continue to produce melanin over the lifespan of an individual. Melanocytes have a lifespan that extends over many years, and they do not divide as frequently as other skin cells like keratinocytes. However, they can be replaced, when necessary, especially in response to certain stimuli such as injury or UV exposure, which can activate stem cells in the skin to differentiate into new melanocytes. Their numbers and function can decrease due to aging, environmental factors, or specific skin conditions like vitiligo. This turnover, while relatively slow, suggests that while melanocytes are durable, they are not entirely permanent and can be subject to renewal and replacement under certain conditions.

Vitiligo is a multifactorial disease affecting melanocytes leading to depigmentation of the skin. The repigmentation in vitiligo can be spontaneous or following

A. Bishnoi · K. B. Meghana · D. Parsad (✉)
Department of Dermatology, Venereology and Leprology, Postgraduate Institute of Medical Education and Research, Chandigarh, India

R. Sarkar, V. Narayan R (eds.), *A Concise Guide to The Management of Vitiligo*,
https://doi.org/10.1007/978-981-95-3857-7_5

treatment. The mechanism of repigmentation is not fully understood. Morphologically, repigmentation can follow perifollicular, marginal, or diffuse patterns. "Repigmentation" and "maintenance of repigmentation" are now considered core outcome domains by "The Vitiligo Global Issues Consensus Conference (VGICC)", through an international e-Delphi consensus and should be included in all vitiligo trials [1].

5.2 Clinical Patterns of Repigmentation

Four classical patterns of repigmentation are described:

(i) *Perifollicular repigmentation*: It is the most common pattern of repigmentation. It appears as small, round, peri-follicular pigmented macules. Earlier, in vivo studies found dormant 3,4-dihydroxy-L-phenylalanine (DOPA)-negative melanocytes in the outer root sheath of hair follicles in both healthy persons and vitiligo patients. Later, the hair follicle bulge was identified as the source of these DOPA-negative melanocytes, as demonstrated in both transgenic mouse models and human skin. Melanocyte precursors move upwards from this site to restore the depigmented epidermis in individuals with vitiligo receiving ultraviolet radiation therapy (UVR). The UV-induced repigmentation process involves several stages: stimulation of keratinocytes and activation of melanocytes following UV light exposure, melanocyte migration (which includes detachment from the basement membrane and keratinocytes inside the hair follicles, cellular movement, and reattachment to the basal layer in the interfollicular epidermis), followed by differentiation that imparts the ability to generate melanin (Fig. 5.1) [2].

(ii) *Marginal repigmentation*: The marginal pattern of repigmentation appears along the edges of the lesions. This occurs due to the activation of functional epidermal melanocytes at the lesion borders. Some researchers have suggested the existence of an epidermal repigmentation reservoir, which consists of immature melanocyte precursors that likely possess the capacity to migrate, differentiate, and potentially proliferate (Fig. 5.2) [3].

(iii) *Diffuse repigmentation*: The diffuse repigmentation pattern is characterized by a generalized darkening across vitiligo patches. This pattern indicates that repigmentation might originate from interfollicular melanocyte precursors, through the reactivation of DOPA-negative melanocytes, which are thought to persist in the center of the depigmented lesions (Fig. 5.3) [4].

(iv) *Combined pattern*: This type does not fit into any particular pattern and consists of at least two patterns of repigmentation together occurring in the lesion (Fig. 5.4).

A new pattern of *medium-spotted repigmentation* pattern was found in places with little to no hair, including the palms, soles, lips, wrists, and ankles, in a recent study of paediatric vitiligo patients [5]. This rare pattern starts as larger spots that

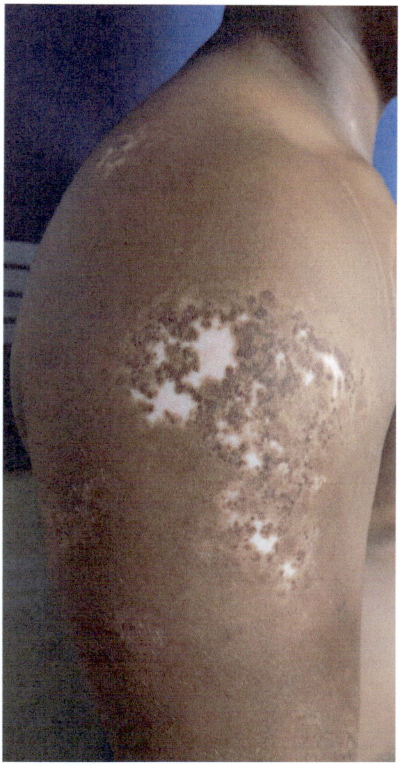

Fig. 5.1 Depigmented patch on arm showing perifollicular repigmentation

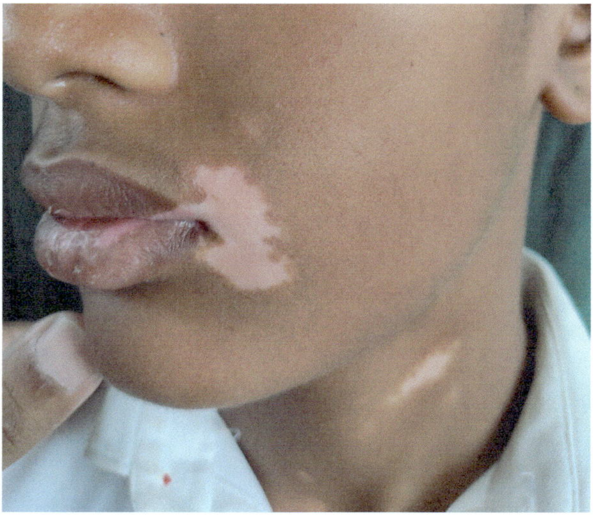

Fig. 5.2 Vitiligo patch on the angle of mouth showing marginal repigmentation

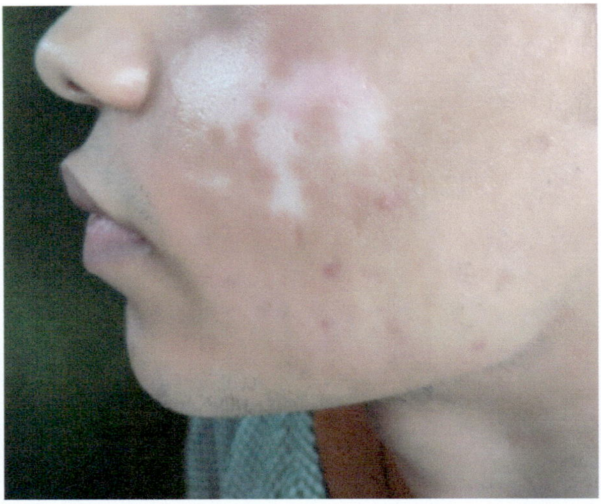

Fig. 5.3 Vitiligo patch on infraorbital region showing diffuse pigmentation

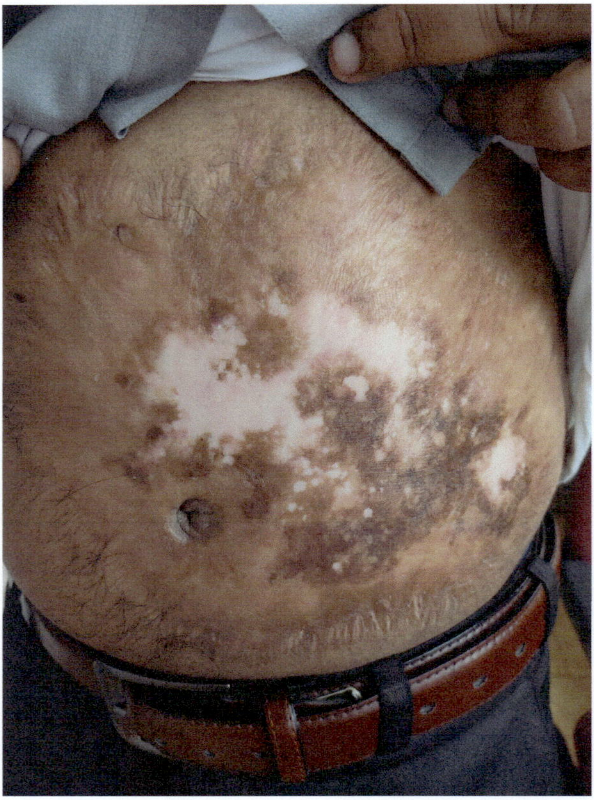

Fig. 5.4 Depigmented patch on abdomen showing combined pattern of repigmentation

are not centered around specific hair follicles. Supporting these findings, an earlier study reported an unusual pattern of repigmentation on a patient's palms, characterized by irregular brown macules following psoralen plus UVA (PUVA) therapy. Along the basement membrane of the repigmented patches, tyrosinase-positive (TYR+) melanocytes were seen; in contrast, the surrounding vitiliginous skin did not contain these cells [6]. In a study comparing various repigmentation patterns, the perifollicular pattern was predominantly seen with PUVA therapy, while topical corticosteroids most frequently led to a diffuse repigmentation pattern [7].

5.3 Favourable Factors for Repigmentation

1. Repigmentation tends to occur more effectively in areas with higher hair follicle density. Repigmentation can take place in areas with either terminal or vellus hair. Theoretically, repigmentation should be more noticeable in areas containing terminal hair because of the greater density of stem cells. However, since the face typically receives the most sun exposure, it usually shows the most significant response to repigmentation efforts.

   Regions such as the face, arms, forearms, thighs, legs, abdomen, and back show quicker responses to treatment, while areas with fewer hair follicles, dorsum of the hands, fingers, feet, and toes, tend to respond more slowly [8]. The potential for treatment success in hairless sites depends on migration of melanocytes from the edges of the lesion, which can migrate approximately 4–5 mm into the depigmented area. It could also occur from the migration of melanocytes from the extrafollicular dermal sources or melanocytes surviving and residing in the depigmented lesions [9].
2. Areas with leukotrichia show poor response to medical treatment and have minimal chances of repigmentation. Leukotrichia may indicate a more severe, prolonged, and active immune-mediated attack by CD8+ cytotoxic T cells on melanocytes, which has gradually progressed from the epidermis down to the bulge [10].
3. It is now known that melanocytes are not completely absent in the vitiligo lesions. Melanocytes were successfully isolated and cultured from both vitiligo and normal skin samples, regardless of disease duration or treatment, although immunohistochemical analysis did not detect intact melanocytes in affected skin. The study also highlighted the findings of melanocyte degeneration in vitiligo, including vacuolation, a dilated endoplasmic reticulum, and granular deposits. Small amounts of melanin granules were found in long-term vitiligo cases, indicating the presence of some functioning melanocytes. Rare, intact melanocytes, though typically amelanotic or poorly melanized, were also observed in lesional skin [11].

5.4 Repigmentation with Various Therapeutic Agents in Vitiligo

5.4.1 Phototherapy

Although vitiligo manifests with complete loss of pigmentation in the epidermis, the pigmentation of hair in the affected patch is often retained, especially in non-segmental disease phenotype. This suggests that the melanocytes in the *hair bulb* and the melanocyte reservoir in the *hair bulge* region inside the depigmented vitiligo skin remain unaffected by the immune attacks [12]. Recent immunostaining studies have confirmed the existence of melanocyte precursors in the hair follicles of depigmented vitiligo areas [13].

Two possible explanations for the preservation of melanocytes/their precursors inside the hair follicle bulge and bulb are as follows: (i) melanocytes are positioned deep within the follicle; autoreactive CD8+ T lymphocytes are unable to recognize the melanocyte-associated antigens and (ii) the hair follicle benefits from immune privilege, which shields melanocytes from cytotoxic T cell attacks [14]. Studies have indicated that melanocyte and keratinocyte stem cells find a somewhat secure location in the bulge area of hair follicles. This bulge, which is a component of the outer root sheath, extends to the base of the permanent section of the hair follicle and acts as the site of attachment for the arrector pili muscle. Additionally, the bulge is recognized as an immune-privileged site, shielding it from harmful immunologic inflammation. Transforming growth factor beta-1 (TGF-β1) is secreted in higher levels by keratinocytes in the bulge, which keeps melanocyte stem cells in a quiescent state by down-regulating the activity of the microphthalmia-associated transcription factor (MITF) [15]. TGF-β1 from this niche also contributes to an immunosuppressive environment, helping to preserve the immune privilege of the bulge region [16].

Three populations of melanocytes are present in successive slices of skin treated with NB-UVB: Dct+/c-Kit−/TYR− (melanocyte stem cells), Dct+/c-Kit+/TYR− (melanoblasts), and Dct+/c-Kit+/TYR+ (mature melanocytes) [13]. Dormant melanocyte stem cells (Dct+/c-Kit−/TYR−) found in the bulge area of hair follicles are immediately activated by NB-UVB and migrate upward through the ORS to the lesional epidermis and eventually differentiate into functional melanocytes (Dct+/c-Kit+/TYR+).

The two main pathways that accelerate the pigmentation and differentiation process are mediated via p53 and Wnt/β-catenin. It is well established that UVR-induced cellular and DNA damage causes p53 activation. p53 regulates melanocyte activation by coordinating the release of paracrine and growth factors from keratinocytes that promote melanogenesis [17] via the microphthalmia-associated transcription factor (MITF). Similarly, in vitiligo, p53 and its downstream effector, α-melanocyte stimulating hormone—a potent inducer of MITF—mediate melanocyte activation by NBUVB. Wnt signaling is also essential for melanocyte development and differentiation. Its activation leads to the stabilization of the β--catenin/

lymphoid enhancer factor (Lef) complex, which in turn causes the transactivation of downstream target genes like MITF [18]. Epidermal Wnt regulates the induction of hair follicles by coordinating molecular signaling between the dermis and epidermis. Hair matrix cell growth requires epithelial Wnt/β-catenin signaling, while bulge stem cells and epidermal proliferation also require β-catenin [19].

In a meta-analysis of 35 studies, long-duration NBUVB phototherapy showed at least a mild response (>25% repigmentation) in 62.1%, 74.2%, and 75.0% subjects at 3, 6, and 12 months, respectively, with marked responses (>75% repigmentation) observed in 13%, 19.2%, and 35.7% [20]. Additionally, it was noted that the NBUVB-induced repigmentation was more stable than PUVA-induced repigmentation [21]. Regarding the pattern of repigmentation, perifollicular pattern is more common with both NBUVB and PUVA, followed by marginal pattern. Several studies have now shown that the NBUVB is more effective than PUVA in inducing repigmentation in vitiligo, and the colour match is better with NBUVB compared to PUVA therapy [22, 23].

5.4.2 Human Models of Repigmentation

Punch Grafts Punch grafts placed on depigmented vitiligo lesions were then treated with UV radiation and khellin. Melanocyte migration ability was demonstrated in immunostaining tests that showed horizontal migration to depigmented regions [24].

Punch Biopsies Skin biopsies from patients treated with NBUVB for 3 and 6 months, as well as from patients with untreated vitiligo, were immunostained with keratinocyte-specific marker (K14), proliferation and/or migration markers (KI-67), and melanocyte markers (DCT, C-KIT, TYR, or PAX3). The melanocyte count was found significantly increased in response to NBUVB, and normal melanocyte population in the epidermis was restored [13].

5.4.3 Repigmented NB-UVB-Treated Skin Versus Normal Skin and Untreated Vitiligo Skin

Through immunostaining techniques and skin biopsy analysis from vitiligo patients, the authors demonstrated that NBUVB treatment led to a modest rise in two populations of immature melanocytes in the hair follicle bulge: a stem cell population marked by C-KIT(−)/DCT(+) and a melanoblast population marked by C-KIT(+)/DCT(+). Melanocyte proliferation following NBUVB treatment was indirectly indicated by an increase in melanocyte numbers across all regions examined and directly measured by the co-expression of KI-67 with C-KIT, DCT, and TYR. The study observed a possible migratory melanocyte population that was marginally present in the bulge but increased in the infundibulum and epidermis. Melanocyte precursors demonstrated differentiation in the upper infundibulum by progressively expressing TYR, a process that accompanied their proliferation and migration, continuing into the epidermis (TYR(+)/MCAM(+)/KI-67(+). No significant differences in melanocyte marker expression were observed between NBUVB-treated vitiligo skin and normal human skin, suggesting that 3 to 6 months of NBUVB therapy restores pigmentation in depigmented skin to normal levels [13].

5.4.4 Corticosteroids

Corticosteroids function through local immunomodulation. Their primary mechanism involves binding to the glucocorticoid receptor, which leads to the suppression of gene expression for numerous cytokines involved in the pathogenesis, and decreases the activity of cytotoxic T lymphocytes [25]. Corticosteroids are considered more effective in stabilizing vitiligo rather than inducing repigmentation. Systemic corticosteroids are prescribed for rapidly spreading active vitiligo and not in stable disease for the purpose of repigmentation alone. To minimize the possibility of adverse effects, pulse treatment with systemic corticosteroids is preferred.

Repigmentation tends to be better in sun exposed areas, while acral regions typically respond poorly [26]. In a meta-analysis conducted by Njoo et al., both potent (56%) and very potent (55%) topical corticosteroids (TCS) demonstrated comparable efficacy in achieving ≥75% repigmentation in treating localized vitiligo [27].

Oral prednisolone was given to patients with active vitiligo in a trial by Kim et al. during the first 2 months at a dose of 0.3 mg/kg of body weight. The results revealed that 70.4% of patients had repigmentation and 87.7% of patients had cessation of the active disease [28]. In a retrospective analysis, 444 active vitiligo patients were treated with low-dose oral mini-pulse treatment regimen. The patients received a dosage of 2.5 mg/day on two consecutive days each week. 91.8% of patients had no longer had disease activity, and the follow-up period showed a 12.25% recurrence rate. Regarding repigmentation, 303 patients (68.3%) showed good improvement, 56 patients (12.6%) exhibited moderate improvement, and 6 patients (1.2%) had excellent outcomes. The repigmentation of the remaining 79 patients (17.9%) showed little improvement [29]. Diffuse pattern of repigmentation was most common pattern observed by topical corticosteroids followed by perifollicular pattern [7].

5.4.5 *Topical Calcineurin Inhibitors*

Topical calcineurin inhibitors act by restoring the disrupted cytokine network in vitiligo patients. By downregulating the transcription of genes producing proinflammatory cytokines such as interleukin (IL)-2, IL-3, IL-4, IL-5, interferon (IFN)-γ, tumour necrosis factor (TNF)-α, and granulocyte-macrophage colony-stimulating factor in T cells, tacrolimus has been demonstrated to limit T-cell activation [30].

Furthermore, tacrolimus has been shown to have direct impacts on melanocyte migration and differentiation during repigmentation [31, 32]. Co-treatment with NB-UVB and tacrolimus enhances melanosome secretion and transfer to keratinocytes [33]. An open-label study of combined treatment with NB-UVB and tacrolimus 0.03% ointment involving 110 patients showed variable response in different regions of the body. The clinical response was defined as over 50% repigmentation. Response rates varied significantly by site, with the highest observed on facial lesions (73%), followed by limbs (68%) and trunk (53.5%). Conversely, the therapeutic impact on extremities and genital areas was notably less effective [34]. TCI has been shown to be effective as monotherapy in a comprehensive review and meta-analysis by Lee et al., with ≥25% repigmentation in 55% of patients, ≥50% repigmentation in 38.5% of patients, and ≥ 75% repigmentation in 18.1% of patients. According to the study, the hands and feet showed the least favourable response, while the face and neck showed the most favourable response, followed by the trunk and extremities [35].

5.4.6 *Topical Vitamin D Analogues*

Topical vitamin D analogues have the potential to restore pigmentation in vitiligo lesions by directly activating melanocytic precursors and melanogenic pathways, as well as by triggering local skin immunosuppression [36]. Despite experimental data suggesting a stimulatory effect of vitamin D compounds on melanocyte pigmentation in humans and animals at the cellular and molecular levels, a thorough review of the literature found no evidence of repigmentation as monotherapy.

Vitamin D analogues appear to have a therapeutic effect when used in conjunction with topical steroids or phototherapy [37]. In an 18-month double-blind study, 19 patients with symmetrical lesions were treated with 8-methoxypsoralen and sunlight exposure. Calcipotriol was applied to one side of the body and a placebo to the other. After 6 months, 70% of patients showed significant improvement with calcipotriol, compared to 35% with the placebo. By the end of study, 76% had marked improvement with calcipotriol, while 53% saw moderate improvement with the placebo. Repigmentation of hands and feet was especially enhanced with the combination of PUVAsol and calcipotriol [38].

In a randomized controlled trial by Kumaran et al., the effectiveness of calcipotriol 0.005% ointment and betamethasone dipropionate 0.05% cream in treating localized vitiligo was evaluated. Administered either alone or together, the results showed 6.7% of patients had marked repigmentation (50–75%) with calcipotriol alone, 13.3% with betamethasone alone, and 26.7% with the combination therapy. The combination treatment resulted in faster repigmentation onset [39].

5.4.7 JAK Inhibitors

JAK inhibitors such as tofacitinib and ruxolitinib function by suppressing the JAK-STAT pathway, leading to inhibition of interferon-gamma (IFN-γ) axis, which is implicated in vitiligo pathogenesis. IL-15 and the IFN-γ/CXCL9/10 pathway are also involved in pathogenesis. Keratinocytes generate IL-15 in response to oxidative stress; this cytokine binds to its receptor, IL-15 receptor, on the cell membrane of tissue-resident memory T cells in the epidermis. In vitiligo lesions, there is an increase in IL-15 levels, which is important for preserving memory T cells and promoting the synthesis of IFN-γ. Furthermore, IL-15 promotes the generation of IFN-γ by natural killer (NK) cells and type 1 innate lymphoid cells (ILC1) in the epidermis by supporting their development, maintenance, and activation [40, 41].

In a phase 2 open-label trial involving 11 patients, Ruxolitinib 1.5% cream was applied twice daily over a 20-week period, with treatment areas covering up to 10% of the body surface or a maximum of 3.75 g per application. This study reported a statistically significant 27% improvement in the overall mean Vitiligo Area Scoring Index (VASI), noting a more favourable response on the face compared to other body areas [42].

Another phase 2 study conducted by Rosmarin et al. explored the effectiveness and safety of ruxolitinib cream across three concentrations (0.15%, 0.5%, and 1.5%), against a placebo over a period of 52 weeks. Patients were assigned to one of four treatment groups, including 1.5% cream applied once or twice daily. At the 24-week checkpoint, those using the 1.5% cream once and twice daily achieved facial VASI reductions of 50% and 45%, respectively, significantly outperforming the 3% improvement observed in the placebo group. The most robust responses were seen with the twice-daily application of the 1.5% cream, achieving reductions of 58% in F-VASI50, 52% in F-VASI75, and 33% in F-VASI90 by the 52-week mark [43].

In the two randomized, double-blind, phase 3 trials that involved 674 patients, ruxolitinib 1.5% cream consistently outperformed the placebo. By week 52, 74.6% of patients achieved a $\geq$ 50% reduction in their facial VASI, while 50.3% saw a $\geq$ 75% reduction. Additionally, over half the patients (51.1%) achieved at least a 50% improvement in their total VASI. Treatment-related adverse events affected 13.7% of patients, primarily manifesting as acne at the application site (4.4%) and pruritus (3.5%) [44].

These studies collectively underscore the significant potential of ruxolitinib cream in managing vitiligo, especially with consistent and higher-concentration applications, and highlight its role in substantial skin repigmentation, particularly on the face. The USFDA now approves topical ruxolitinib 1.5% cream for treatment of non-segmental vitiligo in ≥12 years of age, and is the first medical treatment approved by the FDA for vitiligo [45].

Oral tofacitinib was first used in a female vitiligo patient with approximately 10% depigmentation of body surface area, who had not responded to topical corticosteroid and tacrolimus ointment. A daily dose of 5 mg of oral tofacitinib was given to the patient. After 5 months of therapy, just 5% of the patient's body surface area remained depigmented [46]. In a study of 10 vitiligo patients treated with oral tofacitinib (5–10 mg daily) for an average of 9.9 months, only half achieved repigmentation, *primarily in sun-exposed areas*. Flow cytometry showed a reduction in CD8+ T cells after treatment. Chemokine levels, including CXCL9 and CXCL10, were significantly reduced [47]. Other open-label studies and case series have shown that oral tofacitinib (5 mg twice daily) can lead to variable repigmentation in areas like the face, scalp, and trunk [48, 49].

In a phase 2 trial, patients were randomly assigned to receive daily oral ritlecitinib, (an irreversible inhibitor with a high selectivity for JAK3), with or without a 4-week loading dose (200/50 mg, 100/50 mg, 30 mg, or 10 mg), or a placebo for 24 weeks during the dose-ranging phase. Following this, patients entered a 24-week extension period where they were given 200/50 mg of ritlecitinib daily. The primary measure of effectiveness was the percentage change from the baseline in the Facial-Vitiligo Area Scoring Index (F-VASI) at week 24. Results showed that out of 364 patients treated during the dose-ranging phase, those in the 50 mg ritlecitinib groups, both with a loading dose (−21.2 vs. 2.1; $p < 0.001$) and without (−18.5 vs. 2.1; $p < 0.001$), as well as those in the 30 mg group (−14.6 vs. 2.1; $p = 0.01$), experienced significant improvements compared to placebo. Further improvement in F-VASI was noted during the extension period with 200/50 mg ritlecitinib ($n = 187$) suggesting that a longer treatment duration may be necessary to achieve optimal repigmentation. There were no trends in dose-dependent adverse events, either emergent or serious, throughout the 48-week treatment period [50].

5.4.8 Afamelanotide

Afamelanotide is a synthetic form of α-melanocyte-stimulating hormone (α-MSH). α-MSH is shown to exist in low levels in the lesional skin and circulation in people with vitiligo [51]. In clinical studies, it has mostly been investigated as an adjuvant treatment in conjunction with phototherapy. According to earlier research, α-MSH acts via the melanocortin-1 receptor, which is usually not present in melanoblasts in the early stages. The co-administration of afamelanotide with NB-UVB phototherapy resulted in improved melanoblast development, differentiation and elevated melanocortin-1 receptor expression [52]. In a randomized multicenter trial comparing afamelanotide with NB-UVB therapy versus NB-UVB monotherapy, the combination treatment showed superior results based on the Vitiligo Area Scoring Index (VASI) and Vitiligo European Task Force assessment (VETFa). Patients receiving the combination therapy experienced faster and higher rates of repigmentation, particularly on the face and upper extremities. By day 168, the combination group had a repigmentation rate of 48.64%, compared to 33.26% in the monotherapy group [52]. The patterns were primarily follicular and confluent.

5.4.9 Basic Fibroblast Growth Factor (bFGF)-Derived Peptide

Nada and Rashed et al. highlighted the significance of basic fibroblast growth factor (bFGF) in vitiligo. This growth factor acts as a mitogen, promoting both the proliferation and migration of melanocytes [53]. The rationale behind using bFGF-derived peptides (bFGFrP) for vitiligo treatment stems from the theory that vitiligo is associated with a deficiency in melanocyte growth factors. Clinical trials provide evidence supporting bFGFrP as a viable treatment option to induce repigmentation in vitiligo management. NBUVB exposure triggers cultured keratinocytes to secrete bFGF. Additionally, NBUVB was found to promote melanocyte migration by increasing the expression of phosphorylated focal adhesion kinase (p125FAK) in melanocytes [54]. So combination of NBUVB and bFGF yields better results. When compared to tacrolimus monotherapy, the combination of 0.1% tacrolimus and 0.1% bFGF-related decapeptide solution demonstrated superior outcomes in a multicentric trial. The combination group showed a significantly greater mean response rate (66.75%) in achieving more than 50% of repigmentation when compared to the tacrolimus monotherapy group (46.47%) [55].

5.4.10 Prostaglandins (PG)

Prostaglandins are secreted by many cells like melanocytes, keratinocytes, and Langerhans cells. They serve several important functions in the skin; one among them is biological regulator of melanocyte growth. Latanoprost (PG F2α) when used to treat glaucoma, resulted in periorbital hyperpigmentation and darkening of the iris and eyelashes. The exact process by which prostaglandins cause hyperpigmentation is still unknown. It is hypothesized by stimulating melanocyte growth, modifying the susceptibility of melanocytes to neural signals, and engaging with melanocytes directly or indirectly via stimulating tyrosinase activity through secondary messengers [56]. Patients with stable vitiligo received weekly intradermal injections of prostaglandin E2 (PGE2; group I), PGF2α (group II), or a saline placebo (group III) for 12 weeks, in conjunction with twice-weekly NBUVB phototherapy over 3 months. Groups I and II showed comparable levels of repigmentation, both significantly outperforming group III. However, repigmentation began significantly earlier and patient satisfaction was higher with PGE2 compared to PGF2α. Both diffuse and perifollicular patterns of repigmentation were observed [57]. In a study of 24 individuals with vitiligo, 15 patients showed considerable repigmentation after 6 months of therapy. Patients with localized vitiligo lesions and segmental vitiligo exhibited most improvement [58].

5.4.11 Repigmentation with Surgical Modalities

The main goal in surgical modality of treatment is to restore the melanocytes in a depigmented patch by transferring the functional melanocytes from normal skin. The most important criterion for selection of patient is the stability of the disease. For a given vitiligo patient to undergo surgery, lesional stability of >1 year with global stability of 6–12 months is considered optimal [59]. Even basic dermabrasion can cause depigmented lesions to repigment. It has been proposed that dermabrasion modifies the environment of epidermal cytokines, which may activate dormant outer root sheath melanocytes leading to perifollicular pattern of repigmentation [60]. In suction blister epidermal grafting, melanocytes move easily to the graft bed when epidermal grafts are in touch with the denuded surface of the recipient vitiliginous region for approximately a week, which causes diffuse pattern of repigmentation [61]. Split-thickness skin graft also results in diffuse pattern of repigmentation but carries risk of hyperpigmentation, stuck-on appearance and scars in donor area. In mini punch grafting, grafts of punch size 1.2 mm are used. This promotes the hair follicle reservoir because the mini grafts function as islands of melanocyte reservoirs. The perigraft pigmentation that develops from 1–2 mm minigrafts often spreads 5–10 mm past the graft edge. This technique might create cobblestone appearance in the recipient area [62]. The findings from the 2021 systematic review and meta-analysis by Hyun Jeong Ju et al. reveal that thin skin grafting is the most effective technique, achieving over 90% repigmentation. The repigmentation rate for this method was 72.08%. Suction blister grafting had a repigmentation rate of 61.68%, followed by cultured epidermal cell suspension (CES) at 56.82%, non-cultured epidermal cell suspension (NCES) at 47.51%, punch grafting at 45.76%, and non-cultured follicular cell suspension (NCFS) at 36.24% [63].

5.4.12 Clonal Hypothesis of Repigmentation in Segmental Vitiligo

Segmental vitiligo may involve an autoimmune attack that selectively targets a specific clone of melanocytes in the affected segment. This is supported by the following:

(a) Clonal Selection Hypothesis:

Melanocytes in the skin are not genetically identical; they may arise from different stem cell lineages or neural crest cells. In SV, the immune system may recognize and destroy a particular melanocyte clone that expresses distinct antigens.

(b) Donor Melanocytes as a Different Clone:

Donor melanocytes are typically harvested from unaffected skin (e.g., thigh or gluteal region).

These melanocytes belong to a different clone not targeted by the host immune system in SV.

As a result, when transplanted, they are not recognized as antigenic and can survive, proliferate, and restore pigmentation.

(c) Lack of Recurrence:

The lack of immune attack on donor melanocytes supports the idea that the immune reaction in SV is highly localized and clone-specific. This explains the long-term stability of repigmentation post-surgery in most cases.

5.5 Conclusion

Repigmentation is one of the most important goals in the treatment of vitiligo. Though many treatment options including both medical and surgical are available, there are patients who fail to achieve repigmentation either completely or partially. There is now convincing evidence about the source of melanocytes in hair follicles, in the periphery of the lesion and even in the depigmented lesion. The treatment modality in a given patient should be decided based on the activity of disease, extent of the lesions and the area affected. Patients' acceptance of the result is of utmost importance. The perifollicular pattern of repigmentation being the most common type gives peppering appearance which may not be well acceptable to the patients especially in cosmetically important areas such as the face. Surgical options should be explored in stubborn depigmented patches in stable vitiligo patients. Further understanding of the mechanisms involved in repigmentation will help in exploring novel treatment options for vitiligo.

References

1. Eleftheriadou V, Thomas K, van Geel N, et al. Developing core outcome set for vitiligo clinical trials: international e-Delphi consensus. Pigment Cell Melanoma Res. 2015;28:363–9.
2. Cui J, Shen LY, Wang GC. Role of hair follicles in the repigmentation of vitiligo. J Invest Dermatol. 1991;97(3):410–6.
3. Grichnik JM, Ali WN, Burch JA, et al. KITexpression reveals a population of precursor melanocytes in human skin. J Invest Dermatol. 1996;106(5):967–71.
4. Kanwar AJ, Parsad D. Understanding the mechanism of repigmentation in vitiligo. In: Gupta S, Olsson MJ, Kanwar AJ, et al., editors. Surgical management of vitiligo. 1st ed. Cambridge: Wiley; 2007. p. 14–9.

5. Gan EY, Gahat T, Cario-André M, et al. Clinical repigmentation patterns in peadiatric vitiligo. Br J Dermatol. 2016;175:555–60.
6. Davids LM, du Toit E, Kidson SH, et al. A rare repig mentation pattern in a vitiligo patient: a clue to an epidermal stem-cell reservoir of melanocytes? Clin Exp Dermatol. 2009;34(2):246–8.
7. Parsad D, Pandhi R, Dogra S, Kumar B. Clinical study of repigmentation patterns with different treatment modalities and their correlation with speed and stability of repigmentation in 352 vitiliginous patches. J Am Acad Dermatol. 2004;50(1):63–7.
8. Birlea SA, Spritz RA, Norris DA. Vitiligo. In: Wolff K, Goldsmith LA, Katz SI, et al., editors. Fitzpatrick's dermatology in general medicine. 8th ed. New York: McGraw-Hill; 2012. p. 792–803.
9. Hoerter JD, Bradley P, Casillas A, et al. Extrafollicular dermal melanocyte stem cells and melanoma. Stem Cells Int. 2012;2012:407079.
10. Parsad D. In: Vitiligo Picardo M, Taïeb A, editors. Natural history and prognosis. Heidelberg: Springer; 2010. p. 139–42.
11. Tobin DJ, Swanson NN, Pittelkow MR, Peters EM, Schallreuter KU. Melanocytes are not absent in lesional skin of long duration vitiligo. J Pathol. 2000;191(4):407–16.
12. Falabella R. Vitiligo and the melanocyte reservoir. Indian J Dermatol. 2009;54:313–8.
13. Goldstein NB, Koster MI, Hoaglin LG, Spoelstra NS, Kechris KJ, Robinson SE, et al. Narrow band ultraviolet B treatment for human vitiligo is associated with proliferation, migration, and differentiation of melanocyte precursors. J Invest Dermatol. 2015;135:2068–76.
14. Ito T, Ito N, Saatoff M, Hashizume H, Fukamizu H, Nickoloff BJ, et al. Maintenance of hair follicle immune privilege is linked to prevention of NK cell attack. J Invest Dermatol. 2008;128:1196–206.
15. Nishimura EK, Suzuki M, Igras V, Du J, Lonning S, Miyachi Y, et al. Key roles for transforming growth factor beta in melanocyte stem cell maintenance. Cell Stem Cell. 2010;6:130–40.
16. Meyer KC, Klatte JE, Dinh HV, Harries MJ, Reithmayer K, Meyer W, et al. Evidence that the bulge region is a site of relative immune privilege in human hair follicles. Br J Dermatol. 2008;159:1077–85.
17. Murase D, Hachiya A, Amano Y, et al. The essential role of p53 in hyperpigmentation of the skin via regulation of paracrine melanogenic cytokine receptor signaling. J Biol Chem. 2009;284(7):4343–53.
18. Yamada T, Hasegawa S, Inoue Y, et al. Wnt/b-cate nin and kit signaling sequentially regulate melano cyte stem cell differentiation in UVB-induced epidermal pigmentation. J Invest Dermatol. 2013;133(12):2753–62.
19. Choi YS, Zhang Y, Xu M, et al. Distinct functions for Wnt/b-catenin in hair follicle stem cell proliferation and survival and interfollicular epidermal homeostasis. Cell Stem Cell. 2013;13(6):720–33.
20. Bae JM, Jung HM, Hong BY, et al. Phototherapy for vitiligo: asystematic review and meta-analysis. JAMA Dermatol. 2017;153:666–74.
21. Parsad D, Kanwar AJ, Kumar B. Psoralen-ultraviolet a vs. narrow-band ultraviolet B phototherapy for the treatment of vitiligo. J Eur Acad Dermatol Venereol. 2006;20(2):175–7.
22. Sapam R, Agrawal S, Dhali TK. Systemic PUVA vs. narrowband UVB in the treatment of vitiligo: a randomized controlled study. Int J Dermatol. 2012;51(9):1107–15.
23. Yones SS, Palmer RA, Garibaldinos TM, Hawk JLM. Randomized double-blind trial of treatment of Vitiligo: efficacy of psoralen–UV-A therapy vs narrowband–UV-B therapy. Arch Dermatol. 2007;143(5):578–84.
24. Kovacs D, Abdel-Raouf H, Al-Khayyat M, et al. Viti ligo: characterization of melanocytes in repigmented skin after punch grafting. J Eur Acad Dermatol Venereol. 2015;29(3):581–90.
25. Masuria BL, Batra A, Kothiwala RK, et al. Topical mometasone furoate for the treatment of childhood vitiligo. Indian J Dermatol Venereol Leprol. 1999;65(5):219.
26. Taieb A, Alomar A, Böhm M, Dell'anna ML, De Pase A, Eleftheriadou V, et al. Guidelines for the management of vitiligo: the European dermatology forum consensus. Br J Dermatol. 2013;168(1):5–19.

27. Njoo MD, Spuls PI, Bos JD, Westerhof W, Bossuyt PMM. Nonsurgical Repigmentation therapies in vitiligo: meta-analysis of the literature. Arch Dermatol. 1998;134(12):1532–40.
28. Kim SM, Lee HS, Hann SK. The efficacy of low-dose oral corticosteroids in the treatment of vitiligo patients. Int J Dermatol. 1999;38:546–50.
29. Kanwar AJ, Mahajan R, Parsad D. Low-dose oral mini-pulse dexamethasone therapy in progressive unstable vitiligo. J Cutan Med Surg. 2013;17:259–68.
30. Sisti A, Sisti G, Oranges CM. Effectiveness and safety of topical tacrolimus monotherapy for repig mentation in vitiligo: a comprehensive literature re view. An Bras Dermatol. 2016;91(2):187–95.
31. Lan CC, Chen GS, Chiou MH, et al. FK506 promotes melanocyte and melanoblast growth and creates a favourable milieu for cell migration via keratinocytes possible mechanisms of how tacrolimus ointment induces repigmentation in patients with vitiligo. Br J Dermatol. 2005;153(3):498–505.
32. Jung H, Chung H, Chang SE, et al. FK506 regulates pigmentation by maturing the melanosome and facilitating their transfer to keratinocytes. Pigment Cell Melanoma Res. 2016;29(2):199–209.
33. Anuradha PD. FK506 regulates pigmentation by maturing the melanosome and facilitating their transfer to keratinocytes. Dermatol Ther. 2016;29(6):396
34. Fai D, Cassano N, Vena G. Narrow-band UVB phototherapy combined with tacrolimus ointment in vitiligo: a review of 110 patients. J Eur Acad Dermatol Venereol. 2007;21(7):916–20.
35. Lee JH, Kwon HS, Jung HM, Lee H, Kim GM, Yim HW, Bae JM. Treatment outcomes of topical calcineurin inhibitor therapy for patients with vitiligo: a systematic review and meta-analysis. JAMA Dermatol. 2019;155:929–38.
36. Birlea SA, Costin GE, Norris DA. Cellular and molec ular mechanisms involved in the action of vitamin D analogs targeting vitiligo depigmentation. Curr Drug Targets. 2008;9(4):345–59.
37. Picardo M. Vitamin D analogs. In: Picardo M, Taieb A, editors. Vitiligo. Heidelberg: Springer; 2010. p. 339–42.
38. Parsad D, Saini R, Verma N. Combination of PUVAsol and topical calcipotriol in vitiligo. Dermatology. 1998;197(2):167–70.
39. Kumaran MS, Kaur I, Kumar B. Effect of topical calcipotriol, betamethasone dipropionate and their combination in the treat ment of localized vitiligo. J Eur Acad Dermatol Venereol. 2006;20:269–73.
40. Richmond JM, Strassner JP, Zapata L Jr, et al. Antibody blockade of IL-15 signaling has the potential to durably reverse vitiligo. Sci Transl Med. 2018;10(450):eaam7710.
41. Waldmann TA, Miljkovic MD, Conlon KC. Interleukin-15 (dys)regulation of lymphoid homeostasis: implications for therapy of autoimmunity and cancer. J Exp Med. 2020;217(1):e20191062.
42. Hamzavi I, Jain H, McLean D, Shapiro J, Zeng H, Lui H. Parametric modeling of narrowband UV-B phototherapy for vitiligo using a novel quantitative tool: the vitiligo area scoring index. Arch Dermatol. 2004;140:677–83.
43. Rosmarin D, Pandya AG, Lebwohl M, Grimes P, Hamzavi I, Gottlieb AB, Butler K, Kuo F, Sun K, Ji T, et al. Ruxolitinib cream for treatment of vitiligo: a randomised, controlled, phase 2 trial. Lancet. 2020;396:110–20.
44. Rosmarin D, Passeron T, Pandya AG, Grimes P, Harris JE, Desai SR, et al. Two phase 3, randomized, controlled trials of ruxolitinib cream for vitiligo. N Engl J Med. 2022;387(16):1445–55.
45. Seneschal J, Speeckaert R, Taïeb A, Wolkerstorfer A, Passeron T, Pandya AG, et al. Worldwide expert recommendations for the diagnosis and management of vitiligo: position statement from the international vitiligo task force-part 2: specific treatment recommendations. J Eur Acad Dermatol Venereol. 2023;37(11):2185–95.
46. Craiglow BG, King BA. Tofacitinib citrate for the treatment of vitiligo: a pathogenesis-directed therapy. JAMA Dermatol. 2015;151(10):1110–2.

47. Liu LY, Strassner JP, Refat MA, Harris JE, King BA. Repigmentation in vitiligo using the Janus kinase inhibitor tofacitinib may require concomitant light exposure. J Am Acad Dermatol. 2017;77:675–682.e671.
48. Fang WC, Chiu SH, Lin SY, Huang SM, Lan CE. Evaluation of low-dose tofacitinib combining narrowband UVB therapy for treating vitiligo patients who had failed previous therapy: a pilot study. Photodermatol Photoimmunol Photomed. 2021;37(4):345–7.
49. Song H, Hu Z, Zhang S, Yang L, Liu Y, Wang T. Effectiveness and safety of tofacitinib combined with narrowband ultraviolet B phototherapy for patients with refractory vitiligo in real-world clinical practice. Dermatol Ther. 2022;35(11):e15821.
50. Ezzedine K, Peeva E, Yamaguchi Y, et al. Efficacy and safety of oral ritlecitinib for the treatment of active nonsegmental vitiligo: A randomized phase 2b clinical trial [published correction appears in]. J Am Acad Dermatol. 2023;89(3):639.
51. Cha YC, Lee HJ, Lee SJ, Na GY, Chung SL. The expression of the α-melanocyte stimulating hormone (α-MSH) and melanocortin-1 receptor (MC1R) in the epidermis of the vitiligo. Kor J Dermatol. 2003;41:690–5
52. Lim HW, Grimes PE, Agbai O, et al. Afamelanotide and narrowband UV-B phototherapy for the treatment of vitiligo: a randomized multicenter trial. JAMA Dermatol. 2015;151(1):42–50.
53. Nada HR, Rashed L. Basic fibroblast growth factor & vitiligo. J Egypt Women Dermatol Soc. 2012;9:22–5.
54. Wu CS, Lan CC, Chiou MH, Yu HS. Basic fibroblast growth factor promotes melanocyte migration via increased expression of p125FAK on melanocytes. Acta Derm Venereol. 2006;86:498–502.
55. Ramaiah A, Kar HK, Garg VK, Bajaj N, Gupta L, Madhava AS. A double blind randomized phase IV clinical trial of basic fibroblast growth factor related deca-peptide in vitiligo. J Pigment Disord. 2015;3:0–4.
56. Jiang S, Hao Z, Qi W, Wang Z, Zhou M, Guo N. The efficacy of topical prostaglandin analogs for hair loss: a systematic review and meta-analysis. Front Med (Lausanne). 2023;10:1130623.
57. Neinaa YME, Mahmoud MAE, El Maghraby GM, Ibrahim ZAE. Efficacy of prostaglandin E2 versus prostaglandin F2 alpha assisted with narrowband-UVB in stable vitiligo. Arch Dermatol Res. 2023;315(9):2647–53.
58. Parsad D, Pandhi R, Dogra S, Kumar B. Topical prostaglandin analog (PGE2) in vitiligo–a preliminary study. Int J Dermatol. 2002;41(12):942–5.
59. Majid I, Mysore V, Salim T, Lahiri K, Chatterji M, Khunger N, et al. Is Lesional stability in vitiligo more important than disease stability for performing surgical interventions? Results from a multicentric study. J Cutan Aesthet Surg. 2016;9(1):13–9.
60. Staricco RG. Amelanotic melanocytes in the outer sheath of the human hair follicle. J Invest Dermatol. 1959;33:295–7.
61. Shenoi SD, Srinivas CR, Pai S. Treatment of stable vitiligo with autologous epidermal grafting and PUVA. J Am Acad Dermatol. 1997;36(5 Pt 1):802–3.
62. van Geel N, Ongenae K, Naeyaert JM. Surgical techniques for vitiligo: a review. Dermatology. 2001;202(2):162–6.
63. Ju HJ, Bae JM, Lee RW, Kim SH, Parsad D, Pourang A, Hamzavi I, Shourick J, Ezzedine K. Surgical interventions for patients with vitiligo: a systematic review and meta-analysis. JAMA Dermatol. 2021;157:307–16.

Part II
Clinical Science

Chapter 6
Classification, Clinical Features, Associations, Special Variants

Alpana Mohta

Abstract Vitiligo classification primarily uses the Taieb and Picardo system (2010) and the Bordeaux VGICC system (2012). These classify vitiligo into non-segmental, segmental, mixed, and unclassified types, with subtypes such as acrofacial, mucosal, generalized, universal, and rare variants like vitiligo punctata, follicular, minor, and blue vitiligo. Segmental vitiligo includes unisegmental, bisegmental, and multisegmental forms. Variants include trichrome, quadri-chrome, penta-chrome, follicular, and guttate vitiligo. Vitiligo is associated with autoimmune and immunodeficiency conditions, genetic predispositions, and sometimes family history.

Keywords Vitiligo classification systems · Non-segmental vitiligo · Segmental vitiligo types · Follicular vitiligo · Trichrome vitiligo · Quadrichrome vitiligo · Blue vitiligo · Guttate vitiligo · Autoimmune vitiligo associations · Vitiligo genetic predispositions

6.1 Classification

Currently, two classification systems are used for vitiligo. The first one was introduced in 2010 by Taieb et al. It divides vitiligo into four types: non-segmental (NSV), segmental (SV), mixed (NSV + SV), and unclassified (Table 6.1) [1].

However, in 2012, the Bordeaux VGICC classification and consensus nomenclature was adopted at the suggestion of an international panel of experts at the 2011 International Pigment Cell Conference (IPCC). It divides vitiligo into non-segmental, segmental, and unclassified groups (Table 6.2) [2].

A. Mohta (✉)
Department of Dermatology, Venereology and Leprosy, Sharda Multispeciality Clinic, Bikaner, Rajasthan, India

R. Sarkar, V. Narayan R (eds.), *A Concise Guide to The Management of Vitiligo*,
https://doi.org/10.1007/978-981-95-3857-7_6

Table 6.1 The Taieb and Picardo classification (2010)

Vitiligo type	Subtypes
Non-segmental	Focal
	Acrofacial
	Mucosal
	Generalized
	Universal
Segmental	Focal
	Mucosal
	Unisegmental
	Bisegmental
	Multisegmental
Mixed	Non-segmental vitiligo with segmental vitiligo
Unclassified	Temporary classification of asymmetrical focal, multifocal, or mucosal spots until further observation allows precise classification

Table 6.2 The Bordeaux Vitiligo Global Issues Consensus Conference (VGICC) classification (2012)

Vitiligo type	Subtypes
Non-segmental	Acrofacial
	Mucosal (multifocal)
	Generalized (vitiligo vulgaris)
	Universal
	Mixed (non-segmental vitiligo with segmental vitiligo)
	Rare variants (vitiligo punctata, follicular, minor, marginal and blue vitiligo)
Segmental vitiligo	Unisegmental
	Bisegmental
	Multisegmental
Undetermined or unclassified	Focal
	Mucosal (single isolated lesion)

6.2 Historical Perspective

In 1977, Kong et al. proposed a classification for vitiligo into non-segmental (type A) and segmental (type B), attributing type A to immunologic factors and type B to sympathetic nervous system dysfunction (Table 6.3) [3, 4].

Despite its initial utility, this system has not been broadly accepted due to the inconsistent distribution of segmental vitiligo, which does not always align with dermatomal patterns akin to those seen in herpes zoster. The discovery of neurohormonal influences on melanocytes and the embryological connection between melanocytes and neural cells point against the binary division of vitiligo into groups A and B [5].

Table 6.3 The Kong et al. classification

Attribute	Type A vitiligo	Type B vitiligo
Distribution	Non-dermatomal	Dermatomal
Age of onset	Can occur at any age	Younger onset
Disease progression	Continuous throughout life	Stabilizes within a few years without widespread progression
Association	May be associated with autoimmune diseases	Rarely associated with Sutton's leucoderma, does not koebnerize, or have a history of related autoimmune diseases
Pathogenesis	Linked to autoimmune mechanisms	Linked to sympathetic system dysfunction
Prevalence	3:4	1:4

6.3 Clinical Features

6.3.1 Non-Segmental Vitiligo

According to the VGICC classification, the term non-segmental vitiligo (NSV) serves as a collective designation for all categories of generalized vitiligo. NSV encompasses acrofacial, mucosal, generalized, universal, mixed, and some rare forms of vitiligo.

(a) Acrofacial vitiligo: Involves acral areas (hands and feet) and facial regions (face and head). Frequently appears around the mouth, lips, and fingertips, colloquially known as "lip-tip vitiligo."
(b) Mucosal vitiligo: Targets the mucosa of oral and genital areas. Mucosal regions might also be involved in acrofacial, generalized, or universal forms. However, when only a single mucosal site is involved, it is labeled as "indeterminate" [6].
(c) Generalized vitiligo: Also known as "common vitiligo" or "vitiligo vulgaris." Some symmetrical macules or patches can appear anywhere on the body, with a predilection for hands, fingers, feet, face, and trauma-prone regions.
(d) Universal vitiligo: It is the most common form in adults, often seen following generalized vitiligo, covering 80–90% of the body surface area.
(e) Mixed: Involves both segmental and non-segmental types, with segmental usually appearing first.
(f) Rare variants of vitiligo: These forms were previously considered unclassifiable. They include vitiligo punctata, follicular, minor, and blue vitiligo.

6.3.1.1 Generalized Vitiligo

(a) Clinical Features

Generalized vitiligo manifests as asymptomatic and well-defined round-to-oval, milky-white depigmented macules or plaques, symmetrically distributed bilaterally.

The size of the macules or plaques ranges from a few millimeters to centimeters. Sometimes, the margins may be ill-defined, gradually merging into the normally pigmented surrounding skin. The depigmentation in these areas is purely macular, with the epidermis remaining free from surface changes like atrophy, telangiectasia, hyperkeratosis, etc.

Transient erythema post-UV exposure or during the menstrual phase (Punshi's Sign) may mislead diagnosis. Lesions in individuals with skin of color can have hyperpigmented borders following UV exposure (Fig. 6.1) [7]. Initially, hair in affected areas retains pigmentation, but as the disease progresses, depigmentation occurs, particularly on the scalp, leading to patches of gray or white hair and sometimes total depigmentation [8].

(b) Distribution

Generalized vitiligo can begin anywhere on the body, commonly starting at the fingers, hands, and face as acrofacial vitiligo. Lesions that tend to originate simultaneously from the posterior trunk and acral regions often spread more widely and progressively affect extensor surfaces like metacarpal or metatarsal joints, interphalangeal region, umbilicus, and axillae in a bilaterally symmetrical pattern [8, 9]. Koebner's phenomenon can prompt lesion spread at sites of trauma such as the

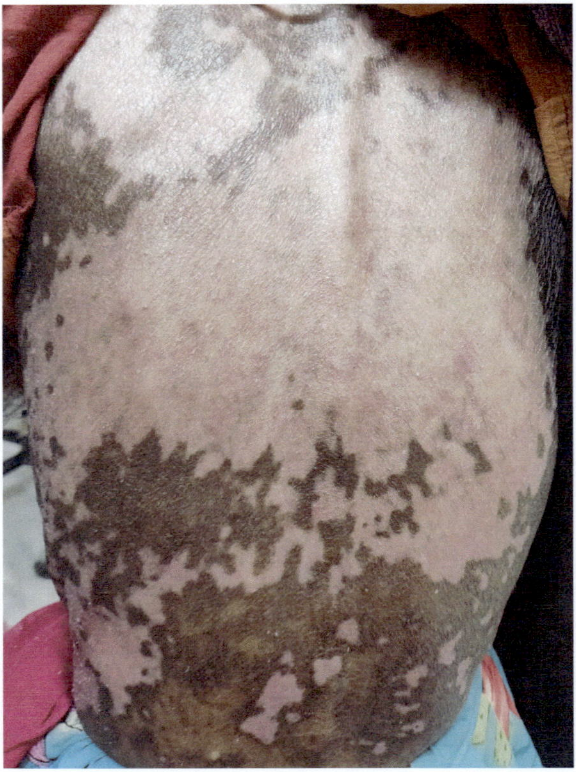

Fig. 6.1 Vitiligo vulgaris over the back of a patient with skin having hyperpigmented borders following being treated with phototherapy

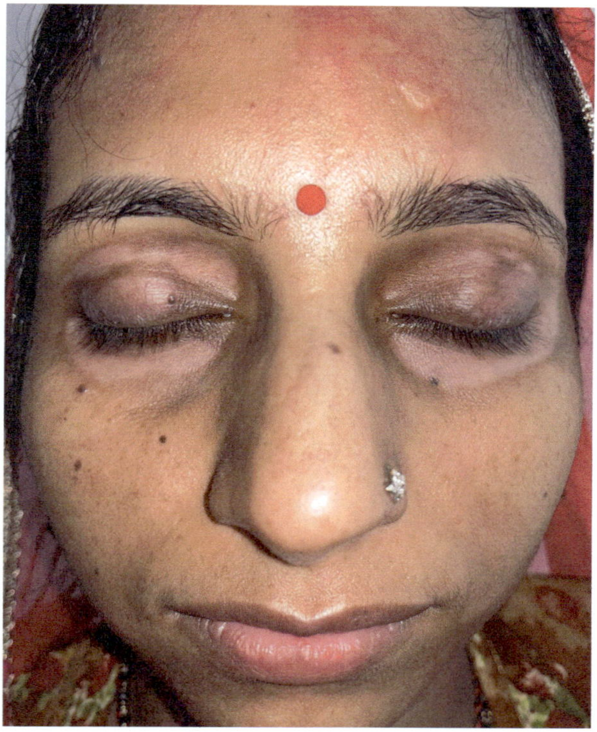

Fig. 6.2 Periocular vitiligo lesions in a patient with vitiligo vulgaris

scalp, palms, soles, knees, shin of the tibia, malleoli, elbows, volar aspect of wrists, lumbosacral area, waistband, and belt areas [10].

Diagnosis in darker skin, especially on palms and soles, can be challenging and may require Wood's lamp examination [11]. Lesions can also appear around the perioral, periocular, perinasal, perianal, and periungual sites, potentially affecting mucosal surfaces of the mouth, lips, distal penis, external genitalia in females, and nipples (Fig. 6.2).

(c) Clinical Variants

Multichrome Vitiligo

Trichrome vitiligo: This is a form of unstable vitiligo with a hypopigmented band bordering the depigmented vitiligo patch and the unaffected pigmented skin (Fig. 6.3) [12]. Cockade-like vitiligo represents a subtype of trichrome vitiligo [13].

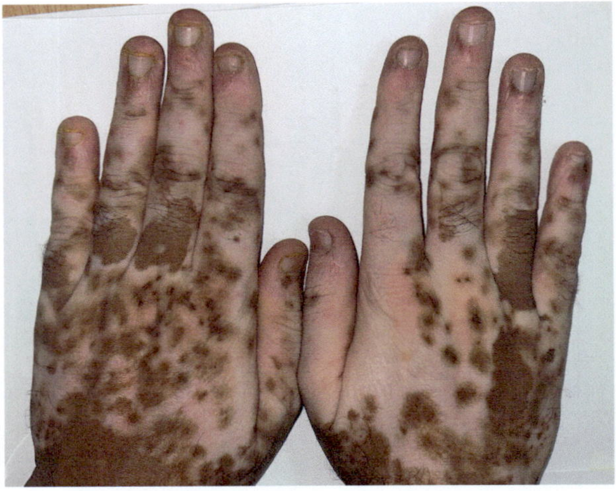

Fig. 6.3 Trichrome vitiligo over the dorsal surface of hands with depigmented, hypopigmented, and normally pigmented skin

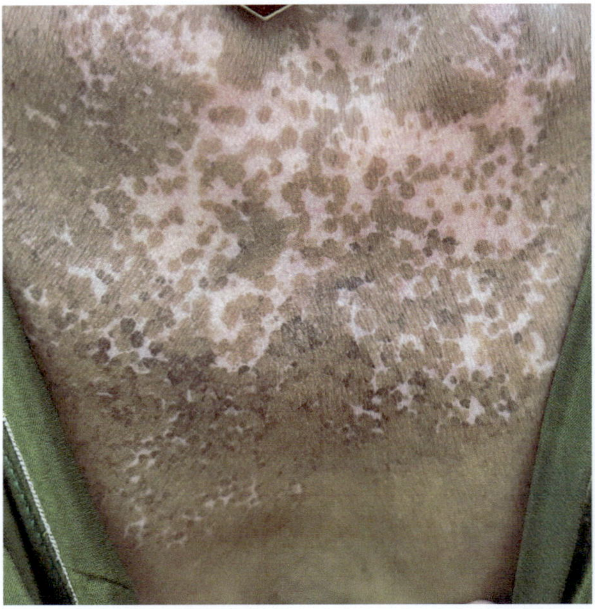

Fig. 6.4 Quadrichrome vitiligo with hyperpigmented regions

Quadri-chrome Vitiligo

Characterized by a fourth color in lesions, mainly seen in darker skin types, it shows macular hyperpigmentation, either perifollicular or marginal, signaling repigmentation (Fig. 6.4).

Penta-Chrome Vitiligo

A very rare variant displaying sequential loss of pigmentation from normal skin color to blue-gray, brown, tan, and ultimately white (complete depigmentation), primarily affecting individuals with darker skin [12].

Blue Vitiligo

Blue vitiligo, first described by Ivker et al. in an HIV-positive patient with Kaposi sarcoma, features blue-tinged depigmented macules [14]. It is characterized histologically by excessive melanophages in the dermis and the absence of melanocytes. The blue hue may result from post-inflammatory hyperpigmentation or drug-induced pigmentation, often following treatments like narrowband UVB or intralesional psoralens [15].

Inflammatory Vitiligo

Inflammatory vitiligo is marked by red, scaly, sometimes itchy, or burning lesions. This condition can arise from aggressive treatments and may coexist with other diseases like HIV, hepatitis C, atopic dermatitis, Sjögren's syndrome, and lichen sclerosus. It often shows both inflammatory and stable patches and is linked to various systemic disorders [12, 16–19].

Marginal Vitiligo (Inflammatory Vitiligo with Raised Borders)

Marginal vitiligo also referred to as inflammatory vitiligo with raised borders (IVRB), is variably regarded in the literature. Some authors classify it as a distinct subtype of inflammatory vitiligo, while others consider it synonymous with inflammatory vitiligo [19, 20].

Marginal vitiligo is characterized by 1–3 cm depigmented patches with raised, erythematous, occasionally hyperpigmented or scaly borders, often pruritic. It may follow vitiligo treatment or exposure to phenolic compounds and can co-localize with alopecia areata. Unlike common vitiligo, IVRB shows dermal lymphocytic infiltrates, lymphocyte exocytosis, occasional eosinophils, focal spongiosis, and interface dermatitis [20].

The closest differential diagnosis is discoid lupus erythematosus (DLE), ruled out by the absence of follicular plugging, typical histology, and negative direct immunofluorescence [20].

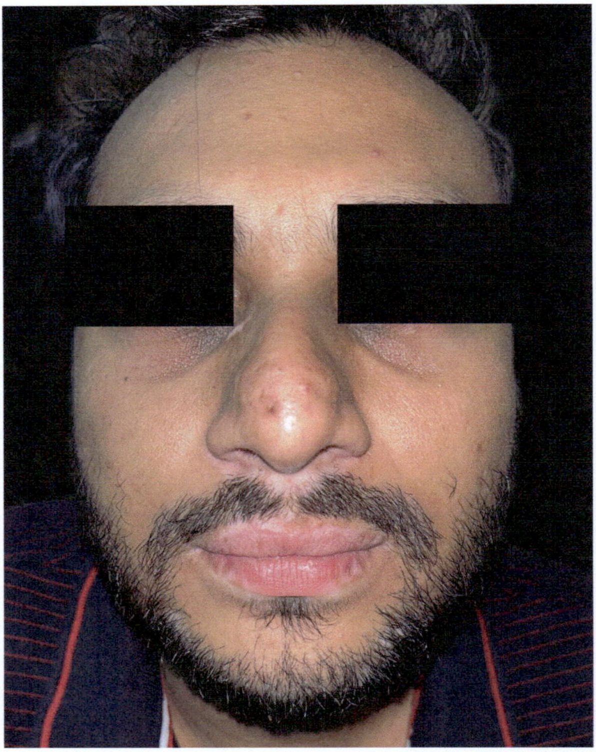

Fig. 6.5 Acrofacial vitiligo with perioral lesions and involvement of upper and lower lips

Acrofacial Vitiligo

Acrofacial vitiligo (AFV) affects acral regions such as hands, feet, face, and head, with prominent depigmentation on distal fingers and perioral areas (Figs. 6.5 and 6.6). AFV can potentially evolve into generalized vitiligo and is strongly linked to mucosal vitiligo, particularly affecting the oral and genital mucosa. [21, 22] However, its association with autoimmune thyroid conditions is weaker than generalized vitiligo [23].

Assessing the exact prevalence of AFV is challenging due to the varying definitions used by researchers. Epidemiological data reveals a significant variation in prevalence rates across different populations: 44% in India, 25.6% in Brazil, 6.8% among Chinese Han and non-Han, and 5.8% in France [21, 23–25].

6.3.1.2 Vitiligo Universalis

Vitiligo universalis (VU) is the most extreme manifestation of non-segmental vitiligo, characterized by comprehensive or almost complete loss of skin pigmentation, and occasionally affects the hair. Epidemiologically, VU is exceedingly uncommon, accounting for approximately 1.3% of all vitiligo cases [26]. This condition is more

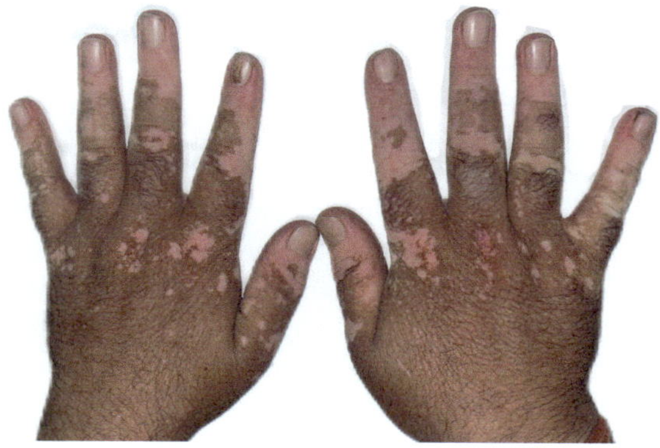

Fig. 6.6 Acral and periungual lesions in the same patient with acrofacial vitiligo

conspicuous in individuals with darker skin tones, predominantly affects adults, and is exceptionally rare in children; for example, only one instance of pediatric VU was documented among 1315 patients with vitiligo in a study by Song et al. [27]

Clinically, VU manifests as total or near-total loss of skin pigmentation, with occasional slight residual pigmentation in areas exposed to sunlight, sometimes trichrome vitiligo. While pigmentation in scalp hair may initially persist, depigmentation often extends to other body hair as the disease progresses. Depigmentation of mucosal tissues is also frequently observed.

6.3.2 *Segmental Vitiligo*

Unlike NSV, segmental vitiligo (SV) manifests early and progresses more swiftly but stays confined within the designated area or segment of the body. The distribution of SV mirrors that observed in other acquired pigmentation anomalies such as nevus spilus, suggesting potential underlying mutations in melanocytes during fetal development or somatic mosaicism [28]. Due to its relatively stable nature and minimal ongoing melanocyte depletion, SV responds better to treatment and serves as an ideal subject for investigating repigmentation strategies.

6.3.2.1 Clinical and Pathological Characteristics

SV usually begins at a younger age compared to NSV, with an average onset of 17.3 years in SV versus 26.59 years in NSV [29]. It predominantly affects the youth, with a 27.9% occurrence rate in children. Notably, 41.3% of SV cases manifest before age 10 and 87.0% before reaching 30 years [4].

The initial presentation of SV frequently manifests as a singular, round-to-oval, hypopigmented, or depigmented macule indistinguishable from focal vitiligo until further characteristic spreading patterns are observed. There is less uniform pigmentation loss compared to NSV. In lighter skin tones, these lesions might not be visible under standard lighting but become apparent under Wood's light. A distribution pattern that is dermatomal or pseudo-dermatomal has been proposed, supporting the neural hypothesis of SV; however, it is common for lesions to span multiple dermatomes and occasionally cross the midline. [30, 31]

Typically, the depigmentation progresses rapidly within a defined segment and then stabilizes, partially or completely depigmenting the area. Transition to a generalized form is uncommon, but when SV and nonsegmental vitiligo coexist, the condition is referred to as "mixed vitiligo," which often presents a more challenging response to treatment, implying a possibly intensified pathogenic process in the SV regions [32].

Regarding anatomical prevalence, over half of the cases involve the head. Following in frequency are the torso, limbs, extremities, and neck, with the neck being more commonly affected in females. SV often presents as a solitary lesion in three-quarters of cases [33]. A depigmented macule presenting initially on the nipple or areola usually signifies the onset of SV since focal NSV is exceedingly rare over these sites.

Typically, there is no distinct preference for either side of the body, though some patients may exhibit lesions in two separate unilateral dermal segments. The distribution frequently coincides with the trigeminal nerve territory, which supports the neural theory underlying SV [34]. Despite the segmental nature of the disease, most cases do not display a recognizable dermatomal or blaschkoid pattern.

In segmental vitiligo, hair depigmentation, known as poliosis or leukotrichia, predominantly manifests within vitiliginous SV macules, seen in 30–100% of patients, especially involving eyebrows, eyelashes, pubic or axillary area. [35, 36] Leukotrichia is a sign of poor prognosis and treatment resistance for SV patients, often necessitating melanocyte transplantation for effective results.

6.3.3 Classification of Segmental Vitiligo

6.3.3.1 Cephalic SV Classification

Kim et al. have divided facial segmental vitiligo into seven subtypes (Table 6.4). There is a predilection for the left side of the face [37]. Type I affects the forehead, scalp, eyelid, and cheek (Fig. 6.7). Type II covers the mouth's angle, ear, cheek, and mandible, possibly reaching the upper neck. Type III spreads from below the lower lip to the chin and medial neck. Type IV features lesions on the right forehead, eyelids, nose, and cheek. Type V, the least common, is confined to the right orbital area and may extend to the temporal region. The mixed type combines features of types II and III.

Table 6.4 Proposed classification of facial segmental vitiligo

Type	Description
I-a	Most common subtype. Begins on one side of the forehead, crosses the facial midline near the glabella, extends to the contralateral eyelid, nose, philtrum, and cheek, sparing the scalp hair
I-b	Appears on one side of the forehead, often affects the scalp hair, with occasional spread to the periorbital region and eyebrows
II	Originates at the mouth's angle, arches toward the ear across the cheek or mandible, commonly reaching the upper neck, with varying curvatures
III	Starts below the lower lip, spreads to include the chin and neck, predominantly affecting the medial neck parts, seldom reaching the upper chest
IV	Features lesions on the right side of the forehead, expanding to the eyelids, nose, and cheek without crossing the midline
V	Least common subtype. Confined to the right orbital area, may extend to the temporal region
Mixed	Commonly combines characteristics of types II and III

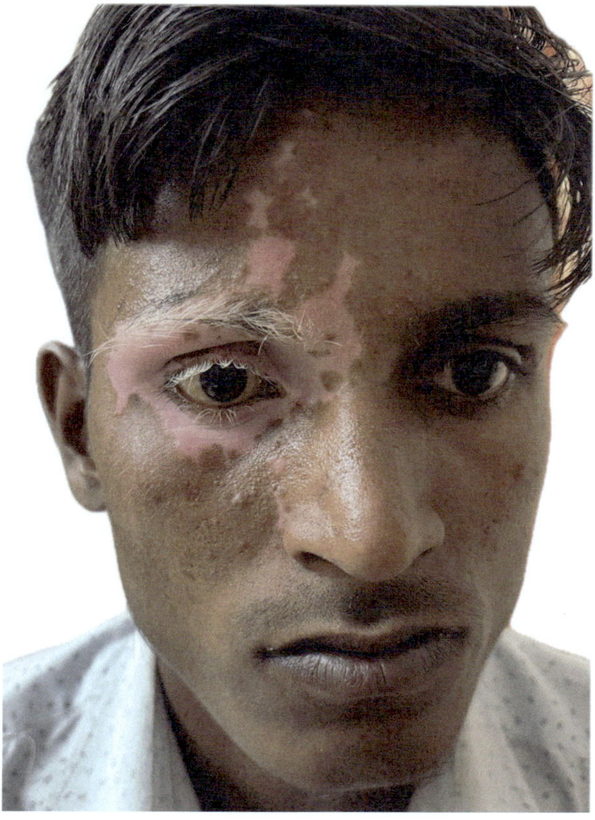

Fig. 6.7 Type I facial segmental vitiligo with leukotrichia involving the eyelashes

6.3.3.2 Truncal SV Classification

Table 6.5 Proposed classification of truncal segmental vitiligo

Type	Pattern	Location	Description
1	Midline or mid-central linear	Trunk midline	Extension of type III SV from the face, crosses the midline
2	Shoulder	Trunk	May extend to the ipsilateral arm
3	High V-shape	thorax	Least common subtype. Descends toward lower midline, follows Blaschko's lines
4	Low V-shape	Thorax	May extend to ipsilateral arm
5	Bandlike	Lateral trunk	Most common subtype. Horizontal distribution
6	Checkerboard	Below waist	Affects upper leg, occurs on both anterior and posterior lower trunk, spares lateral regions

Van Geel et al. have categorized truncal SV into six patterns: midline, shoulder, high V-shape on the thorax, low V-shape on the thorax, bandlike, and checkerboard (Table 6.5) [38]. A combination of these patterns often manifests on both the anterior and posterior aspects of the lower trunk, although sparing the lateral regions. Unlike facial SV, there is no predominant left- or right-side distribution in truncal subtypes, although younger patients more frequently exhibit left-sided trunk lesions (Fig. 6.8).

6.4 Special Variants

6.4.1 Follicular Vitiligo

Leukotrichia consistently appears alongside skin depigmentation, commonly associated with segmental vitiligo, with a prevalence rate ranging from 49% to 100% [39]. It serves as a negative prognostic factor for vitiligo repigmentation due to melanocyte depletion within hair follicles. In nonsegmental vitiligo, body hair typically remains unaffected at the outset, but hair depigmentation may develop as the disease progresses.

In 2012, a distinct presentation of vitiligo was reported, characterized only by the involvement of hair follicles, leading to the proposal of a new variant termed "follicular vitiligo." Follicular vitiligo can occur independently or concurrently with skin depigmentation, potentially at the same or different body sites. It may also precede visible skin lesions by several months, an early indicator of further depigmentation [40].

Identified initially by Ezzedine and colleagues, this subtype targets melanocyte reservoirs in the hair follicles, resulting in early hair depigmentation without impacting the surrounding skin. Supported by clinical and histopathological evidence, follicular vitiligo may exhibit a complete absence of melanocytes in the basal layer and within hair follicles. Observations of cells bearing mast cell markers within these

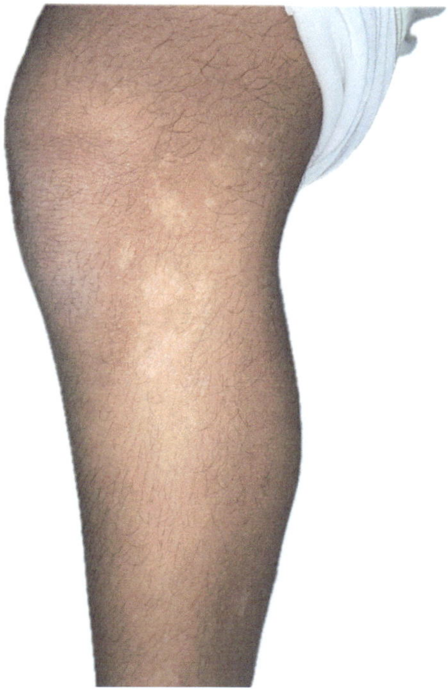

Fig. 6.8 Segmental vitiligo over left leg

infiltrates suggest a potential link between follicular vitiligo and alopecia areata, indicating a shared pathogenic pathway. [40, 41]

6.4.2 Guttate Vitiligo

Guttate vitiligo (vitiligo guttata), also known as vitiligo punctata, confetti leukoderma, or leukoderma punctata, manifests as numerous small hypopigmented and achromic macules ranging from 0.5 to 1.5 mm in diameter (Fig. 6.9). These lesions predominantly appear on the sun-exposed regions of the limbs. This variant is considered a phototoxic reaction to phototherapy characterized by the degeneration of keratinocytes and melanocytes. This entity is clinically and histopathologically indistinguishable from guttate hypomelanosis [42, 43].

6.4.3 Vitiligo Minor

Hypochromic vitiligo, or vitiligo minor, is a rare form seen primarily in dark-skinned individuals, characterized by hypopigmented lesions without prior inflammation (Fig. 6.10). Hypopigmented macules often appear at the onset or during the

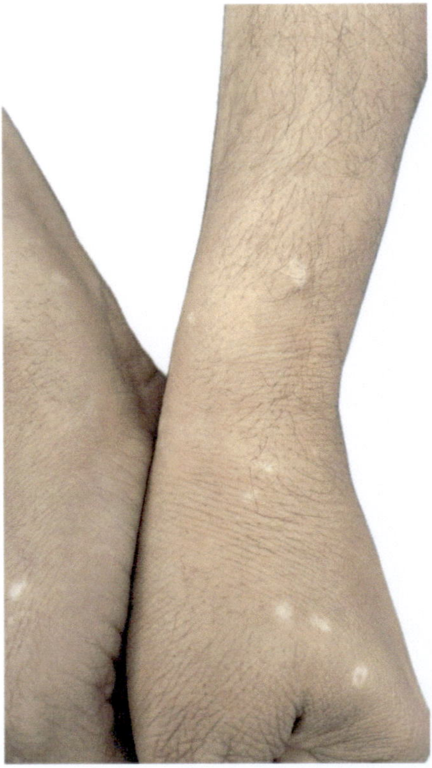

Fig. 6.9 Guttate vitiligo over wrist and dorsum of hand

active spread of NSV. It is more common in patients with Fitzpatrick skin type V or VI. It mainly affected seborrheic regions and involved multiple discrete hypopigmented macules on the scalp, chest, limbs, and trunk [44].

Vitiligo minor is often a diagnosis of exclusion after other mimickers like cutaneous T cell lymphoma (CTCL), pityriasis alba, indeterminate leprosy, post-inflammatory hypopigmentation, and nevus depigmentosus have been ruled out. The absence of inflammation, scaling, hypoesthesia, skin infiltration, leukotrichia, and Wood's lamp examination helps establish the clinical diagnosis.

6.5 Associations

Extensive genome-wide association studies (GWAS) have identified that approximately 90% of the genetic loci associated with vitiligo susceptibility are related to immune system components, with many of these loci overlapping with other autoimmune and inflammatory diseases. [45, 46]

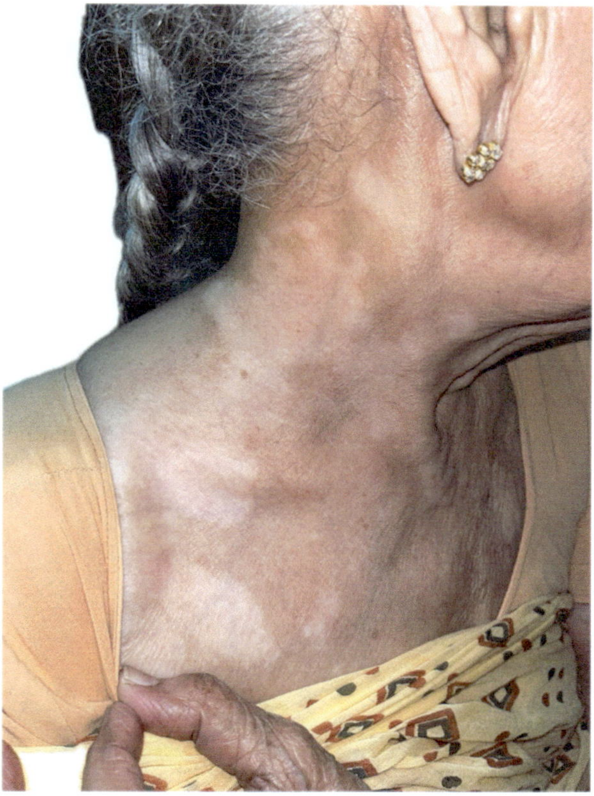

Fig. 6.10 Hypopigmented macules of vitiligo minor with fuzzy borders indicating progressive disease

6.5.1 Autoinflammatory and Autoimmune Diseases

Shared genetic loci vitiligo susceptibility genes and other autoimmune diseases suggest commonality in pathogenic mechanisms, potentially involving the same high-risk alleles across conditions like thyroid disease (Hashimoto's thyroiditis and Graves' disease), type 1 diabetes, alopecia areata, pernicious anemia, and rheumatoid arthritis [47].

Additionally, the presence of atopic diseases such as atopic dermatitis and asthma has been reported in a significant subset of vitiligo patients, suggesting a potential shared genetic predisposition [48].

6.5.2 Immunodeficiencies

T-cell and combined immunodeficiencies are frequently associated with autoimmunity and vitiligo. Notably, HIV infection, a leading cause of acquired immunodeficiency, has been linked to the emergence of vitiligo, either at the onset of HIV or during immune reconstitution following antiviral therapies. Common variable immunodeficiency (CVID) has also shown potential links with vitiligo [49].

6.5.3 Vogt-Koyanagi-Harada Syndrome

Numerous autoimmune and autoinflammatory conditions are associated with vitiligo, often co-occurring in patients with Vogt-Koyanagi-Harada (VKH) syndrome. The transition from VKH to Vitiligo Universalis (VU) can blur the lines between these disorders. VKH syndrome may initially present with extracutaneous symptoms, such as visual and auditory impairments, alopecia, and central nervous system anomalies, before the appearance of skin depigmentation. Additionally, VU may be linked to other autoimmune diseases like autoimmune thyroiditis and alopecia areata after the onset of vitiligo. [50, 51]

6.5.4 Monogenic Diseases

There is a genetic overlap between vitiligo and disorders like piebaldism and autoimmune polyendocrine syndromes (APS). Inherited immunodeficiencies like ataxia-telangiectasia and Nijmegen breakage syndrome and monogenic disorders characterized by organ-specific autoimmune responses and chromosomal or mitochondrial dysfunctions are also frequently associated with vitiligo [49].

6.5.5 Auditory and Ocular Involvement

A study conducted in Turkey revealed that, though minor, hearing loss is frequently observed in patients with non-segmental vitiligo (NSV), with approximately 14% experiencing at least mild hyperacusis [52]. Ocular pigmentation remains intact, although associated complications like uveitis may result in blindness. Ocular and auditory symptoms in patients with extensive vitiligo may be attributed to the depletion of melanocytes within these sensory organs, a characteristic prominently associated with Vogt-Koyanagi-Harada syndrome.

6.5.6 Family History

About 12% of SV cases have a familial history of vitiligo [53]. Unlike NSV, SV is less often linked with systemic autoimmune conditions but frequently coincides with localized skin disorders like linear morphea. SV exhibits inflammation with erythematous borders and hypopigmentation, marked by CD8+ T lymphocyte migration toward the basal layer and flow cytometry demonstrating these cells' anti-melanocyte activity. Increased halo nevi and NSV occurrences further emphasize the immune mechanisms in SV [31, 54].

6.6 Conclusion

In summary, the classification and understanding of vitiligo have evolved significantly over the decades, providing structured frameworks for categorizing the disease. Recognizing clinical subtypes is crucial not just for academic learning but also for predicting the prognosis and treatment response. While non-segmental vitiligo can have an aberrant and unfavorable course, segmental vitiligo is an excellent model to study repigmentation therapies owing to its stability and sectoral loss of melanocytes. Moreover, the associations with autoimmune, genetic, and immunodeficiency conditions point to the complex and multifactorial nature of vitiligo as an autoimmune disease that can be targeted by immunomodulators. Future research should aim to identify and modify the factors that trigger the depigmentation process across the skin.

References

1. Taieb A, Picardo M. Epidemiology, definitions and classification. In: Picardo M, Taieb A, editors. Vitiligo. Heidelberg: Springer; 2010. p. 13–24.
2. Ezzedine K, Lim HW, Suzuki T, et al. Revised classification/nomenclature of vitiligo and related issues: the vitiligo global issues consensus conference. Pigment Cell Melanoma Res. 2012;25(3):E1–13.
3. Koga M. Vitiligo: a new classification and therapy. Br J Dermatol. 1977;97(3):255–61.
4. Koga M, Tango T. Clinical features and course of type A and type B vitiligo. Br J Dermatol. 1988;118(2):223–8.
5. Hann SK, Yu H, Lan CE, et al. Segmental Vitiligo. In: Picardo M, Taïeb A, editors. Vitiligo. Cham: Springer; 2019.
6. Faria AR, Tarlé RG, Dellatorre G, et al. Vitiligo–Part 2–classification, histopathology and treatment. An Bras Dermatol. 2014;89(5):784–90.
7. Madke B, Nayak C. Eponymous signs in dermatology. Indian Dermatol Online J. 2012;3(3):159–65.
8. Joge RR, Kathane PU, Joshi SH. Vitiligo: a narrative review. Cureus. 2022;14(9):e29307.
9. Costin GE, Hearing VJ. Human skin pigmentation: melanocytes modulate skin color in response to stress. FASEB J. 2007;21(4):976–94.
10. Zhang Y, Ding X, Wang F, et al. Clinical significance of Koebner's phenomenon in vitiligo: a hospital-based epidemiological investigation from China. Chin Med J. 2023;136(4):502–4.
11. Abdi P, Anthony MR, Farkouh C, et al. Non-invasive skin measurement methods and diagnostics for vitiligo: a systematic review. Front Med (Lausanne). 2023;10:1200963.
12. Sehgal VN, Srivastava G. Vitiligo: compendium of clinico-epidemiological features. Indian J Dermatol Venereol Leprol. 2007;73:149–56.

13. Dupré A, Christol B. Cockade-like vitiligo and linear vitiligo a variant of fitzpatrick's trichrome vitiligo. Arch Dermatol Res. 1978;262(2):197–203.
14. Ivker R, Goldaber M, Buchness MR. Blue vitiligo. J Am Acad Dermatol. 1994;30(5 Pt 2):829–31.
15. Jassi R, Mehta N, Ramam M, Bhari N. Blaschkoid blue vitiligo. Int J Dermatol. 2019;58(2):e45–6.
16. Tsuboi H, Yonemoto K, Katsuoka K. Vitiligo with inflammatory raised borders with hepatitis C virus infection. J Dermatol. 2006;33:577–8.
17. Weisberg EL, Le LQ, Cohen JB. A case of simultaneously occurring lichen sclerosus and segmental vitiligo: connecting the underlying autoimmune pathogenesis. Int J Dermatol. 2008;47:1053–5.
18. Sugita K, Izu K, Tokura Y. Vitiligo with inflammatory raised borders, associated with atopic dermatitis. Clin Exp Dermatol. 2006;31:80–2.
19. Tanioka M, Takahashi K, Miyachi YI. Narrowband ultraviolet B phototherapy for inflammatory vitiligo with raised borders associated with Sjögren's syndrome. Clin Exp Dermatol. 2009;34(3):418–20.
20. Trikha R, McCowan N, Brodell R. Marginal vitiligo: an unusual depigmenting disorder. Dermatol Online J. 2014;21(3):13030/qt7q9852nr.
21. Mchepange UO, Gao XH, Liu YY, et al. Vitiligo in north-eastern China: an association between mucosal and acrofacial lesions. Acta Derm Venereol. 2010;90:136–40.
22. Attili VR, Attili SK. Acral vitiligo and lichen sclerosus- association or a distinct pattern?: a clinical and histopathological review of 15 cases. Indian J Dermatol. 2015;60:519.
23. Silva de Castro CC, do Nascimento LM, Olandoski M, et al. A pattern of association between clinical form of vitiligo and disease-related variables in a Brazilian population. J Dermatol Sci. 2012;65:63–7.
24. Agarwal S, Ojha A, Gupta S. Profile of vitiligo in Kumaun region of Uttarakhand, India. Indian J Dermatol. 2014;59:209.
25. Ezzedine K, Diallo A, Léauté-Labrèze C, et al. Pre- vs. post-pubertal onset of vitiligo: multivariate analysis indicates atopic diathesis association in pre-pubertal onset vitiligo. Br J Dermatol. 2012;167:490–5.
26. Mahajan VK, Vashist S, Chauhan PS, et al. Clinico-epidemiological profile of patients with vitiligo: a retrospective study from a tertiary care center of North India. Indian Dermatol Online J. 2019;10(1):38–44.
27. Song MS, Hann SK, Ahn PS, et al. Clinical study of vitiligo: comparative study of type a and type B vitiligo. Ann Dermatol. 1994;6:22–30.
28. Kwon HS, Jung HM, Lee JH, Kim GM, Bae JM. A case of segmental vitiligo along Blaschko's lines. Ann Dermatol. 2018;30(6):747–8.
29. Sarma N, Chakraborty S, Poojary S, et al. A Nationwide, multicentric case-control study on vitiligo (MEDEC-V) to elicit the magnitude and correlates. Indian J Dermatol. 2020;65(6):473–82.
30. Park JH, Jung MY, Lee JH, et al. Clinical course of segmental vitiligo: a retrospective study of eighty-seven patients. Ann Dermatol. 2014;26(1):61–5.
31. Speeckaert R, Lambert J, Bulat V, et al. Autoimmunity in segmental vitiligo. Front Immunol. 2020;11:568447.
32. Ezzedine K, Gauthier Y, Léauté-Labrèze C, et al. Segmental vitiligo associated with generalized vitiligo (mixed vitiligo): a retrospective case series of 19 patients. J Am Acad Dermatol. 2011;65:965–71.
33. Lerner AB. Vitiligo. J Invest Dermatol. 1959;39:285–310.
34. Tanioka M, Yamamoto Y, Katoh M, et al. Vitiligo vulgaris and autoimmune diseases in Japan: a report from vitiligo Clinic in Kyoto University Hospital. Dermatoendocrinol. 2009;1(1):43–5.
35. Lee DY, Kim CR, Park JH, et al. The incidence of leukotrichia in segmental vitiligo: implication of poor response to medical treatment. Int J Dermatol. 2011;50(8):925–7.

36. Raju BP, Nagaraju U. Profile of childhood vitiligo with associated ocular abnormalities in South India. Indian J Paediatr Dermatol. 2016;17(3):179–85.
37. Kim DY, Oh SH, Hann SK. Classification of segmental vitiligo on the face: clues for prognosis. Br J Dermatol. 2011;164:1004–9.
38. van Geel N, Bosma S, Boone B, et al. Classification of segmental vitiligo on the trunk. Br J Dermatol. 2014;170:322–7.
39. Gan EY, Cario-André M, Pain C, et al. Follicular vitiligo: a report of 8 cases. J Am Acad Dermatol. 2016;74(6):1178–84.
40. Ezzedine K, Amazan E, Seneschal J, et al. Follicular vitiligo: a new form of vitiligo. Pigment Cell Melanoma Res. 2012;25:527–9.
41. Cabrera R, Reculé F, Hojman L, et al. Follicular vitiligo: dermatoscopic features of a new subtype of vitiligo. An Bras Dermatol. 2019;94(1):120–1.
42. Falabella R, Escobar CE, Carrascal E, et al. Leukoderma punctata. J Am Acad Dermatol. 1988;18(3):485–94.
43. Loquai C, Metze D, Nashan D, et al. Confetti-like lesions with hyperkeratosis: a novel ultraviolet-induced hypomelanotic disorder? Br J Dermatol. 2005;153:190–3.
44. Ezzedine K, Mahé A, van Geel N, et al. Hypochromic vitiligo: delineation of a new entity. Br J Dermatol. 2015;172(3):716–21.
45. Spritz RA. Six decades of vitiligo genetics: genome-wide studies provide insights into autoimmune pathogenesis. J Invest Dermatol. 2012;132:268–73.
46. Spritz RA. Recent progress in the genetics of generalized vitiligo. J Genet Genomics. 2011;38:271–8.
47. Yuan J, Sun C, Jiang S, et al. The prevalence of thyroid disorders in patients with vitiligo: a systematic review and meta-analysis. Front Endocrinol (Lausanne). 2019;9:803.
48. Acharya P, Mathur M. Association of atopic dermatitis with vitiligo: a systematic review and meta-analysis. J Cosmet Dermatol. 2020;19(8):2016–20.
49. Seneschal J, Morice-Picard F, Taïeb A. Vitiligo, associated disorders and comorbidities (autoimmune-inflammatory disorders, immunodeficiencies, rare monogenic diseases). In: Picardo M, Taïeb A, editors. Vitiligo. Cham: Springer; 2019.
50. Vukojević M, Vukojevic N, Vuković A, et al. Vitiligo as a first sign of Vogt-Koyanagi-Harada disease. Acta Dermatovenerol Croat. 2023;31(4):229–31.
51. Prignano F, Betts CM, Lotti T. Vogt-Koyanagi-Harada disease and vitiligo: where does the illness begin? J Electron Microsc. 2008;57(1):25–31.
52. Aydogan K, Turan OF, Onart S, et al. Audiological abnormalities in patients with vitiligo. Clin Exp Dermatol. 2006;31:110–3.
53. Passeron T, Ortonne JP, Kumarasinghe P, et al. Vitiligo/nonsegmental vitiligo including Acrofacial and Universalis. In: Picardo M, Taïeb A, editors. Vitiligo. Cham: Springer; 2019.
54. van Geel N, De Lille S, Vandenhaute S, et al. Different phenotypes of segmental vitiligo based on a clinical observational study. J Eur Acad Dermatol Venereol. 2011;25:673–8.

Chapter 7
The Natural History and Prognosis of Vitiligo

Christian Gan and Michelle Rodrigues

Abstract The natural history and prognosis of vitiligo can be difficult to predict. Baseline patient characteristics including family history, the type and location of vitiligo and clinical markers of disease activity must be understood by the treating clinician in order to plan treatment and address patient expectations. The non-segmental subtype and acral involvement suggest a risk of future autoimmune thyroid disease. Dermoscopy findings and serum or lesional biochemical markers may also serve as predictors of disease activity. The extent of depigmentation, the involvement of the hair follicle unit and repigmentation patterns provides prognostic information on repigmentation. It is important for the practicing clinician to identify prognostic factors that can indicate progressive and active disease, as early treatment initiation in these patients will help prevent uncontrolled or irreversible disease activity.

Keywords Vitiligo · Prognosis · Prognostic factors · Depigmentation · Koebner phenomenon · Trichrome lesions · Confetti depigmentation · Repigmentation · Leukotrichia

---

C. Gan
Department of Dermatology, St Vincent's Hospital, Melbourne, Australia

M. Rodrigues (✉)
Department of Dermatology, The Royal Children's Hospital, Melbourne, VIC, Australia

Department of Paediatrics, The University of Melbourne, Parkville, VIC, Australia

Chroma Dermatology, Pigment and Skin of Colour Centre, Melbourne, VIC, Australia
e-mail: michelle.rodrigues@unimelb.edu.au

R. Sarkar, V. Narayan R (eds.), *A Concise Guide to The Management of Vitiligo*,
https://doi.org/10.1007/978-981-95-3857-7_7

7.1 Introduction

The development of vitiligo is multifactorial and as such its natural progression and prognosis can be erratic. Descriptions of the natural clinical course of vitiligo can include a spectrum from focal to generalized skin involvement, stable to rapidly progressive depigmentation, or lesions that demonstrate periods of inactivity followed by periods of slow or swift depigmentation [1, 2]. However, there have been significant efforts to better characterize the natural progression of vitiligo lesions in the literature, which has led to advances in how clinicians can project a patient's disease course based on the presence of prognostic factors [3]. The prognostic information can be gleaned from patient demographics as well as cutaneous clues within and around vitiliginous lesions.

This chapter describes the key clinical and biochemical markers seen in active, progressive vitiligo, the significance of baseline demographics in predicting natural disease outlook, and how these characteristics have contributed to the way clinicians prognosticate and stratify vitiligo lesions. Disease associations and their risk in patients who have vitiligo as well as factors important to prognosticate the probability of repigmentation will also be described.

7.2 Classification of Vitiligo as a Predictor of Natural History and Prognosis: Segmental Versus Non-segmental Vitiligo

Segmental vitiligo occurs in a minority of patients and describes unilateral vitiligo lesions that develop into a linear or block pattern [3]. These distribution patterns differentiate segmental vitiligo from focal variants [4]. Other features seen in but not exclusive to segmental vitiligo include early age of disease onset (41.3% before the age of 10 years), irregular margins, leukotrichia, and islands of pigment within vitiligo [5, 6]. Common areas of involvement include the face, trunk, neck, extremities, and scalp in descending order of frequency [6].

Segmental vitiligo carries a unique pattern of disease evolution, with most cases demonstrating progressive disease during the initial 12–24 months from disease onset, often refractory to treatment [5]. However, once the disease stabilizes, further progression is rare though disease quiescence is not guaranteed [6]. In particular, involvement of the trunk, face, and neck is more likely to demonstrate reactivation years later [7]. Segmental vitiligo features fewer vitiliginous lesions and a reduced body surface area of involvement compared with non-segmental vitiligo [8]. Early leukotrichia is more common in segmental vitiligo and results in a poor response to medical treatment [9].

Mixed vitiligo describes a few cases that present as segmental vitiligo but later extend beyond typical distribution patterns and include bilateral skin involvement and resemble non-segmental vitiligo distribution patterns. The presence of halo naevi, leukotrichia, and an initial truncal lesion may be indicators of progression to mixed vitiligo [3].

7.3 Clinical Markers of Vitiligo Disease Activity and Their Utility as Indicators of Prognosis

In contrast to other cutaneous inflammatory dermatoses, vitiligo lesions lack typical signs of inflammation and instead present with unique clinical signs of disease activity [10]. The presence of activity markers indicates likely disease spread and a need for prompt treatment [1, 10]. Confetti-like lesions, Koebner phenomenon, and trichrome lesions represent three common prognostic signs of disease activity, in approximate descending order of frequency [10].

Most cases of vitiligo extend contiguous to the initial site of onset [11]. However, koebnerization manifests as depigmentation in areas of trauma, such as from pressure, friction, or sunburn, and can occur in both new and longstanding disease [3]. Koebnerization tends to affect the dorsal hands [12].

The Koebner phenomenon (Fig. 7.1) is more common in progressive disease compared with stable disease (67.3% had vs. 44.2% respectively) [13] It is also seen more commonly in recent disease activity (e.g. <12 months), and in those with greater body surface area involvement. This increases the risk of further depigmentation despite treatment [14]. Subtypes of KP including KP assessed by history (type 1) and by clinical examination (type 2) reveal clues to its presence [11, 14]. Interestingly, koebnerization over friction areas (type 2A) has been associated with the development of systemic autoimmune diseases [14].

The presence of the Koebner phenomenon in vitiligo appears to be more likely in patients who develop vitiligo at a younger age, who have a disease duration over 3

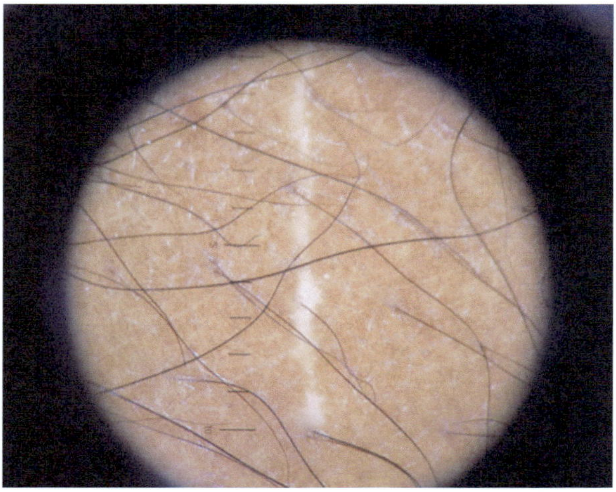

Fig. 7.1 Dermoscopy view of koebnerization in vitiligo as seen by evolving linear depigmentation over a previous scratch site

years, and involvement over the forehead and scalp areas, eyelids, wrists, genital and belt areas, knees, and tibial crests [5, 14, 15]. Pooled results also suggest an association between the Koebner phenomenon, confetti-depigmentation, and itch [16].

Confetti depigmentation (Fig. 7.2) is characterized by clusters of pinpoint depigmented macules at the periphery of pre-existing lesions [3]. This pattern of depigmentation carries associations with higher vitiligo disease activity scores, K-VSCOR scores, CD8+ T cell inflammatory infiltrate in the papillary dermis and an absence of melanin on histopathology [17]. The area affected by confetti vitiligo can later progress into complete depigmentation without adequate treatment [10]. Confetti lesions are also more likely to present alongside trichrome and hypochromic lesions [16].

Trichrome lesions (Fig. 7.3) describe the presence of a tan zone of hypopigmentation between the depigmented vitiliginous lesion and unaffected skin [18]. Trichrome vitiligo represents a transitional pigmentary state that is predictive of lesion expansion, and the hypopigmented zone can indicate the future disease borders once lesions stabilize [1]. Biopsy findings of trichrome areas show corresponding changes in melanin granule density and inflammatory cell infiltration, but preserved melanocyte numbers [19]. Interestingly, biopsies of normal perilesional skin surrounding trichrome zones demonstrate vacuolar changes in the basal layer and inflammatory infiltration that suggest ongoing vitiligo evolution despite an absence of clinical depigmentation [19]. Most trichrome lesions have been observed over truncal, sun-protected lesions and the axillae [12, 19]. Patients with trichrome vitiligo demonstrated greater vitiligo assessment severity index score (VASI) improvements following narrowband UV-B phototherapy and topical tacrolimus [1].

Each prognostic marker carries a risk of vitiligo progression by itself, but the presence of multiple clinical markers is further predictive of disease progression, and is associated with greater CXCL10 serum levels, higher VASI scores, and less VASI improvement with treatment [1].

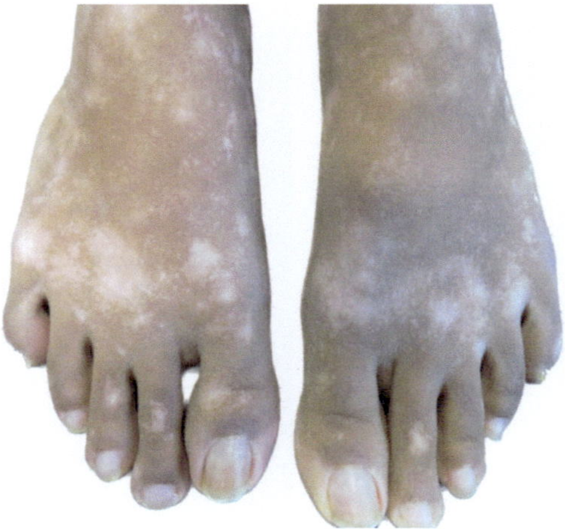

Fig. 7.2 Confetti depigmentation demonstrated by small macular depigmentation around the periphery of larger vitiligo lesions

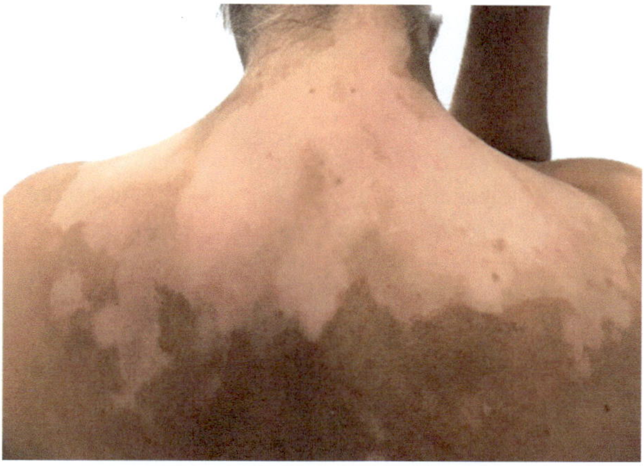

Fig. 7.3 Trichrome lesions as demonstrated by the presence of a tan zone of hypopigmentation between fully depigmented vitiliginous patches and unaffected skin

Inflammatory vitiligo is rare and commonly associated with non-segmental vitiligo. Vitiliginous lesions are accompanied by scale, erythema, and pruritus. These cases appear to be associated with future clinical progression, rapid enlargement of lesions, greater inflammatory cell infiltrates on biopsy, and systemic autoimmunity [16, 18]. Inflammatory vitiligo is predominantly associated with non-segmental vitiligo [16].

Halo naevi describe pigmented naevi with a rim of depigmentation. In a subset of cases, halo naevi are associated with generalized/non-segmental vitiligo, and can appear prior to the development of vitiligo [20]. However, there appears to be no correlation between their presence and the prognosis or disease activity of vitiligo [20]. Patients who have both vitiligo and halo naevi seem to have a lower prevalence of additional associated autoimmune diseases than those who have only vitiligo, but this patient subgroup still carries greater rates of associated autoimmune diseases than those who only have halo naevi [20, 21]. This distinction may be related to the presence of various human leukocyte antigen (HLA) haplotypes that can all precipitate vitiligo development but carry different risks of developing other autoimmune diseases [21].

7.4 Location of Vitiliginous Lesions

Mucosal involvement describes vitiligo in the oral or genital region and may be associated with progressive disease [3]. It can be isolated or as part of generalized vitiligo [4].

The presence of localized periorificial area involvement is associated with a greater risk of new lesion development that tends to arise in areas of mechanical stress [22]. In these patients the areas of mechanical stress included parts of the face involved in physical motions such as blinking, speaking, and chewing [22].

7.4.1 *Bedside Tools*

7.4.1.1 Dermoscopy

There is evidence to support the use of dermoscopy to identify active vitiligo, with poor prognostic findings including ill-defined borders, satellite lesions, comet-tail appearances (micro-koebnerization), broken pigment networks, and leukotrichia [23, 24]. In contrast, stable lesions can be identified by a well-defined border and either an absent or regular reticular network [23, 24].

Many of the dermoscopy signs can be likened to the aforementioned clinical markers of disease progression such as confetti lesions, koebnerization, and trichrome lesions seen on naked eye assessment. There are contradictions in the literature regarding the significance of perifollicular pigmentation or depigmentation as both an active or stable prognostic factor, and unfortunately there is an absence of consensus criteria on the significance of dermoscopy findings in vitiligo to date in relation to diagnosis and staging [24].

7.4.1.2 Baseline Demographic Findings Predictive of Prognosis

A family history of vitiligo has been established as a predictive factor for vitiligo development, vitiligo progression, and poor treatment response [25–27]. It may also be related to early onset in children. A large global study across 17 countries identified 57.1% of patients had a family history of vitiligo [28].

Age of onset overall is not always positively correlated to disease progression; in fact some retrospective studies suggest that childhood vitiligo may carry a slower disease progression [11, 25]. However, in childhood populations, the literature suggests that patients with very early onset vitiligo (<3 years old) are more likely to develop more extensive body surface area involvement and disease progression [29]. Another study revealed that compared with those over 10, those diagnosed under 10 years of age had more extensive involvement (>10% BSA), male sex, a prolonged clinical course, and the presence of koebnerization or halo naevi [30].

The patient's age may also be predictive of the distribution of future lesions. If knees, hips, and ankles are spared at a young age (<20 years), these areas appear less likely to be affected in the future disease course; however, this has not been observed for hand, wrist, arm, and elbow involvement [11]. Vitiligo distributed over the knees, hips, and ankles overall appears to be less likely to further spread and/or expand [11].

Sex does not have a clear correlation with vitiligo prognosis [25]. Gender may be predictive of lesion distribution as involvement of feet, elbows, hips, trunk, and axilla are more frequently observed in women, versus hands and genitals in men [11].

In pregnant patients with vitiligo, observational studies suggest that vitiligo lesions remain stable during the pregnancy and up to 6 months post-delivery, with some patients demonstrating clinical improvement; a cross-sectional study found 66.66% (63.15% 6 months post-partum) of pregnant women with vitiligo noted stability of their condition and 12.8% (5.25% 6 months post-partum) noted improvement [31, 32]. The implications of having vitiligo during pregnancy remain unclear; some papers suggest vitiligo may confer an increase in miscarriage rates; however, significant confounders likely exist including the inherent autoimmune predisposition implicated in vitiligo patients. No association of specific perinatal complications has been identified [31, 33].

Skin phototype does not predict progression of vitiligo but more patients with darker Fitzpatrick skin types appear to achieve cosmetically acceptable repigmentation on the face compared to those with phototypes I and II with vitiligo [34]. Expert consensus statements have suggested that darker skin phototypes may experience an increased efficiency in rate of repigmentation [35].

7.4.1.3 Chemical Biomarkers Prognostic of Vitiligo Severity and Progression

Clinical features of vitiligo disease activity remain the gold standard predictor of future expansion of lesions, particularly in the absence of a biomarker [10]. The C-X-C motif chemokine ligand 10 (CXCL10) plays a pivotal role in T cell trafficking and function and is a key component in the interferon-γ-JAK-STAT-CXCL10 pathway that drives autoimmunity in vitiligo [3]. CXCL10 interacts with the C-X-C motif chemokine receptor 3 on cytotoxic CD8 T cells to recruit these cells into the affected skin and precipitate melanocyte destruction [36]. Serum CXCL10 levels have been associated with greater Vitiligo Area Scoring Index (VASI) scores, were later reduced after successful treatments, and may represent a novel biomarker to indicate progressive and/or active disease [36]. CXCL10 levels also correlate strongly with the presence of clinical markers for active disease such as trichrome sign, Koebner phenomenon, and confetti depigmentation [1].

A minimally invasive non-scarring skin biopsy technique utilizing suction blisters has been tested as a method to evaluate for progressive vitiligo [37]. Suction blisters produce blister fluid with interstitial skin cells. C-X-C motif chemokine ligand 9 (CXCL9) was extracted from lesional blister fluid as a biomarker [37]. Lesional CXCL9 levels were significantly associated with clinically active disease, defined in this study by a recency of new lesions, presence of confetti depigmentation, and/or trichrome lesions [37]. The study identified CXCL9 as a more sensitive and specific marker compared to CXCL10 for disease activity [37]. The upregulation of CXCL9 appears first in new vitiligo lesions, later followed by an upregulation of CXCL10 [38].

7.4.1.4 Disease Associations

Disease associations include thyroid disorders, chronic urticaria, rheumatoid arthritis, pernicious anemia, type 1 diabetes, psoriasis, Addison's disease, and alopecia areata [39–41]. Studies have reported up to 35% of vitiligo cases also have other comorbid autoimmune disorders [39, 40]. Thyroid disorders carry the strongest association with reports in 20–25% of cases, and clinical signs consistent with thyroid disease in 43% [4, 39, 42].

Studies have attempted to identify prognostic factors that may carry clues to predict future autoimmune disease development, especially as vitiligo usually precedes other autoimmune conditions such as thyroid dysfunction [11]. A strong association exists between thyroid disorders and acral lesions. Gray hair and abdominal lesions have been reported as a possible indicator of pernicious anemia but this association is not as well established [39].

The segmental variant of vitiligo is less likely to be associated with other autoimmune diseases.

7.4.1.5 Predictors of Re-pigmentation

Repigmentation naturally occurs from the hair follicle unit, the border of vitiligo lesions, or from unaffected melanocytes within depigmented areas [43]. The most significant source of repigmentation is from the hair follicle unit as melanocytes can be present here in large numbers and migrate to the epidermis [43]. The specific repigmentation pattern differs based on the disease state of the underlying lesion; perifollicular and marginal (from unaffected skin at the border of lesions) repigmentation patterns are more commonly observed in completely depigmented, stable lesions while diffuse repigmentation is more frequently seen in incompletely depigmented lesions, sun-exposed areas, and in actively enlarging or newly developed lesions [44]. The diffuse repigmentation pattern is believed to reflect the resuscitation of impaired but surviving melanocytes as opposed to other repigmentation patterns which require the migration of melanocytes from epidermal reservoirs into the depigmented skin [44].

Vitiligo lesions in areas of the body with greater hair follicle density as well as greater frequency of UV exposure, such as the forehead, are more likely to repigment faster [45]. Many studies exploring repigmentation following phototherapy report greater results over the face than the body [34]. Naturally, areas of the body lacking hair such as the palms and soles are much less likely to demonstrate repigmentation [34]. Likewise, the presence of leukotrichia (Fig. 7.4) represents melanocyte reservoir exhaustion, and suggests that subsequent repigmentation with or without treatment may be unlikely [43].

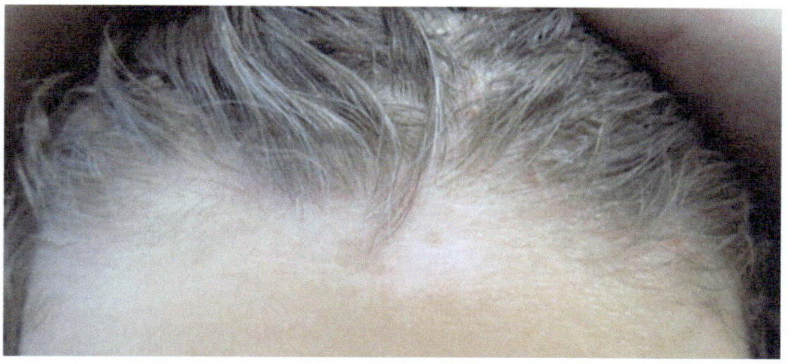

Fig. 7.4 Leukotrichia overlying patches of vitiligo on the forehead

7.5 Conclusion

The natural history and prognosis of vitiligo can still be aptly and succinctly described as unpredictable, and it is important to manage these expectations with patients. To predict the natural history and prognosis of vitiligo requires an understanding of and ability to identify key clinical prognostic factors that suggest more aggressive disease. Distribution, morphology, baseline characteristics, and more recently dermoscopic and biochemical factors can all be predictive of future spread or stability. Nevertheless, the presence of negative prognostic findings does not mean patients' vitiligo cannot be treated. Rather, they should highlight the importance of identifying disease activity and offering appropriate management early in the disease course.

Acknowledgements Thank you to Ms. Yebin Yang for assistance with selection of clinical images to accompany this chapter.

Declarations: *Funding*: No funding was received

- *Acknowledgements*: None
- *Conflict of Interests to declare*: Dr. Michelle Rodrigues is a primary investigator for Pfizer and MSD and has been a consultant for Pfizer and Abbvie. Dr Christian Gan has no conflict of interest to declare.

References

1. Zhang L, Chen S, Kang Y, Wang X, Yan F, Jiang M, et al. Association of clinical markers with disease progression in patients with vitiligo from China. JAMA Dermatol. 2020;156(3):288–95.
2. Yaghoobi R, Omidian M, Bagherani N. Vitiligo: a review of the published work. J Dermatol. 2011;38(5):419–31.
3. Rodrigues M, Ezzedine K, Hamzavi I, Pandya AG, Harris JE. New discoveries in the pathogenesis and classification of vitiligo. J Am Acad Dermatol. 2017;77(1):1–13.
4. Ezzedine K, Lim HW, Suzuki T, Katayama I, Hamzavi I, Lan CC, et al. Revised classification/nomenclature of vitiligo and related issues: the vitiligo global issues consensus conference. Pigment Cell Melanoma Res. 2012;25(3):E1–13.
5. Khaitan BK, Kathuria S, Ramam M. A descriptive study to characterize segmental vitiligo. Indian J Dermatol Venereol Leprol. 2012;78(6):715–21.

6. Hann SK, Lee HJ. Segmental vitiligo: clinical findings in 208 patients. J Am Acad Dermatol. 1996;35(5, Part 1):671–4.
7. Park JH, Jung MY, Lee JH, Yang JM, Lee DY, Park KK. Clinical course of segmental vitiligo: a retrospective study of eighty-seven patients. Ann Dermatol. 2014;26(1):61–5.
8. Mazereeuw-Hautier J, Bezio S, Mahe E, Bodemer C, Eschard C, Viseux V, et al. Segmental and nonsegmental childhood vitiligo has distinct clinical characteristics: a prospective observational study. J Am Acad Dermatol. 2010;62(6):945–9.
9. Lee DY, Kim CR, Park JH, Lee JH. The incidence of leukotrichia in segmental vitiligo: implication of poor response to medical treatment. Int J Dermatol. 2011;50(8):925–7.
10. Aboul-Fettouh N, Hinojosa J, Tovar-Garza A, Pandya AG. The majority of patients presenting with vitiligo have a clinical sign of activity. J Am Acad Dermatol. 2017;77(4):774–5.
11. Speeckaert R, van Geel N. Distribution patterns in generalized vitiligo. J Eur Acad Dermatol Venereol. 2014;28(6):755–62.
12. Delbaere L, van Causenbroeck J, Duponselle J, Van Goethem C, Speeckaert R, van Geel N. Hot spots for clinical signs of disease activity in vitiligo. Exp Dermatol. 2024;33(1):e14975.
13. Zhang Y, Ding X, Wang F, Li M, Du J. Clinical significance of Koebner's phenomenon in vitiligo: a hospital-based epidemiological investigation from China. Chin Med J. 2023;136(4):502–4.
14. van Geel N, Speeckaert R, De Wolf J, Bracke S, Chevolet I, Brochez L, et al. Clinical significance of Koebner phenomenon in vitiligo. Br J Dermatol. 2012;167(5):1017–24.
15. Diallo A, Boniface K, Jouary T, Seneschal J, Morice-Picard F, Prey S, et al. Development and validation of the K-VSCOR for scoring Koebner's phenomenon in vitiligo/non-segmental vitiligo. Pigment Cell Melanoma Res. 2013;26(3):402–7.
16. van Geel N, Grine L, De Wispelaere P, Mertens D, Prinsen CAC, Speeckaert R. Clinical visible signs of disease activity in vitiligo: a systematic review and meta-analysis. J Eur Acad Dermatol Venereol. 2019;33(9):1667–75.
17. Sosa JJ, Currimbhoy SD, Ukoha U, Sirignano S, O'Leary R, Vandergriff T, et al. Confetti-like depigmentation: a potential sign of rapidly progressing vitiligo. J Am Acad Dermatol. 2015;73(2):272–5.
18. Goh B-K, Pandya AG. Presentations, signs of activity, and differential diagnosis of vitiligo. Dermatol Clin. 2017;35(2):135–44.
19. Hann S-K, Kim Y-S, Yoo JH, Chun Y-S. Clinical and histopathologic characteristics of trichrome vitiligo. J Am Acad Dermatol. 2000;42(4):589–96.
20. van Geel N, Vandenhaute S, Speeckaert R, Brochez L, Mollet I, De Cooman L, et al. Prognostic value and clinical significance of halo naevi regarding vitiligo. Br J Dermatol. 2011;164(4):743–9.
21. de Vijlder HC, Westerhof W, Schreuder GM, de Lange P, Claas FH. Difference in pathogenesis between vitiligo vulgaris and halo nevi associated with vitiligo is supported by an HLA association study. Pigment Cell Res. 2004;17(3):270–4.
22. Kim DH, Cho SI, Hwang J, Jeong J, Kim S, Lee SH. Periorificial lesions associated with poor prognosis in patients with localized vitiligo: a retrospective study of 126 patients. J Am Acad Dermatol. 2022;87(4):927–30.
23. Bhat YJ, Khare S, Nabi N. Dermoscopy of disorders of hypopigmentation. Pigm Int. 2022;9(1)
24. Yang Y, Morriss S, Rodrigues M. Dermoscopy in vitiligo, diagnostic clues and markers of disease activity: a review of the literature. Clin Exp Dermatol. 2024;49:llad365.
25. Hann SK, Chun WH, Park YK. Clinical characteristics of progressive vitiligo. Int J Dermatol. 1997;36(5):353–5.
26. Dave S, Thappa DM, Dsouza M. Clinical predictors of outcome in vitiligo. Indian J Dermatol Venereol Leprol. 2002;68(6):323–5.
27. Nejad SB, Qadim HH, Nazeman L, Fadaii R, Goldust M. Frequency of autoimmune diseases in those suffering from vitiligo in comparison with normal population. Pak J Biol Sci. 2013;16(12):570–4.

28. Hamzavi IH, Bibeau K, Grimes P, Harris JE, van Geel N, Parsad D, et al. Exploring the natural and treatment history of vitiligo: perceptions of patients and healthcare professionals from the global VALIANT study. Br J Dermatol. 2023;189(5):569–77.
29. Mu EW, Cohen BE, Orlow SJ. Early-onset childhood vitiligo is associated with a more extensive and progressive course. J Am Acad Dermatol. 2015;73(3):467–70.
30. Mahajan VK, Verma YR, Mehta KS, Chauhan PS, Sharma R, Sharma A, et al. Adults with a more extensive body involvement, moderate to extremely severe vitiligo and a prolonged clinical course have an early onset in childhood in addition to other prognostic factors as compared to individuals with later-onset vitiligo. Australas J Dermatol. 2021;62(1):e24–e8.
31. Abdelhafez MMA, Ahmed KAM, Ping Pang NT, Pg Baharuddin DM, Than WW, Kadir F, et al. Vitiligo and pregnancy: how do each affect the other? Ann Med Surg (Lond). 2021;70:102833.
32. Webb KC, Lyon S, Nardone B, West DP, Kundu RV. Influence of pregnancy on vitiligo activity. J Clin Aesthet Dermatol. 2016;9(12):21–5.
33. Hung CT, Huang HH, Wang CK, Chung CH, Tsao CH, Chien WC, et al. Pregnancy outcomes in women with vitiligo: a Taiwanese nationwide cohort study. PLoS One. 2021;16(3):e0248651.
34. Nicolaidou E, Antoniou C, Stratigos AJ, Stefanaki C, Katsambas AD. Efficacy, predictors of response, and long-term follow-up in patients with vitiligo treated with narrowband UVB phototherapy. J Am Acad Dermatol. 2007;56(2):274–8.
35. Gan EY, Eleftheriadou V, Esmat S, Hamzavi I, Passeron T, Böhm M, et al. Repigmentation in vitiligo: position paper of the vitiligo global issues consensus conference. Pigment Cell Melanoma Res. 2017;30(1):28–40.
36. Wang XX, Wang QQ, Wu JQ, Jiang M, Chen L, Zhang CF, et al. Increased expression of CXCR3 and its ligands in patients with vitiligo and CXCL10 as a potential clinical marker for vitiligo. Br J Dermatol. 2016;174(6):1318–26.
37. Strassner JP, Rashighi M, Ahmed Refat M, Richmond JM, Harris JE. Suction blistering the lesional skin of vitiligo patients reveals useful biomarkers of disease activity. J Am Acad Dermatol. 2017;76(5):847–55.e5.
38. He S, Xu J, Wu J. The promising role of chemokines in vitiligo: from oxidative stress to the autoimmune response. Oxidative Med Cell Longev. 2022;2022:8796735.
39. Silverberg J, Silverberg, N. Clinical predictors of comorbid autoimmune disease in vitiligo. J Am Acad Dermatol 2013;68(4, Supplement 1):AB188.
40. Al-smadi K, Imran M, Leite-Silva VR, Mohammed Y. Vitiligo: a review of Aetiology, pathogenesis, treatment, and psychosocial impact. Cosmet [Internet]. 2023;10(3)
41. Zhang Z, Xu S-X, Zhang F-Y, Yin X-Y, Yang S, Xiao F-L, et al. The analysis of genetics and associated autoimmune diseases in Chinese vitiligo patients. Arch Dermatol Res. 2009;301(2):167–73.
42. AL-smadi K, Imran M, Leite-Silva VR, Mohammed Y. Vitiligo: a review of aetiology, pathogenesis, treatment, and psychosocial impact. Cosmet. 2023;10(3):84.
43. Falabella R. Vitiligo and the melanocyte reservoir. Indian J Dermatol. 2009;54(4):313–8.
44. Yang K, Xiong X, Pallavi G, Ling Y, Ding F, Duan W, et al. The early repigmentation pattern of vitiligo is related to the source of melanocytes and by the choice of therapy: a retrospective cohort study. Int J Dermatol. 2018;57(3):324–31.
45. Sangha AM. Dermatological conditions in skin of color-: debunking vitiligo myths. J Clin Aesthet Dermatol. 2022;15(9 Suppl 1):S10–s1.

Chapter 8
Dermoscopy and Noninvasive Methods of Evaluation

Priyansh Gupta and Vinay Keshavamurthy

Abstract Evaluation of vitiligo can be aided by noninvasive diagnostic methods, which help confirm the diagnosis, assess disease activity, evaluate treatment response, and support research efforts. Commonly used noninvasive methods include dermoscopy, reflectance confocal microscopy, Wood's lamp examination, and digital imaging, with or without assessment by artificial intelligence or computer software. Less common methods include colorimetry, spectrophotometry, digital planimetry, and infrared or ultraviolet light photography. The latest methods include third harmonic generation microscopy, multiphoton microscopy, and optical coherence tomography.

The Wood's lamp is the most commonly used noninvasive diagnostic tool due to its affordability, wide availability, and ease of use. Dermoscopy has gained popularity because of its portability, ease of image capture and storage, and the extensive published literature supporting its use. However, dermoscopy requires expertise, has a slow learning curve, and the cost of a dermoscope is high. Reflectance confocal microscopy is much more expensive than dermoscopy but offers better histopathological and disease activity correlation. It can also be used in combination with other methods. Additionally, various imaging techniques have been developed that can be used alongside computer software or artificial intelligence-based applications.

Keywords Dermatoscopy · Dermoscopy · Noninvasive · Skin imaging · Vitiligo

---

P. Gupta · V. Keshavamurthy (✉)
Department of Dermatology, Venereology and Leprology, Postgraduate Institute of Medical Education and Research, Chandigarh, India

R. Sarkar, V. Narayan R (eds.), *A Concise Guide to The Management of Vitiligo*,
https://doi.org/10.1007/978-981-95-3857-7_8

8.1 Introduction

Vitiligo is an autoimmune disease characterized by the loss of functional melanocytes from the epidermis. Evaluation of vitiligo includes confirming the diagnosis and assessing disease activity. Assessing disease activity is crucial not only for medical management but also for selecting the right candidates for surgical treatment.

Noninvasive evaluation methods include dermoscopy, Wood's lamp examination, reflectance confocal microscopy, and digital photography with computerized evaluation. These methods can also be used in combination, such as pairing dermoscopy or Wood's lamp with confocal microscopy. In this chapter, we briefly discuss the various noninvasive evaluation methods and the characteristic findings observed in vitiligo patients.

8.2 Dermoscopy

Vitiligo is primarily a clinical diagnosis, and imaging modalities are not routinely used for diagnosis or follow-up. However, dermoscopy can serve as an auxiliary tool for confirming the diagnosis, assessing vitiligo activity, and monitoring treatment response. Dermoscopy is the most commonly used method for evaluating vitiligo lesions due to its widespread availability. The advent of hand-held devices has made this method a go-to option for dermatologists. There are several reports describing the dermoscopic features of vitiligo in a cross-sectional manner [1–5]. The characteristic features seen in vitiligo include diffuse white glow (Fig. 8.1),

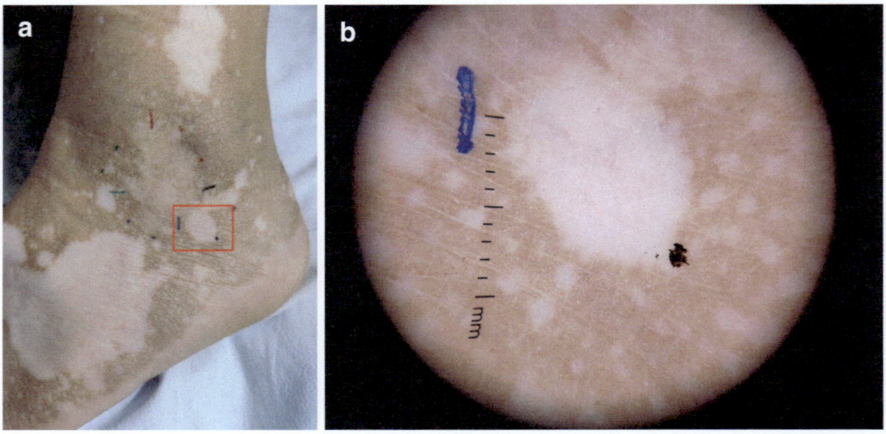

Fig. 8.1 (**a**) Clinical image of a vitiligo patch over left foot marked clockwise with different colored ball point pens. (**b**) Dermoscopy of the lesion highlighted with a red box in **a** showing well-defined margins with diffuse white glow (absent pigment network) in the center and satellite lesions in the surrounding skin giving tapioca sago appearance (Dermlite DL4 10× polarized mode)

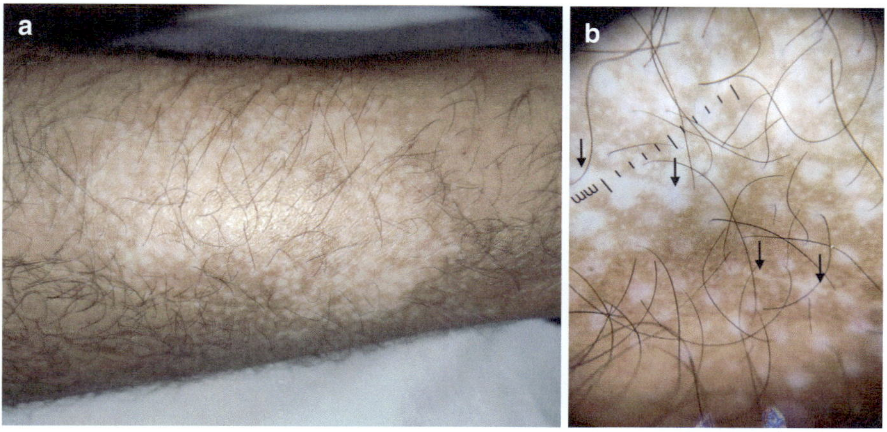

Fig. 8.2 (**a**) Clinical image of a patch of follicular vitiligo over leg. (**b**) Dermoscopic image of the same lesion showing absent pigment network limited to the perifollicular region with sparing of the rest of the area. In addition, linear depigmentation suggestive of micro-koebnerization can also be noted, black arrow (Dermlite DL4 10× polarized mode)

pigment network changes (reduced or absent pigment network, Figs. 8.1, 8.2, 8.3, 8.4, 8.5, and 8.6), trichrome pattern (Fig. 8.4b), perifollicular pigment changes (perifollicular depigmentation, Fig. 8.2b; perifollicular repigmentation, Fig. 8.6b and perifollicular pigment retention), marginal changes like perilesional or marginal pigmentation (Fig. 8.3b), ill-defined (Fig. 8.4b) or well-defined margins (Fig. 8.1b), satellite lesions (Fig. 8.1b) or micro-Koebner phenomenon (Figs. 8.2b and 8.5b), intralesional or perilesional erythema with telangiectasia (Fig. 8.3b). Some rare features include tapioca sago appearance or confetti-like lesions (Fig. 8.1b), pigmentary islands, starburst pattern, comet tail and reverse pigment network. Although there is a lack of standardization among these dermoscopic features with lots of discrepancy, the most accepted definitions have been summarized in Table 8.1 [6, 7].

8.2.1 *Disease Activity with Dermoscopy*

Studies have tried to correlate the observed dermoscopic features with disease activity [1–6, 8–11]. In the study by Chuh and Zawar [1], it was found that residual perifollicular pigmentation signifies either focally active or repigmenting vitiligo. Meng et al. [8, 12] recruited 176 patients with disorders of hypopigmentation of which 97 patients were suffering from vitiligo. Residual perifollicular pigmentation was seen only in patients with vitiligo and was not present in 79 cases diagnosed with depigmented disorders other than vitiligo. Even among patients with vitiligo, residual perifollicular pigmentation was seen in 91.94% (57/62) of patients with active spreading vitiligo and 62.86% (22/35) of those with inactive or stabilized disease. Other dermoscopic features seen in vitiligo patients were marginal

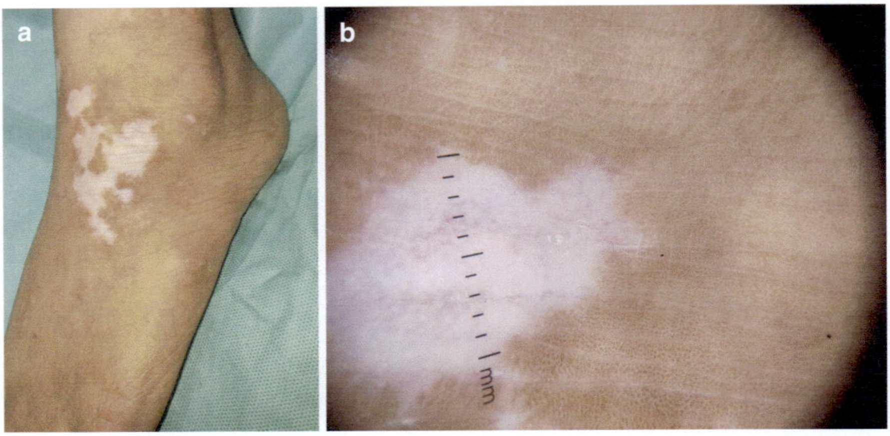

Fig. 8.3 (**a**) Clinical image of a vitiligo patch over left foot. (**b**) Dermoscopy of the same lesion showing diffuse white glow in the center and perilesional hyperpigmentation suggestive of repigmenting vitiligo. In addition, telangiectasia can also be noted in the lesion (Dermlite DL4 10× polarized mode)

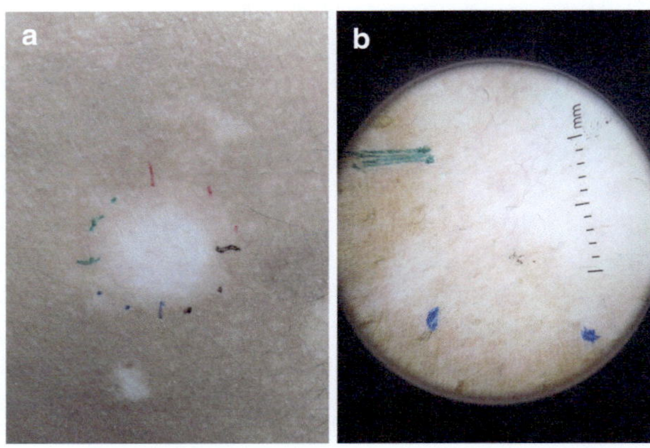

Fig. 8.4 (**a**) Clinical image of an active patch of vitiligo over abdomen. (**b**) Dermoscopy showing diffuse white glow, trichrome lesions with ill-defined margins (Dermlite DL4 10× polarized mode)

hyperpigmentation, telangiectasias and early reservoirs of pigmentation. The reported dermoscopic findings associated with stable or repigmenting vitiligo include perilesional and perifollicular hyperpigmentation, islands of normal reticular pigment network, and marginal reticular pigment network. Thatte et al. [2] studied 30 patients with progressive vitiligo and evaluated dermoscopic features in both polarized and ultraviolet light. Dermoscopic features associated with progressive vitiligo included altered pigment network, marginal and perifollicular hyperpigmentation seen in polarized mode, and diffuse white glow seen in ultraviolet light. In a study by Jha et al. [4], the most constant dermoscopic feature of vitiligo includes perifollicular pigment changes. It was also observed that perifollicular depigmentation was most commonly encountered in stable vitiligo while perifollicular pigmentation was the predominant dermoscopic feature of progressive vitiligo. Pigment

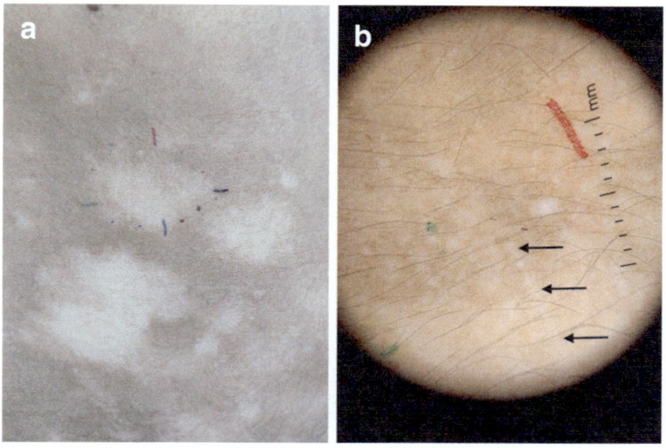

Fig. 8.5 (**a**) Clinical image of an active patch of vitiligo with trichrome pattern seen clinically. (**b**) Dermoscopy showing, in addition to the trichrome pattern, ill-defined margins, satellite lesions, and micro-koebnerization, which is not evident on clinical image (Dermlite DL4 10× polarized mode)

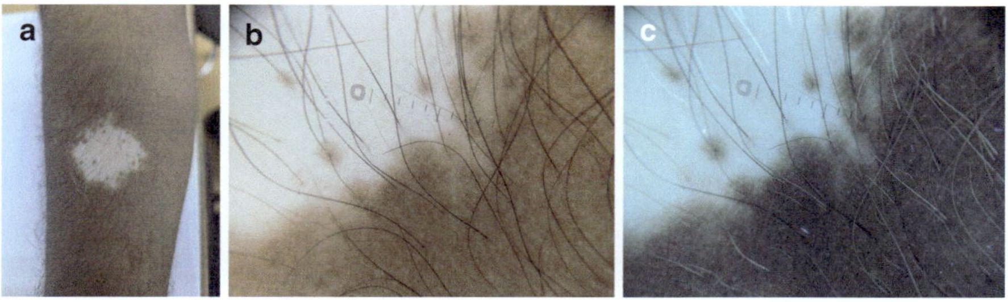

Fig. 8.6 (**a**) Clinical and (**b**) dermoscopic images of a patch of vitiligo showing perifollicular and marginal pigmentation that became more apparent on UV dermoscopy (**c**) (Dermlite DL5 10×, UV mode)

network changes were seen in 32 cases (91.4%) of progressive or active vitiligo in the same study. Other than these features some specific morphological features like salt and pepper pigmentation, comet tail appearance, trichrome vitiligo, and starburst appearance are considered to be suggestive of active or progressive vitiligo. Comet tail appearance is thought to be a dermoscopic counterpart of Koebner's phenomenon seen clinically. A newly described dermoscopic feature, i.e., the "tapioca sago" appearance was also reported in this study [3]. This "tapioca sago" appearance is found in the perilesional, clinically normal skin, and is considered to be a marker of active vitiligo [3]. A recently conducted longitudinal study with a novel imaging method and relying on a multitude of factors to assess disease activity concluded pigment network changes, perifollicular depigmentation, ill-defined margins, and satellite lesions as markers of disease activity [6]. In contrast, perifollicular repigmentation was found to be a feature of stabilized or repigmenting vitiligo. The trichrome pattern was seen in both active as well as stabilized/repigmenting vitiligo. Confetti-like depigmentation has also shown to be a hot spot of disease activity signs [13]. Another study [7], with a large sample size of 200 vitiligo patches and follow-up of 6 months showed well-defined borders as a marker of static vitiligo and ill-defined borders, trichrome pattern, satellite lesions, and

Table 8.1 Common dermoscopic features seen in vitiligo irrespective of activity and their accepted definition

Dermoscopic feature	Definition
Margins—ill-defined	When at least 25% of the margins are ill-defined If less than 25% margins are ill-defined, lesion is considered to have well-defined margins Note: A single lesion cannot have both ill-defined as well as well-defined margins at a particular point of time
Perilesional hyperpigmentation	Accentuated of pigment network of at least 25% perilesional skin
Perifollicular changes (a) Perifollicular depigmentation (b) Perifollicular pigment retention (c) Perifollicular repigmentation	Loss of pigment network around at least 25% the hair follicles within the lesion Retention of perifollicular pigment network in at least 25% of the hair follicles when there is loss of pigment network in the rest of the patch It refers to the reappearance of pigment network around hair follicles, which previously had a complete loss of pigment network in at least 25% of the hair follicles
Pigment network changes (a) Reduced pigment network (a) Absent pigment network	Diminished pigment network in interfollicular area No pigment network in interfollicular areas
Leukotrichia	Presence of depigmented hair in at least 25% of total hair follicles
Micro-Koebner phenomenon	Linearly arranged areas of depigmentation, which are not easily perceived by naked eye examination
Satellite lesions	White structureless areas of size >1 mm in diameter in the perilesional skin, which may or may not be apparent on clinical examination

Adopted from Gupta et al. [6]

micro-Koebner's phenomenon as markers of active vitiligo. Perifollicular pigmentation and perilesional hyperpigmentation were found as markers of repigmenting vitiligo.

In our opinion, the gold standard method to determine the activity of a vitiligo patch is serial clinical and photographic monitoring of the vitiligo patch. However, dermoscopic assessment helps in assessing disease activity and can be handy in a busy practice (Table 8.2). One novel method of imaging inspired from Mohs' micrographic surgery can be useful especially for the imaging of smaller lesions [14]. Dermoscopy can also be used in combination with other clinical, biochemical and physiological markers to better assess disease activity [15].

Table 8.2 Summary of dermoscopic features of active and stable vitiligo

Active vitiligo	Stable/repigmenting vitiligo	Features not specific to disease activity
Perifollicular depigmentation	Perifollicular repigmentation	Perifollicular pigment retention
Pigment network changes		Leukotrichia
Ill-defined border		Trichrome vitiligo
Satellite lesions and micro-koebnerization		

8.2.2 *Newer Methods*

Another technique namely ultraviolet (UV) dermoscopy has also been used for assessment of vitiligo. Compared to conventional dermoscopy, UV dermoscopy incorporates wavelengths of 360–390 nm which produce different fluorescence of skin lesions. In vitiligo, absent melanin leading to non-absorption of UV light produces bright blue-white patches. The UV dermoscopic features are similar to those seen by conventional dermoscopy [12]. Advantages over the standard technique include better visualization of border and perifollicular changes, enhancement of pigmented and depigmented junctional zone (Fig. 8.6).

A modification of conventional dermoscopy is blue light dermoscopy. Its use is based on the principle that UV light is most absorbed by melanin in the spectrum. The blue light being closest to the UV spectrum helps in better demarcation of depigmented and normally pigmented skin. Unstable vitiligo lesion will show hypopigmented ill-defined margins on blue light dermoscopy [16]. Limitations of the technique include difficulty in capturing images and auto-focusing [12, 16, 17].

8.3 Reflectance Confocal Microscopy

RCM is a noninvasive tool based on repetitive imaging providing real-time images of almost cellular resolution. The principle of RCM is that the melanin appears refractile. In active vitiligo, RCM demonstrated complete loss of melanin in lesional skin characterized by the loss or disruption of architecture of bright dermal papillary rings normally seen at dermo-epidermal junctions. In addition, highly refractile inflammatory cells are seen within papillary dermis in lesional as well as adjacent normally appearing skin. Partial loss of rings and ill-defined margins can also be seen in adjacent normally appearing skin [18]. In stable phase, RCM demonstrates complete loss of melanin in lesional skin and clear border. The content of melanin and dermal papillary rings in adjacent normally appearing skin show no changes. Repigmenting vitiligo shows dendritic and highly refractile melanocytes. The diagnosis of vitiligo by RCM is reliable and found to be consistent with histopathological diagnosis [19].

Studies have been done to correlate dermoscopic features with those of RCM [20]. A recent study used a combination of RCM and dermoscopy in assessment of disease activity in vitiligo, which was compared to assessment by RCM and dermoscopy alone. The combination approach showed higher sensitivity and specificity [21]. Dermoscopic features with a good treatment response in repigmenting vitiligo were telangiectasia, increased lesional pigment, and perifollicular pigmentation, while leukotrichia, absent pigment network, and perilesional hyperpigmentation were associated with poor treatment response. Under RCM, the presence of increased pigment granules and dendritic melanocytes and incompletely disappearing pigment rings were associated with good treatment response.

8.4 Wood's Lamp

Before the widespread use of the dermoscope, Wood's lamp examination was the most common noninvasive method for evaluation of vitiligo lesions. However, with widespread availability of the dermoscope, newer dermoscopes with inbuilt UV light, and difficulty in establishing a dark room, UV dermoscopic assessment is preferred over Wood's lamp.

The Wood's lamp principle involves projection of 365 nm wavelength UV light on the lesion which causes fluorescence of underlying collagen in the absence of melanin in vitiligo, appearing as a blue-white area. It helps in better demarcation of depigmented and normally pigmented skin (Fig. 8.7). Sharply demarcated borders are features of stable vitiligo while the presence of hypochromic islands is considered to be a feature of repigmenting vitiligo [22]. However, whether such hypochromic islands can also be seen in incompletely depigmented progressive vitiligo still remains a question to be answered. There have been attempts to classify vitiligo lesions on the basis of Wood's lamp findings [23].

Recently, Wood's lamp has been used in combination with reflectance confocal microscopy. Lesions are categorized as grade 1: stable stage, grade 2: slowly progressive stage and grade 3: rapidly progressive lesions. Porcelain white with clear borders were seen in grade 1, off-white color with clear border in grade 2 and trichromatic, confetti-like lesions, hypopigmented with blurred margins or inflammatory sign were seen in grade 3. RCM findings include melanocytes and lymphocytes at lesion border in rapidly progressive lesions, lymphocytic infiltration at the border or some phagocytic melanocytes outside the border in slowly progressive lesions and comparatively fewer inflammatory cells in stable or repigmenting vitiligo [24].

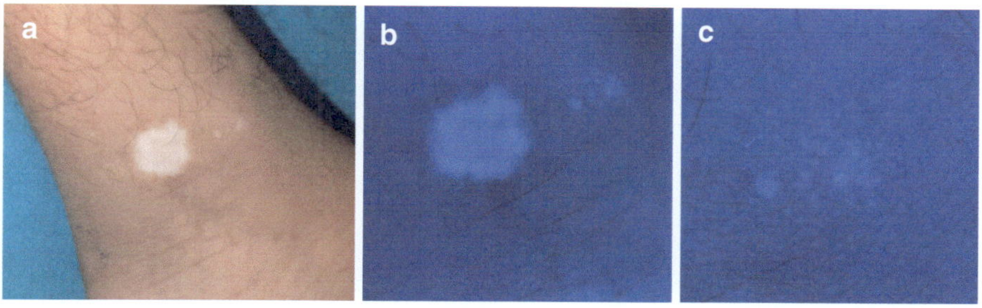

Fig. 8.7 (**a**) Clinical image of the left ankle of the patient showing a large depigmented patch and a few small grouped satellite lesions. (**b**) Wood's lamp examination of the lesion showing better demarcation of the border as well as the hyperpigmented margins. (**c**) Similarly, the smaller satellite macules appear to be better appreciated under Wood's lamp

A novel alternative method to Wood's lamp is generating a blue screen background on a smartphone. However, it is not UV light but rather short-wavelength visible light. It is useful in resource-poor settings. 365 nm Wood's lamp is also recommended to eliminate the blue appearance of normal structures under standard broadband Wood's lamp [25].

8.5 Visible Light and Digital Photography

This method includes obtaining images using a digital camera. It is a semi-objective measurement of the extent of vitiligo. Serial imaging of vitiligo lesions is helpful in assessing disease activity as well as treatment response. However, it is not devoid of bias especially the method of imaging as the camera, background, exposure, distance, and angle should be uniform for every visit. The use of this technique in patients with innumerable lesions is doubtful where assessment might be difficult. However, it requires a lot of expertise in the technical part and is not devoid of limitations. Computer-aided imaging analysis is helpful for comprehensive quantification [26]. However, the method is expensive and requires extensive training for diagnostic interpretations. Additionally, the method lacks standardization. Various other types of imaging include infrared photography and ultraviolet photography. Some applications like vitiligo extent score (VES) or VES plus are used to measure the extent of vitiligo (severity) and utilize computers for image analysis.

8.6 Artificial Intelligence

Artificial intelligence (AI) assisted diagnostic tools can contribute to the accurate diagnosis of vitiligo. Examples include ResNet and Swin transformer deep learning models [27]. The major attention of AI-assisted diagnostic tools is to achieve a more accurate classification of medical images. However, lack of interpretability undermines the reliability of deep learning methods, thus limiting their use in clinical practice. The major advantage of AI-assisted tools is that even non-dermatologist physicians or laypersons can use them for the classification of skin lesions. AI is also used in image-processing applications.

8.7 Spectrophotometry

It involves exposing the epidermal surface to white light. Backscattered photos are then detected from various layers of skin tissue. Thus, melanin index, relative melanin indexes are estimated which are statistically low in vitiligo patches as compared to normal skin [26].

8.8 Reflectance Colorimetry

It is a noninvasive instrument used to quantify the skin color and thus assess progression and response to treatment. It measures luminance value and melanin index. This method can assess repigmentation around a month before it is clinically apparent. It is less time-intensive and more standardized [26].

8.9 Third-Harmonic Generation Microscopy

Third-harmonic generation (THG) microscopy operates on the principle that discontinuities at material surfaces generate a new wave in the forward direction at the third harmonic. This wave is detected by a pixel detector and camera. Like other nonlinear optical techniques, THG microscopy offers excellent 3D sectioning capabilities. Since all materials possess nonvanishing third-order susceptibilities, THG microscopy can be used as a versatile imaging technique without requiring fluorescence labeling or staining. It can produce high-resolution, real-time images, although the method is not yet standardized. However, its application is limited by a lack of specificity and availability. [28, 29]

8.10 Multiphoton Microscopy

Multiphoton microscopy is a noninvasive technique that utilizes laser-induced excitation of low-energy photons to achieve high-resolution imaging of melanocyte distribution and density. It offers deeper tissue penetration and enables real-time imaging. However, the field of view is limited, and the method has yet to be standardized [30].

8.11 Optical Coherence Tomography.

It detects infrared ray reflections to generate high-resolution images of the target tissue. This quick method offers real-time, wide-field imaging. However, its application is limited by a steep learning curve and restricted availability due to high costs. [31]

8.12 Others

8.12.1 Digital Planimetry

Digital photography with planimetry, also known as image digitization, is an imaging modality wherein each pixel of the image is sampled and quantified in terms of brightness, which is stored in a computer's bitmap image [32].

8.12.2 Point Counting of Digital Images

It is a simple and accurate method of assessment of surface area of polygonal lesions where the lesion is projected over a transparent paper with points (+) on it. The number of intersections is counted and then multiplied by the representative area of the grid to estimate the total area of the lesions [32].

The key uses, advantages, and disadvantages of commonly used methods have been summarized in Table 8.3.

Table 8.3 Key features of commonly used noninvasive methods of evaluation for vitiligo

Method	Uses	Advantages	Disadvantages	Comments
Dermoscopy	Confirmation of diagnosis Assessment of disease activity Monitoring of treatment response	Hand-held and portable with chargeable battery Image capturing Extensive literature	Slow learning curve High cost Standardization of terms is lacking	Most common method used currently UV dermoscopy or blue light dermoscopy newer advancements
Reflectance confocal microscopy	Confirmation of diagnosis Assessment of disease activity and treatment response	Real time imaging Almost equivalent to histopathological examination	Learning curve slow requiring lot of expertise Costly set up Limited availability	Combination with dermoscopy or Wood's lamp has better sensitivity and specificity
Wood's lamp	Confirmation of diagnosis Assessment of disease activity	Low cost Easy availability	Capturing image is difficult Limited features can be demonstrated as compared to dermoscopy	Blue light background on smartphone in resource poor settings
Visible light and digital photography	Disease activity	Serial imaging—gold standard for assessing disease activity	Subjectivity adds to the bias Requires lot of expertise Difficult to do and follow when multiple lesions are present Lacks standardization	Computer-aided imaging analysis for comprehensive quantification
Artificial intelligence	Diagnosis Disease activity Treatment response	Accurate diagnosis and assessment Minimal expertise is required	Very costly Limited literature is available Not validated	Indispensable in coming future

8.13 Conclusion

Although the diagnosis of vitiligo is clinical with diagnostic confusion arising rarely, the different methods of assessing vitiligo aid not only in diagnosis but also in the assessment of disease activity and treatment response. The above-discussed, noninvasive methods can be used alone or in combination for assessing vitiligo. Though, characteristic findings have been discussed, their validation may require further studies or head-to-head comparison of different methods.

Clinical Pearls

1. Dermoscopy is the most common noninvasive method used for assessing vitiligo and it can potentially be useful in assessing disease activity or treatment response. The dermoscopic features of stable vitiligo are perifollicular repigmentation and unstable vitiligo are pigment network changes, perifollicular depigmentation, satellite lesions, and micro-koebnerization and ill-defined margins.
2. RCM has recently emerged as a method with studies showing better correlation with histopathological findings. In active vitiligo, RCM demonstrated complete loss of melanin in lesional skin characterized by the loss or disruption of architecture of bright dermal papillary rings normally seen at dermo-epidermal junction. In the stable phase, RCM demonstrates a complete loss of melanin in lesional skin and clear borders. Repigmenting vitiligo shows dendritic and highly refractile melanocytes.
3. Wood's lamp evaluation may be a useful method especially in combination with RCM.
4. Artificial intelligence is an evolving tool for the assessment of digital images.

Acknowledgments We thank the patient for granting permission for clinical photography.

Conflict of Interest None.

Funding Source None.

References

1. Chuh AAT, Zawar V. Demonstration of residual perifollicular pigmentation in localized vitiligo–a reverse and novel application of digital epiluminescence dermoscopy. Comput Med Imaging Graph. 2004;28(4):213–7.
2. Thatte S, Khopkar U. The utility of dermoscopy in the diagnosis of evolving lesions of vitiligo. Indian J Dermatol Venereol Leprol. 2014;80(6):505–8.
3. Kumar Jha A, Sonthalia S, Lallas A, Chaudhary RKP. Dermoscopy in vitiligo: diagnosis and beyond. Int J Dermatol. 2018;57(1):50–4.
4. Jha AK, Sonthalia S, Lallas A. Dermoscopy as an evolving tool to assess vitiligo activity. J Am Acad Dermatol. 2018;78(5):1017–9.
5. Nirmal B, Antonisamy B, Dincy Peter CV, George L, George AA, Dinesh GM. Cross-sectional study of dermatoscopic findings in relation to activity in vitiligo: BPLeFoSK criteria for stability. J Cutan Aesthet Surg. 2019;12(1):36–41.
6. Gupta P, Vinay K, Bishnoi A, Kumaran MS, Parsad D. A prospective observational study to sequentially determine the dermoscopic features of vitiligo and its association with disease activity in patients on medical treatment: dermoscopy and disease activity in vitiligo. Pigment Cell Melanoma Res. 2023;36(1):33–41.
7. Kamath C, Dhurat R, Shah B, Sharma R, Kowe PA, Chamle S. Monitoring of vitiligo patches over six months to validate dermoscopic findings of lesional stability. Dermatol Pract Concept. 2023;13(4):e2023277.
8. Ru-Song M, Guang Z, RuiKang C, Xiao M, Zhiguo J. Application of polarized light dermoscopy in the early diagnosis of vitiligo and its differential diagnosis from other depigmented diseases. Chin J Dermatol. 2009;42(12):810–3.

9. Wang LM, Lu WJ, Yuan JT, Zeng BB, Li D, Zhang F, et al. Utility of dermoscopy for evaluating the therapeutic efficacy of tacrolimus ointment plus 308-nm excimer laser combination therapy in localized vitiligo patients. Exp Ther Med. 2018;15(4):3981–8.
10. Errichetti E, Zelin E, Pinzani C, Kyrgidis A, Lallas A, Stinco G. Dermoscopic and clinical response predictor factors in nonsegmental vitiligo treated with narrowband ultraviolet B phototherapy: a prospective observational study. Dermatol Ther (Heidelb). 2020;10(5):1089–98.
11. Dev A, Vinay K, Bishnoi A, Kumaran MS, Dogra S, Parsad D. Dermatoscopic assessment of treatment response in patients undergoing autologous non-cultured epidermal cell suspension for the treatment of stable vitiligo: a prospective study. Dermatol Ther. 2021;34(5):e15099.
12. Yuan M, Xie Y, Zheng Y, Zhang Z, Yang C, Li J. Novel ultraviolet-dermoscopy: early diagnosis and activity evaluation of vitiligo. Skin Res Technol. 2023;29(1):e13249.
13. Delbaere L, van Causenbroeck J, Duponselle J, Van Goethem C, Speeckaert R, van Geel N. Hot spots for clinical signs of disease activity in vitiligo. Exp Dermatol. 2024;33(1):e14975.
14. Gupta P, Dev A, Vinay K, Bishnoi A, Kumaran MS, Parsad D. Validating a novel technique of dermatoscopic imaging or sequential comparison of target lesions in vitiligo. Dermatol Pract Concept. 2024;14(1):e2024003.
15. Yang Y, Morriss S, Rodrigues M. Dermoscopy in vitiligo, diagnostic clues and markers of disease activity: a review of the literature. Clin Exp Dermatol. 2024;49:969.
16. Nirmal B. Utility of blue light in dermoscopy for diagnosing stable lesions in vitiligo. Dermatol Pract Concept. 2021;11(1):e2021141.
17. Böhm M, Schunter JA, Fritz K, Salavastru C, Dargatz S, Augustin M, et al. S1 guideline: diagnosis and therapy of vitiligo. J Dtsch Dermatol Ges. 2022;20(3):365–78.
18. Lai LG, Xu AE. In vivo reflectance confocal microscopy imaging of vitiligo, nevus depigmentosus and nevus anemicus. Skin Res Technol. 2011;17(4):404–10.
19. van Geel N, Grine L, De Wispelaere P, Mertens D, Prinsen CAC, Speeckaert R. Clinical visible signs of disease activity in vitiligo: a systematic review and meta-analysis. J Eur Acad Dermatol Venereol. 2019;33(9):1667–75.
20. Godínez-Chaparro JA, Roldán-Marín R, Soto-Mota A, Calzada-Mendoza CC. Dermatoscopic patterns in childhood vitiligo and their association with reflectance confocal microscopy findings. Dermatol Pract Concept. 2023;13(4):e2023306.
21. Wang HF, Zhai ZF, Wang CY, Zhou XF, Deng XF, Huang H, et al. A new assessment method of vitiligo by combination of dermoscopy and reflectance confocal microscopy. Clin Cosmet Investig Dermatol. 2023;16(12):3615.
22. Wang YJ, Chang CC, Cheng KL. Wood's lamp for vitiligo disease stability and early recognition of initiative pigmentation after epidermal grafting. Int Wound J. 2017;14(6):1391.
23. Kimura Y, Tanemura A, Kurosaki Y, Takafuji M, Yokoi K, Kiyohara E, et al. Clinical observation and proposed classification of Vitiliginous patches by a wood's lamp. J Cosmet Dermatol Sci Appl. 2020;10(4):204–11.
24. Hou Y, Wei Z, Jiang Q, Chen H, Chen L, Wu J. In-depth study of Wood's lamp examination combined with reflective confocal laser scanning microscopy for the guidance of vitiligo staging and treatment. J Cosmet Dermatol. 2024;23(4):1472–9.
25. Bae JM, Lee RW. 365-nm narrowband wood's lamp for vitiligo and hypopigmentation disorders. J Am Acad Dermatol. 2020;83(4):e283–4.
26. Abdi P, Anthony MR, Farkouh C, Chan AR, Kooner A, Qureshi S, et al. Non-invasive skin measurement methods and diagnostics for vitiligo: a systematic review. Front Med (Lausanne). 2023;10(7):1200963.
27. Zhong F, He K, Ji M, Chen J, Gao T, Li S, et al. Optimizing vitiligo diagnosis with ResNet and Swin transformer deep learning models: a study on performance and interpretability. Sci Rep. 2024;14(1):1–15.
28. Liao Y-H, , Shih Y-T, Chen W-S, Jee S-H, Sun C-K. In vivo third-harmonic generation microscopy study on vitiligo patients. J Biomed Opt 2019;25(1):014504.
29. Lévêque-Fort S, Georges P. Microscopy | nonlinear microscopy. In: Encyclopedia of modern optics, Five-Volume set; 2005. p. 92–103.

30. Vicente JR, Durkin A, Shrestha K, Balu M. In vivo imaging with a fast large-area multiphoton exoscope (FLAME) captures the melanin distribution heterogeneity in human skin. Sci Rep. 2022;12(1):1–10.
31. Zavattaro E, Kaliyadan F, Ruggiero A, Abdi P. Non-invasive skin measurement methods and diagnostics for vitiligo: a systematic review. Front Med (Lausanne). 2023;10(7):1200963.
32. Aydin F, Senturk N, Sahin B, Bek Y, Yuksel EP, Turanli AY. A practical method for the estimation of vitiligo surface area: a comparison between the point counting and digital planimetry techniques. Eur J Dermatol. 2007;17(1):30–2.

Chapter 9
Stability, Quality of Life, and Outcome Measures in Vitiligo

Apoorva Sharma, K. B. Meghana, and Muthu Sendhil Kumaran

Abstract Vitiligo is the most common acquired pigmentary disorder encountered in dermatology clinics. It affects individuals across all ages and genders, with a particularly profound effect on those with darker skin tones. It can significantly reduce quality of life, often resulting in psychological challenges such as mental health issues and social withdrawal. The treatment is challenging due to the unpredictable course of the disease. It is therefore important to monitor the activity for appropriate treatment and to measure outcomes that matter to patients and doctors. The chapter summarizes the concept of stability and its importance in treatment and various tools to assess the outcome and quality of life in these patients.

Keywords Stability · Repigmentation · Vitiligo surgery · Quality of life

9.1 Introduction

Vitiligo has a significant effect on the social and psychological aspects of life especially in patients with skin of color like the Indian population. It is important to assess the disease activity and quality of life in all patients to tailor appropriate treatment on an individual basis. Stability of the disease is defined when there are no new lesions and there is no increase in size of preexisting lesions and is important to choose appropriate treatment. There are various disease-specific tools to assess the outcome and quality of life in vitiligo.

A. Sharma · K. B. Meghana · M. S. Kumaran (✉)
Department of Dermatology, Venereology and Leprology, Postgraduate Institute of Medical Education and Research (PGIMER), Chandigarh, India

R. Sarkar, V. Narayan R (eds.), *A Concise Guide to The Management of Vitiligo*,
https://doi.org/10.1007/978-981-95-3857-7_9

9.2 Stability

The course of vitiligo disease is often prolonged and has an uncertain prognosis. Although in most patients the disease activity ceases after a certain period of time on initiating treatment, most continue to experience a prolonged course of disease activity despite aggressive treatment.

9.3 Definition of Stability

There are no standard criteria available to define stability of vitiligo; the duration of stability is important in making decisions regarding surgical intervention. As per consensus recommendations by the IADVL Dermatosurgery Task Force, stability is defined as "a patient reporting no new lesions, no progression of existing lesions, and absence of Koebner phenomenon during past one year." [1] Surgery is indicated only when there is no improvement with medical treatment and the patient meets the above criteria.

9.4 Importance of Disease Stability

Stability of the vitiligo is the most important factor in patient selection for vitiligo transplant surgery. Surgery is indicated in almost all cases of non-segmental, segmental and acro-facial vitiligo when the disease becomes stable as 100% repigmentation might not be achieved with medical management alone. Also the outcome of the surgery is better in patients with stable disease compared to those with unstable vitiligo [1]. Stability is also important in prognostication of vitiligo. Once it becomes stable, the aim of further treatment should be complete repigmentation of left over depigmented lesions. In vitiligo, it is common for a patient to experience depigmentation in certain areas while repigmentation occurs in most. It has been observed that after grafting procedures, the recipient site might depigment while the donor site shows repigmentation or vice versa; these suggest that disease stability in vitiligo may not always be uniform across a given patient, but vary from lesion to lesion. Hence a few researchers take lesional stability rather than global whole-body stability for deciding on vitiligo surgery. Hence as of now, the criteria for stability is debatable, but going as per given vitiligo task force recommendations global stability for 1 year or more still stands more preferable. For a given vitiligo patient to undergo surgery, lesional stability of >1 year even with global stability of 6–12 months is considered optimal [2]. It is especially important in patients with resistant lesions and great social concerns where delay in the treatment can be avoided.

9.5 Stability in Segmental Versus Non-segmental Vitiligo

In segmental vitiligo, disease remains active usually for a duration of 6 months to 2 years and becomes stable thereafter, even without intervention [3]. In non-segmental vitiligo, the duration of stability is not always predictable and it can reactivate even after a prolonged period of stabilization [4]. Hence a longer duration of monitoring is required among non-segmental vitiligo patients. Also, these patients require treatment with immunosuppressants often for a longer time compared to segmental vitiligo to attain disease stability.

9.6 Clinical Markers of Stability

There are many clinical signs that predict the activity of vitiligo. The commonest clinical predictors are as follows:

(i) No history of new lesions in at least the past 1 year and being off any immunosuppressive treatment in past 1 year
(ii) No increase in size or extension of preexisting lesions
(iii) The absence of Koebner phenomenon
(iv) Vitiligo disease activity score (VIDA)
(v) Test grafting

Koebner phenomenon, defined as "the development of vitiligo at sites of traumatized skin," indicates active disease. Njoo et al. have further classified the Koebner phenomenon into two categories: "Koebner phenomenon by history (KP-h)" and "experimentally induced Koebner phenomenon (KP-e)." The Koebner phenomenon experimental (KP-e) was evaluated by inducing a small injury to clinically unaffected skin using a 2-mm punch biopsy. Three months post-procedure, the biopsy site and surrounding area were examined for signs of depigmentation, indicating a positive KP-e result. Notably, a clear distinction between KP-h (historical Koebner) and KP-e was observed, with KP-h demonstrating positive and negative predictive values of 89% and 52%, respectively, when KP-e was considered the gold standard [5].

The VIDA score was introduced by Njoo et al. to assess the activity level of vitiligo in patients who had not received any therapies for at least 6 months. This scoring system rates disease activity from +4 to −1, representing a gradual decline in activity levels. Patients with a score of 0 were classified as having stable disease for 1 year, while those with a score of −1 also experienced spontaneous repigmentation [5].

Falabella et al. introduced this test to identify suitable candidates for surgical intervention in vitiligo. It involves placing a small number of grafts (1–2 mm) in the center of depigmented lesions, followed by dressing with micropore for a few weeks with subsequent exposure to sunlight for 1 mins daily for 3 months. The test is considered positive if clear repigmentation occurs beyond 1 mm from the edge of the implant under Wood's light examination [6]. However, with further studies there might be a better way to assess disease stability based on serological markers and ultrastructural studies.

9.7 Biochemical Markers for Stability

Though the pathogenesis of vitiligo is attributed mainly to auto-immunity, its pathogenesis is still complex with interplay between immune system and cytokines. Serological or tissue biomarkers can help in early diagnosis of the disease or to determine the activity of the disease when clinical signs are inconclusive. These markers also help in studies for research purpose and designing more targeted therapies. In active vitiligo, there is an increase in the number of CD3, CD4, and CD8 cells in lesional, marginal, and non-lesional skin [7]. The concentration of CXCL9 in suction blister fluid from the active borders of vitiligo lesions serves as a highly accurate biomarker for active disease, with a sensitivity of 100% and specificity of 93% [8]. Studies have confirmed elevated CXCL9 levels in vitiligo skin using immunohistochemistry, correlating with the disease activity. Similarly, non-lesional skin in patients with active vitiligo has increased CXCL10 mRNA levels compared to those with stable disease. "Nucleotide-binding domain and leucine rich repeat containing family, pyrin domain containing protein 1" (NLRP1) and hsp70 are other markers found to be elevated in active vitiligo lesions [9, 10].

There is a decrease in circulating levels of the CD4/CD8 ratio in vitiligo patients compared to controls [11]. T-regulatory cells (Tregs) have decreased functioning in active vitiligo i.e., they produce lower levels of TGF-β1 compared to those with stable vitiligo [12]. Also the serum levels of CXCL12, a CXCR4 ligand, were found to be higher compared to controls in a study. The highest levels of CXCL12 were observed in patients who had experienced disease progression in recent months [13]. IL-17 has consistently demonstrated higher levels in vitiligo patients compared to healthy controls, with an association to the extent of the affected body surface area. However, the association between IL-17 levels and disease activity is less consistent in the studies [14]. Interferon-gamma (IFN-γ) and interleukin-1 beta (IL-1β) are two main cytokines that have been implicated in the pathogenesis of vitiligo. A large study found that serum IFN-γ levels were higher in vitiligo patients than in controls and were elevated in active vitiligo compared to stable cases. IL-1β consistently showed elevated levels in vitiligo patients and a correlation with disease activity [15, 16]. The sensitivity and specificity of these markers are yet to be explored. Promising results have been shown by CXCL9 levels in blister fluid from the active border of the lesion. Serological biomarkers are easy to perform while tissue biomarkers are invasive and repeated biopsies are cumbersome.

9.8 Quality of Life

Vitiligo impacts profoundly on quality of life, leading to psychological distress, social stigma, and isolation. Studies have shown that vitiligo can negatively affect self-esteem, body image, and interpersonal relationships. Patients with vitiligo often experience anxiety, depression, and embarrassment due to societal perceptions of beauty. The severity of social impact may vary depending on the individual's occupation, like people working in sectors like sales, media etc. where the interaction with other people is more often experience a greater distress. In India and possibly other regions, individuals of all genders and ages who have vitiligo encounter significant psychological and social challenges. This issue is particularly pronounced among young women and children [17].

The chronicity of the disease, the need for long-term treatment, the absence of consistently effective therapies, and the unpredictable progression of vitiligo can be profoundly demoralizing for patients. Dermatology Life Quality Index (DLQI) is a non-specific, validated, and widely used questionnaire in dermatology for various skin disorders. It takes into account the patient's daily activity, feelings, personal relationships, and treatment. The tool employs a 4-point rating scale for each item, scoring from 0 to 3, resulting in a cumulative score between 0 and 30. Higher total scores correspond to greater impairment in quality of life [18]. The Children's Dermatology Life Quality Index (CDLQI) by Lewis-Jones and Finlay aimed to create a simple, practical questionnaire to assess the impact of skin diseases on the quality of life in children aged 3–16 years. The questionnaire covers the symptoms, emotions, social life, school impact, sleep disturbance, and treatment effects [19]. The quality of life is more impaired in older children, as when the child grows and is exposed to the stigma by the society. There are several disease-specific questionnaires available to assess quality of life. Three important scores relevant to vitiligo in the Indian context are the Vitiligo Quality of Life (VitiQoL), Vitiligo Impact Scale-22 (VIS-22), and Family Vitiligo Impact Scale.

(i) *Vitiligo Quality of Life Index (VitiQoL)*

The VitiQoL questionnaire is a standard tool developed to measure how vitiligo affects a person's quality of life. Consisting of 16 questions, it explores different facets of the condition's impact, including emotional well-being, social experiences, self-image, and the influence on everyday life. Clinicians use this instrument to pinpoint which aspects of living with vitiligo matter most to each patient, enabling them to tailor care accordingly. VitiQoL provides information about both recent and ongoing quality-of-life issues, as it includes the last 4 weeks. As a validated and reliable measure, it is widely recognized for both research and clinical assessment. Its easy design makes VitiQoL easy to implement in routine care and in clinical studies, helping standardize the way the burden of vitiligo is evaluated [20].

(ii) *Vitiligo Impact Scale-22 (VIS-22)*

The Vitiligo Impact Scale (VIS) was developed to address the unique issues faced by vitiligo patients. Originally, the final version of the VIS included 27 items. This questionnaire was designed to assess the impact of vitiligo on various aspects of a patient's life, with 21 items relevant to all participants. An additional five items were tailored specifically for married individuals, and one item was designed for those who were not married, creating some variation in the total number of items considered for each participant. The revised version, known as the VIS-22, consists of 22 items that cover a broad range of topics related to the experience of living with vitiligo. The VIS-22 covers a broad range of topics including feelings of depression, social interactions, anxiety levels, perceptions about the condition, considerations related to treatment, confidence, education, work life, and family relationships. Each question is rated on a scale from 0 to 3, where 0 means "not at all" and 3 represents "very much." The overall score from the VIS-22 ranges from 0 to 66, with higher scores indicating a greater impact of vitiligo on the individual's quality of life. This scale helps to quantify the psychological and social effects of the condition, providing valuable insights for healthcare providers and researchers to better understand and address the needs of patients with vitiligo [21]. It is a validated tool for Indian patients and sensitive to minimum changes. Its generalizability to other populations is limited as of now.

(iii) *Vitiligo Impact Patient Scale (VIPs)*

The Vitiligo Impact Patient Scale (VIPs) is a quality-of-life assessment tool created to capture the wide-ranging effects of vitiligo on emotional well-being and daily function. The instrument includes 29 questions: 19 of these apply to everyone, while 3 are specifically for lighter skin tones and another 7 for those with darker skin. The total score reflects the degree of impact, with possible scores running from 0 to 110 for individuals with fair skin and from 0 to 130 for those with dark skin. Higher scores indicate a greater burden from the disease. The VIPs has undergone validation, demonstrating strong internal consistency and reliability. It also addresses experiences such as social difficulties, mood changes, anxiety, and symptoms of depression. Evaluating these psychological and social domains is essential in understanding how vitiligo shapes patient well-being [22].

(iv) *Family Vitiligo Impact Scale*

The Family Vitiligo Impact Scale serves as a valuable tool in evaluating the familial impact of the disease, allowing healthcare providers to better understand the challenges faced by patients and their families. By assessing various dimensions of the patient's life, including the emotional and social repercussions of vitiligo, this scale provides insights into how the condition affects family dynamics and relationships. It also helps family members identify areas where they may need additional support or resources to improve their coping mechanisms. Family members can gain a clearer understanding of the specific challenges associated with vitiligo, enabling them to develop more effective strategies for managing the emotional and psychological impacts of the disease. [23]

9.9 Outcome Measures

Due to different outcome measures reported across various trials and studies the interpretation of results with treatment becomes challenging. The Vitiligo European Task Force (VETF) and other international groups collaborated to establish a consensus on essential domains for vitiligo clinical trials using a web-based Delphi process. They addressed the question of "what to measure" and achieved agreement on core domains crucial for such trials. Three outcome domains/domain items were identified as "essential" for measurement in all vitiligo trials: "repigmentation, maintenance of repigmentation, and side effects." Additionally, four other outcomes were deemed "recommended" for measurement, where relevant and applicable in vitiligo trials: "cosmetic acceptability of the results, cessation of spreading, tolerability or burden of treatment, and quality of life." [24]

9.10 Clinician-Reported Outcome Measures for Extent and Repigmentation

The most accepted clinical outcome by physicians is the reduction in the extent of depigmentation observed between two points, usually calculated as the degree or percentage of repigmentation.

1. *Vitiligo Area Scoring Index (VASI)*

Introduced in 2004, the VASI was tailored for assessing repigmentation in vitiligo trials, similar to the Psoriasis Area Severity Index (PASI). Today, VASI stands as the most widely used tool in scientific literature and clinical trials for evaluating vitiligo, particularly in terms of repigmentation and treatment efficacy. It quantifies depigmentation extent across five body regions, each represented by hand units, with values ranging from 0 to 100%. The original article has templates of different levels of residual depigmentation that simulate the actual vitiligo lesions with varied levels of depigmentation. It is an easy score to calculate and does not require any expensive tools but it is subjective in nature [25].

$$\text{VASI} = \text{``All body sites} \sum [\text{hand units}] \times [\text{residual depigmentation}]\text{''}$$

2. *Facial Vitiligo Area Scoring Index (F-VASI)*

Facial vitiligo is known to have a particularly negative effect on a person's quality of life, making precise measurement of facial depigmentation essential in clinical care and research. To specifically quantify facial involvement, the Facial Vitiligo Area Scoring Index (F-VASI) was introduced and validated in 2022. This tool builds upon the established VASI score but adapts it for facial lesions using fingertip units (FTUs) instead of hand units. An FTU is defined as the area from one crease to the next on the finger, covering the distal phalanx. For each facial vitiligo lesion, the total number of FTUs involved is counted, with the full face comprising up to 112 FTUs. Each FTU represents approximately 0.9% of total facial skin and only 0.03% of overall body surface area. The F-VASI score is then calculated by multiplying the number of FTUs affected by the degree of depigmentation for each spot, ranging from no pigment loss to complete depigmentation. This approach is also useful for measuring dispersed small lesions, such as those found on the face or genitals. However, its accuracy can vary in children and individuals with higher body mass, where the representation of FTU may not consistently reflect actual skin area [26].

3. *Vitiligo Extent Score (VES)*

The Vitiligo Extent Score (VES) is a clinical tool developed to monitor changes in vitiligo by assessing area affected, disease activity, and extent of repigmentation over time through repeated body surface area estimations. VES is well-suited for both routine care and research trials. The assessment uses standardized photographs for 19 separate anatomical regions, with each region displayed across six possible levels of depigmentation severity—ranging from 0 (no skin involved) to 6 (up to 75% or more area affected). This approach enables clinicians to quantify even subtle differences in pigment loss consistently over multiple visits, improving reliability in measuring disease progression or treatment response [27]. To improve the assessment of treatment results, especially regarding perifollicular repigmentation that often occurs with UVB therapy, a perifollicular evaluation component was added to the standard VES. This adjustment led to the creation of VESplus, which offers enhanced specificity for tracking the perifollicular response pattern commonly seen in treated vitiligo lesions [28]. Though it is user-friendly and quick to perform, it is still subjective in nature and does not include photos of segmental vitiligo lesions.

4. *Vitiligo Extent Score for a Target Area (VESTA)*

VESTA is designed to objectively measure how much a target vitiligo lesion has improved in terms of repigmentation. The assessment utilizes separate scoring for marginal repigmentation and perifollicular repigmentation, referencing photographic guides that illustrate a spectrum of changes for each feature. There are 12 defined categories for marginal and perifollicular regrowth, representing nearly the entire range from no repigmentation up to almost full restoration. By combining the scores for both aspects, clinicians can determine an overall repigmentation percentage for a single lesion. Importantly, the VESTA score is limited to zones where baseline photographs are available and cannot be used to measure the overall extent of vitiligo on the body [29].

9.11 Clinician-Reported Outcome Measures for Activity

- *Vitiligo Signs of Activity Score (VSAS)*

The VSAS is a standardized scoring tool to assess three clinical signs of vitiligo activity: the presence of the Koebner phenomenon, confetti-like spots, and hypochromic borders. If any of these signs are identified on examination, it indicates ongoing disease activity, which often prompts intensifying therapy. The majority of the sites are based on the classical anatomic units, of the Vitiligo Extent Score (VES). In a given location, the presence of any one of the three indications is coded 1, and the absence of any of the three signs results in a score ranging from 0 to 15. Every body part affects the overall score in the same way [30].

- *Vitiligo Disease Activity Score (VDAS) and Vitiligo Disease Improvement Score (VDIS)*

VDAS and VDIS offer evaluation of vitiligo progression and improvement. These tools are valuable for tracking changes in vitiligo over time, through evaluations spaced about 6 months apart, which makes them particularly useful in everyday patient management. It is important to separately document both worsening and improvement using distinct instruments, as both processes can happen at the same time in different areas or even within the same area in a single patient. These tools, assessed every 6 months across 15 anatomical regions like VSAS, provide clinicians with insights into deterioration or repigmentation. The detailed version includes VDIS60 and VDAS60, measuring improvement or worsening degree on a 3-4-point scale for each body part, with scores ranging from 0 to 60 [31].

- *Vitiligo European Task Force assessment Tool (VETFa)*

The VETFa integrates three factors: extent of skin affected, stage, and disease activity. It estimates surface area involvement using both the hand unit method, where a patient's palm equates to 1% of total body surface and the rule of nines to categorize regions of the body. Staging is based on the degree of color loss, through Wood's lamp examination, and classifies lesions into one of four stages depending on residual pigmentation. Disease progression is analyzed on a scale from −1 to +1 based on changes in lesional borders, with −1 indicating regression, 0 stability, and + 1 progression [32]. Though it is very good to assess all three domains, it is time-consuming and availability of Wood's lamp in clinics is an issue.

9.12 Patient-Reported Outcome Measures (PROM)

Patient-reported outcomes reflect individuals' own perspectives regarding their disease, its management, and how it affects their daily lives and overall well-being. These outcomes provide valuable insights into the impact of vitiligo on patients beyond clinical measurements and also help in understanding the outcome that matters the most to them.

- *Vitiligo Disease Activity Score (VIDA)*

VIDA scale is a six-point system designed to evaluate the progression of vitiligo over time. The scoring relies on the patient's recollection of their disease activity. Vitiligo is considered active if there is an enlargement of current lesions or the development of new ones. A low VIDA score indicates less activity. Grading is based on the activity of disease as follows:

- +4—last 6 weeks or less
- +3—last 6 weeks to 3 months
- +2—last 3–6 months
- +1—last 6–12 months
- 0—stable for 1 year or more
- −1—stable with spontaneous re-pigmentation for 1 year or more

The VIDA is seen as the "gold standard" for evaluating vitiligo disease activity and correlates with response to therapy; however, it relies on patient's memory is the major drawback [33].

- *Vitiligo Noticeability Scale (VNS)*

The Vitiligo Noticeability Scale (VNS) is a newer patient-reported measure designed to assess how visible vitiligo patches are posttreatment. According to validated score interpretations, a VNS rating of 4 or 5 is considered indicative of successful treatment, while a score of 3 suggests a partial therapeutic response. Scores of 1 or 2 reflect an unsuccessful outcome. The VNS has demonstrated reliability and is well-regarded as a patient-centered tool for evaluating cosmetically acceptable repigmentation. It captures the patient's own evaluation of how effective the treatment was in restoring pigment. Most research involving VNS has been conducted in populations with darker skin tones (phototypes IV–VI); therefore, further studies are needed to confirm its applicability across a broader range of skin types [34].

- *Self-Assessment Vitiligo Extent Score (SA-VES)*

A self-assessment method using the VES, called the SA-VES. Compared to clinician-assessed Vitiligo Extent Scores (VES), a strong agreement was observed. Importantly, the SA-VES did not overestimate or underestimate disease visibility. The SA-VES offers advantages in providing detailed information on involved body areas, which significantly influences disease impact and treatment response. It is convenient for the patient to self-monitor and is available as a mobile app and online calculator. Over estimation by the patient is a major drawback of this scale [35].

9.13 Conclusion

Vitiligo is a chronic disease with major psychological impact especially in skin of color patients. Hence it is pertinent to closely execute a holistic management plan including monitoring disease and its activity; equally important is to assess the mental burden on the patient as well as family members. Patient-reported outcome measures are designed to assess various aspects of the patient's quality of life, including emotional well-being, social interactions, self-esteem, and treatment satisfaction. These measures provide insights into how patients perceive their condition and its impact on their daily lives, beyond the clinical evaluation of skin lesions. They can also guide clinical trials and research by providing evidence on the effectiveness of interventions from the patient's viewpoint, highlighting the importance of incorporating patient-centered assessments in the management of vitiligo. With the use of well-designed scales and scores, the assessment becomes easier and less time-consuming.

References

1. Parsad D, Gupta S. IADVL Dermatosurgery task force. Standard guidelines of care for vitiligo surgery. Indian J Dermatol Venereol Leprol. 2008;74:S37–45.
2. Majid I, Mysore V, Salim T, Lahiri K, Chatterji M, Khunger N, et al. Is Lesional stability in vitiligo more important than disease stability for performing surgical interventions? Results from a multicentric study. J Cutan Aesthet Surg. 2016;9(1):13–9.
3. Rodrigues M, Ezzedine K, Hamzavi I, Pandya AG, Harris JE. New discoveries in the pathogenesis and classification of vit iligo. J Am Acad Dermatol. 2017;77:1–13.
4. Taneja, Neha; Sreenivas, V 1; Sahni, Kanika; Gupta, Vishal; Ramam, M.. Disease stability in segmental and non-segmental vitiligo. Indian Dermatol Online J2022 13.(1):60–63.
5. Njoo MD, Das PK, Bos JD, Westerhof W. Association of the Köbner phenomenon with disease activity and therapeutic responsiveness in vitiligo vulgaris. Arch Dermatol. 1999;135:407–13.
6. Falabella R, Arrunategui A, Barona MI, Alzate A. The minigrafting test for vitiligo: detection of stable lesions for melanocyte transplantation. J Am Acad Dermatol. 1995;32:228–32.
7. Abdallah M, Lotfi R, Othman W, Galal R. Assessment of tissue FoxP3+, CD4+ and CD8+ T-cells in active and stable nonsegmental vitiligo. Int J Dermatol. 2014;53:940–6.
8. Strassner JP, Rashighi M, Ahmed Refat M, Richmond JM, Harris JE. Suction blistering the lesional skin of vitiligo patients reveals useful biomarkers of disease activity. J Am Acad Dermatol. 2017;76:847–855.e5.
9. Marie J, Kovacs D, Pain C, Jouary T, Cota C, Vergier B, et al. Inflammasome activation and vitiligo/nonsegmental vitiligo progression. Br J Dermatol. 2014;170:816–23.
10. Doss RW, El-Rifaie A-AA, Abdel-Wahab AM, Gohary YM, Rashed LA. Heat shock Protein-70 expression in vitiligo and its relation to the disease activity. Indian J Dermatol. 2016;61:408–12.
11. Dwivedi M, Laddha NC, Arora P, Marfatia YS, Begum R. Decreased regulatory T-cells and CD4(+) /CD8(+) ratio correlate with disease onset and progression in patients with generalized vitiligo. Pigment Cell Melanoma Res. 2013;26:586–91.
12. Lin M, Zhang B-X, Shen N, Dong X-J, Zhang C, Qi X-Y, et al. Regulatory T cells from active nonsegmental vitiligo exhibit lower suppressive ability on CD8+CLA+ T cells. Eur J Dermatol. 2014;24:676–82.

13. Speeckaert R, Ongenae K, van Geel N. Alterations of CXCL12 in serum of patients with vitiligo. J Invest Dermatol. 2017;137(7):1586–8.
14. Singh RK, Lee KM, Vujkovic-Cvijin I, Ucmak D, Farahnik B, Abrouk M, et al. The role of IL-17 in vitiligo: a review. Autoimmun Rev. 2016;15:397–404.
15. Ala Y, Pasha MK, Rao RN, Komaravalli PL, Jahan P. Association of IFN-γ: IL-10 cytokine ratio with nonsegmental vitiligo pathogenesis. Autoimmune Dis. 2015;2015:423490.
16. Laddha NC, Dwivedi M, Mansuri MS, Singh M, Patel HH, Agarwal N, et al. Association of neuropeptide Y (NPY), interleukin-1B (IL1B) genetic variants and correlation of IL1B transcript levels with vitiligo susceptibility. PLoS One. 2014;9:e107020.
17. Parsad D, Dogra S, Kanwar AJ. Quality of life in patients with vitiligo. Health Qual Life Outcomes. 2003;1:58.
18. Finlay AY, Khan GK. Dermatology life quality index (DLQI): a simple practical measure for routine clinical use. Clin Exp Dermatol. 1994;19:210–6.
19. Lewis-Jones MS, Finlay AY. The children's dermatology life quality index (CDLQI): initial validation and practical use. Br J Dermatol. 1995;132(6):942–9.
20. Lilly E, Lu PD, Borovicka JH, et al. Development and validation of a vitiligo-specific quality-of-life instrument (VitiQoL). J Am Acad Dermatol. 2013;69:e11–8.
21. Gupta V, Ramam M. Vitiligo impact scale (VIS)-22: a measure of the psycho-social burden of vitiligo. Indian J Dermatol Venereol Leprol. 2022;88:691–5.
22. Salzes C, Abadie S, Seneschal J, Whitton M, Meurant JM, Jouary T, et al. The vitiligo impact patient scale (VIPs): development and validation of a vitiligo burden assessment tool. J Invest Dermatol. 2016;136(1):52–8.
23. Agrawal S, Satapathy S, Gupta V, Sreenivas V, Khaitan BK, Ramam M. Family vitiligo impact scale: a scale to measure the quality-of-life of family members of patients with vitiligo. Indian J Dermatol Venereol Leprol. 2021;88:32–9.
24. Eleftheriadou V, Thomas K, van Geel N, Hamzavi I, Lim H, Suzuki T, Vitiligo Global Issues Consensus Group, et al. Developing core outcome set for vitiligo clinical trials: international e-Delphi consensus. Pigment Cell Melanoma Res. 2015;28(3):363–9.
25. Hamzavi I, Jain H, McLean D, Shapiro J, Zeng H, Lui H. Parametric modeling of narrowband UV-B phototherapy for vitiligo using a novel quantitative tool: the vitiligo area scoring index. Arch Dermatol. 2004;140(6):677–83.
26. Bae JM, Zubair R, Ju HJ, Kohli I, Lee HN, Eun SH, et al. Development and validation of the fingertip unit for assessing facial vitiligo area scoring index. J Am Acad Dermatol. 2022;86(2):387–93.
27. van Geel N, Lommerts J, Bekkenk M, Wolkerstorfer A, Prinsen CAC, Eleftheriadou V, et al. Development and validation of the vitiligo extent score (VES): an international collaborative initiative. J Invest Dermatol. 2016;136(5):978–84.
28. van Geel N, Wolkerstorfer A, Lommerts JE, Ezzedine K, Eleftheriadou V, Hamzavi I, Harris J, Picardo M, Taieb A, Prinsen CAC, Bekkenk M, Speeckaert R. Validation study of the vitiligo extent score-plus. J Am Acad Dermatol. 2018;78(5):1013–5.
29. Bae JM, Oh SH, Kang HY, Ryoo YW, Lan CE, Xiang LH, East Asia Vitiligo Association, et al. Development and validation of the vitiligo extent score for a target area (VESTA) to assess the treatment response of a target lesion. Pigment Cell Melanoma Res. 2019;32(2):315–9.
30. van Geel N, Passeron T, Wolkerstorfer A, Speeckaert R, Ezzedine K. Reliability and validity of the vitiligo signs of activity score (VSAS). Br J Dermatol. 2020;183(5):883–90.
31. van Geel N, Depaepe L, Vandaele V, Mertens L, Van Causenbroeck J, De Schepper S, Van Coile L, Van Reempts A, De Vos AS, Papeleu J, Hoorens I, Mertens D, Wolkerstorfer A, Lommerts JE, Speeckaert R. Assessing the dynamic changes in vitiligo: reliability and validity of the vitiligo disease activity score (VDAS) and vitiligo disease improvement score (VDIS). J Eur Acad Dermatol Venereol. 2022;36(8):1334–41.
32. Taïeb A, Picardo M, VETF Members. The definition and assessment of vitiligo: a consensus report of the vitiligo European task force. Pigment Cell Res. 2007 Feb;20(1):27–35.

33. Njoo MD, Das PK, Bos JD, Westerhof W. Association of the Köbner phenomenon with disease activity and therapeutic responsiveness in vitiligo vulgaris. Arch Dermatol. 1999;135(4):407–13.
34. Batchelor JM, Tan W, Tour S, Yong A, Montgomery AA, Thomas KS. Validation of the vitiligo noticeability scale: a patient-reported outcome measure of vitiligo treatment success. Br J Dermatol. 2016;174(2):386–94.
35. van Geel N, Lommerts JE, Bekkenk MW, Prinsen CA, Eleftheriadou V, Taieb A, International Vitiligo Score Working Group, et al. Development and validation of a patient-reported outcome measure in vitiligo: the self assessment vitiligo extent score (SA-VES). J Am Acad Dermatol. 2017;76(3):464–71.

Chapter 10
Psychological and Ancillary Support in Vitiligo

Apoorva Sharma and Sunil Dogra

Abstract Vitiligo affects a person's psychological and social well-being including social relationships, mental health, and career chances. The effects that vitiligo has may even include sleep difficulties and interference with interpersonal relationships. Vitiligo has been shown to have a detrimental effect on marriages in certain situations; in other cases, the development of skin depigmentation has been used as justification for divorce. This confluence of social and emotional difficulties emphasises how critical it is to address vitiligo's effects in their entirety and provide psychological and ancillary support for the same.

Keywords Vitiligo · Psychological · Ancillary

10.1 Introduction

Vitiligo has a significant and independent effect on a patient's well-being and quality of life. It can cause a wide range of complicated emotional reactions, including anxiety, despair, and diminished self-confidence. An individual's overall quality of life can be severely reduced by these mental responses, which affect both the person and those in their immediate vicinity. The quality of life (QoL) of family members and close relatives is significantly impacted by vitiligo, according to a study done in 2013 by Bin Saif et al., 91.5% of individuals reported having QoL consequences as a result of knowing someone who had vitiligo [1].

A. Sharma · S. Dogra (✉)
Department of Dermatology, Venereology and Leprology, Postgraduate Institute of Medical Education and Research (PGIMER), Chandigarh, India

R. Sarkar, V. Narayan R (eds.), *A Concise Guide to The Management of Vitiligo*,
https://doi.org/10.1007/978-981-95-3857-7_10

10.2 Factors Associated with Psychosocial Burden

Factors that were significantly associated with higher psychosocial or overall QoL burden were female sex, lesion location in visible areas or genitals, younger age (particularly those aged <30 years and more so in adolescents) and extensive body area involvement [2, 3].

Unmarried and/or single relationship status, longer disease duration (particularly duration >5 years), progressive disease, Fitzpatrick skin phototype IV–VI, lower education status (particularly high school or lower level of education), non-segmental vitiligo (vs segmental or focal vitiligo), non-Caucasian race, positive family history of vitiligo, being employed (compared with being students, unemployed, or retired), and higher socioeconomic level were also significantly associated with increased burden. Four studies reported that comorbid depression significantly reduced overall QoL [3, 4]. Management strategies including camouflage, cognitive behavioural therapy, phototherapy, and depigmentation cream (in patients with extensive vitiligo) were associated with decreased vitiligo-associated burden.

10.3 Psychological Effects of Vitiligo

Patients with vitiligo have a continuous burden because of the condition's unpredictable development and requirement to conceal it with clothes or makeup. Strong psychological effects can be seen in patients who report thinking about their illness frequently during the day and feeling self-conscious when they look in the mirror, even with their lesions covered. Their dissatisfaction with their appearance which is the root of this bad self-perception, commonly leads to anxiety, depression, and low self-esteem (Fig. 10.1).

Vitiligo was listed by Pt. Jawaharlal Nehru, the country's first prime minister, as one of the country's three main medical issues, along with leprosy and malaria. It is also connected to some religious beliefs in India. A person who performed "Guru Droh" in his previous life is reported to have vitiligo in this life, according to certain religious writings in India where reincarnation is believed. As a result, vitiligo sufferers in India experience greater societal issues than those in other nations. There is a real sense of this among young single women. The reason behind this is arranged marriages. Consequently, the likelihood of a young lady with vitiligo getting married is low. A married woman who develops vitiligo after marriage is likely to experience marital issues and may even file for divorce [5].

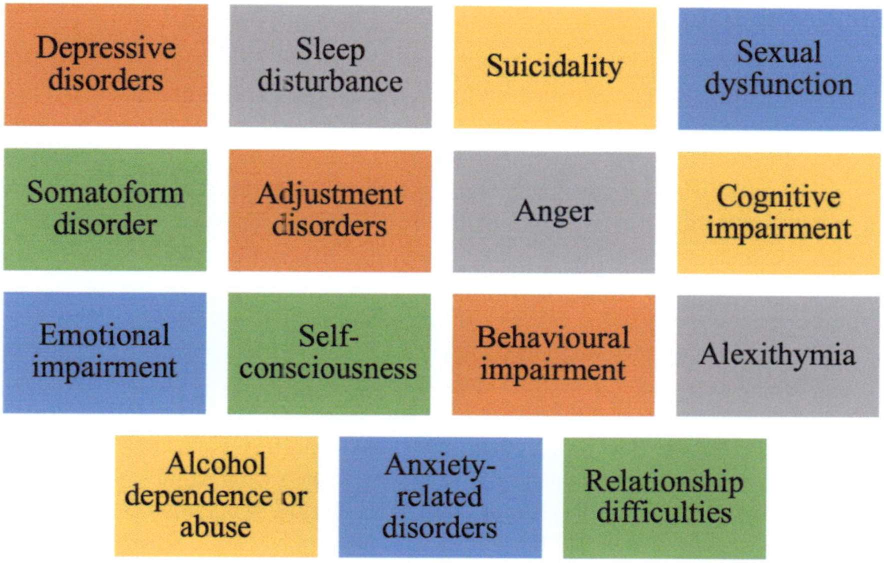

Fig. 10.1 Psychological effects of vitiligo

10.3.1 Psychosocial Vulnerability

Vitiligo is a visible illness to others, unlike most internal disorders, and persons who have it may experience emotional and social implications. In addition to learning to cope with the physical changes they are experiencing, patients need to be psychologically ready for the chance that their illness could worsen or spread at any time, leaving them feeling somewhat powerless and uncertain [6]. Patients suffering from vitiligo frequently experience dread and anxiety about the possibility of developing new lesions because there is no single identifiable cause for the disorder. The unpredictable nature of the disease course, which can be both progressive and episodic, causes psychological stress for numerous individuals.

In a study based in India, psychiatric morbidity was discovered in 28 vitiligo patients, with a clinic prevalence rate of 25% (95% confidence interval 20.3–29.3%). Adjustment disorder was diagnosed in most of the patients. There was a substantial correlation found between dysfunction resulting from sickness and psychiatric morbidity [7]. People may eventually experience a variety of mental health conditions together, such as depression, which has been shown to be five times more common in vitiligo patients than in controls [8]. In actuality, cyclic antidepressants are frequently prescribed to vitiligo sufferers to address their depression [9]. Further research on the psychological state of vitiligo patients revealed that they experience psychological disturbances and feelings of disfigurement, as well as anxiety, sadness, low self-esteem, sleep difficulties, and sexual dysfunction [10]. Numerous factors, including the degree of skin involvement and its distribution, can exacerbate the disease experience.

10.3.2 Self-Esteem

The intricate relationship between vitiligo's physical disparities and social stigma, which has a substantial impact on an individual's self-esteem, highlights the psychosocial impact of the condition. In their 2010 study, Thompson et al. explore the experiences of British South Asian women who live with vitiligo [11]. The study highlights the critical role that cultural norms, societal perceptions, and beauty standards play in determining how people with vitiligo experience their emotions.

Thompson et al. provided insight into the difficulties that people with vitiligo encounter, particularly in the British South Asian society, where they deal with negative responses, misunderstandings about the condition, and prejudice because of their changed look. The research conducted by Ezzedine et al. resonates with them. Through a comprehensive assessment of the literature, Ezzedine et al.'s study explores the psychological implications of vitiligo and offers a more comprehensive knowledge of how people with vitiligo frequently deal with prejudice and social stigma resulting from misconceptions and cultural beauty standards [3]. The unifying theme throughout these studies emphasises how social bias is a worldwide phenomenon and how it can negatively affect someone's sense of self-worth.

Remarkably, research such as that conducted by Thompson et al. and Ezzedine et al. suggests that vitiligo sufferers' low self-esteem and lack of confidence are caused by this stigma. These people may have a negative self-perception as a result of the societal bias they encounter, which may affect how they see themselves and their role in society. Furthermore, the influence of distinct cultural norms and societal beauty ideals intensifies inside particular cultural contexts, increasing the pressure on people to conform to established appearance standards. This heightened focus on fitting in with societal norms may exacerbate the marginalisation that vitiligo sufferers already experience. Establishing support systems that are sensitive to cultural differences and specifically designed to tackle these particular difficulties is therefore becoming increasingly urgent.

10.3.3 Depression and Anxiety

Vitiligo has psychosocial ramifications for mental health, with anxiety and depression being major issues. A systematic review and meta-analysis by Kussainova et al. highlighted the connection between anxiety and vitiligo [12]. Thirty-six percent of vitiligo patients overall had anxiety, according to their study. Similar to this, Lai et al. carried out a comprehensive review and meta-analysis concentrating on the connection between depression and vitiligo [13]. According to their research, vitiligo patients had a markedly increased chance of developing clinical depression or depressive symptoms in comparison to individuals who did not have a depigmenting illness. Up to 25% of vitiligo patients exhibited clinical depression, and about one-third of them reported having poor overall health or sad symptoms.

These studies are important because they shed insight on the psychological effects of vitiligo and illustrate how the condition's visible aspect increases the risk of anxiety and despair. Given this, it becomes essential to implement interventions that deal with both the physical and psychological aspects of vitiligo. The research by Kussainova et al. and Lai et al. highlights the need for holistic ways to support people in overcoming the difficulties presented by vitiligo by illuminating these links.

In a study by Kruger et al. [14] 23 controls and 96 patients with vitiligo were included. It used the Dermatology Life Quality Index (DLQI), Adjustment to Chronic Skin Disorders Questionnaire (ACS), Beck Depression Inventory (BDI), and extra items to assess quality of life (QoL), coping, depression, and stigmatisation. Eighty-seven of the 96 patients (90%) reported queries or approaches, while 23/96 patients (24%) reported hurtful remarks. Sixty-four out of ninety-six (66.7%) had covered up their white spots or avoided situations due to vitiligo. Sixty patients (62.5%) suggested that psychological stress had an impact on how the disease progressed. With the exception of BDI (6.8/7.3), patients outperformed controls on all measures (DLQI = 4.9/1.6, ACS-social anxiety/avoidance = 36.9/22.1, ACS-helplessness = 27.3/16.0, ACS-anxious-depressive mood = 19.4/15.6). Pro-pseudocatalase PC-KUS treatment decreased sadness, anxious-depressive mood, and social anxiety/avoidance [14].

10.3.4 Financial Burdens

Patients with vitiligo frequently experience financial hardship as a result of having to miss work to attend PUVA sessions and other hospital visits. Vitiligo lesions over exposed locations might limit career options by negatively affecting an applicant's chances of getting hired during an interview. Childhood-onset vitiligo has been linked to severe psychological trauma that may have a lifelong impact on these children's sense of self-worth. Children who have vitiligo typically limit or avoid sports and frequently miss important school days. It could be necessary for parents of children with vitiligo to take time off work in order to routinely accompany them to medical visits. Children with vitiligo can either cope with the condition effectively or suffer greatly from it, frequently based on the mindset of their parents, siblings, relatives, teachers, friends, baby sitters etc.

10.4 Coping Mechanisms in Vitiligo Patients

The use of camouflage, concealing clothing and altered body movements were the most frequently mentioned coping strategies in studies. Additional coping mechanisms encompassed acceptance of vitiligo, avoidance behaviour, and counselling or support groups.

In a study by Shourick et al., a shared-medical decision tool was tested in 30 French and 10 US adult patients with vitiligo who reported high satisfaction rates for the use of this tool during consultation. This shared decision-making tool for vitiligo may help patients to better define the aim they would like to improve treatment adherence and success for vitiligo [15].

10.5 Perceptions Regarding Vitiligo

Thirteen publications addressed the topic of views towards vitiligo. Of them, seven examined how patients perceived their condition, while six examined how other people perceived patients with vitiligo. Aspects of attitudes and behaviours related to vitiligo knowledge or beliefs were examined in multiple papers [2].

Many people had the misconception that vitiligo is contagious or that it is brought on by outside factors (such as the "evil eye", witchcraft/sorcery, evil spirits/Jinn, chance/fate), that cleanliness is lacking, or that germs or viruses are infecting people. Participants with enough understanding about vitiligo compared to those with insufficient knowledge reported a lower prevalence of negative attitudes and a higher prevalence of positive attitudes in three studies that examined attitudes towards patients with vitiligo. About 6–94% of participants in four studies indicated that they would be willing to date or marry someone who had vitiligo. The reasons given for not wanting to marry were the effect that vitiligo had on appearance, social reasons, and the belief that vitiligo is inherited or contagious [2].

10.6 Counselling and Psychological Support: Education and Awareness

Studies reveal a relationship between increased educational attainment and patients' capacity to understand their illness rationally, which in turn lessens the stress that the illness causes [16]. In order to treat vitiligo, psychological intervention must first inform patients about their course of illness and therapy. Patients' comprehension of the illness can be improved, their worry and dread can be much reduced, and their resolve to actively treat the condition can be strengthened with increased knowledge about the disorder and its standard therapy [17]. Because of their own beliefs and ideas that vitiligo is incurable or greatly impacted by their behaviour, some people may choose not to get a professional diagnosis [18].

Higher educated patients had significantly better health-related quality of life (HRQoL) than patients with less common medical disorders, according to a recent study [19]. The idea that vitiligo is a minor or cosmetic ailment can be understood by increasing knowledge of the QOL issues associated with the disorder as well as deeper understanding of its underlying causes and relationships to other systemic conditions [20].

It is also important to note that well-known people who have openly coped with vitiligo, like Big Krizz Kaliko, Michael Jackson, Lee Thomas, and Winnie Harlow, have been essential in encouraging education and increasing public awareness of the condition. These significant individuals serve as motivating role models and demonstrate that vitiligo need not stand in the way of a person's quest for happiness and achievement. Their experiences highlight the value of psychological support, acceptance of oneself, and the possibility that people with vitiligo can lead happy lives in spite of the difficulties the disease presents.

10.7 Camouflage

For vitiligo, camouflage is a good supplementary treatment. Benefits are felt right away, and it may be taught in a single day. For people suffering with vitiligo, camouflaging lesions can offer a much-needed safe haven, because the condition's recovery might take months or years to manifest. An Italian group conducted the first paediatric camouflage study, evaluating 15 kids between the ages of 7 and 16, four of whom had vitiligo [21]. After completing a camouflage training session, each person returned to the clinic after 15 days to evaluate their skill and how it affected their quality of life. The employment of camouflage reduced psychological distress, albeit it was not stated to what extent. Additional restrictions on interpreting this research include a brief follow-up period and a lack of subset data for vitiligo-only analysis.

Dihydroxyacetone (DHA), a sunless tanner that has been used successfully in people with vitiligo, may be a more practical option than camouflaging every day [22, 23]. Less money and more durability are two benefits of using a sunless tanner versus concealing with cosmetics. When applied topically, it is thought to be harmless. Higher DHA concentrations have been shown to work better on skin tones with darker pigmentation.

The effects of medical tattooing, skin stains, and bleaching treatments like monobenzone can be used as temporary and permanent camouflaging alternatives.

10.8 Psychotherapy Including Cognitive Behavioral Therapy (CBT)

A number of procedures are used in psychotherapy to detect behavioural, emotional, and cognitive symptoms that are the focus of psychotherapeutic interventions. These methods are applied in accordance with the target behaviour that needs to be addressed and the disorder of interest. A subtype of psychotherapy called CBT focuses on how cognitive processes affect behaviour. It is a problem-focused approach that seeks to recognise and modify cognitive distortions, stay away from upsetting circumstances, and engage in behaviour that lessens stress [24]. It has been demonstrated that adults with vitiligo experience higher rates of anxiety and depression than people without the condition. Preliminary research has also suggested that depression may arise in children with vitiligo [25]. CBT is especially useful for treatment of depressive and anxiety disorders [26] and can thus theoretically be used to treat the psychiatric effects of vitiligo.

Shah et al. investigated a self-help intervention that used strategies drawn from behaviour change theories and cognitive behavioural models of social anxiety. A brochure containing guided imagery-based relaxation techniques, symptom monitoring, and psychoeducation was given to intervention participants. An improved brochure with particular "if-then" scenarios was given to a portion of the intervention group in an effort to promote the usage of the self-help resources [27].

For instance, "I will visualise a beach scene to boost my confidence if I'm nervous at a party". The Brief Fear of Negative Evaluation Scale, which assesses cognitive components of social anxiety, served as the main outcome measure. People can continue to manage their symptoms outside of the clinic with the support of self-help strategies. Children benefit from the usage of "if-then" scenarios because they may find them easier to understand and provide a valuable coping strategy during a crisis. With these resources, parents may also practise enacting the "if-then" situations with their kids at home. People who have gone through similar situations in life can meet together in support groups and draw strength from each other. They also lessen emotions of hopelessness and loneliness and provide participants with a sense of camaraderie [28].

10.9 Support Groups and Social Media

A patient-driven non-profit organisation, Vitiligo Support International provides resources for vitiligo education, research, awareness, advocacy, and community forums [29]. It includes the vitiligo experiences and coping mechanisms of other children with the condition. Additionally, it facilitates parent-to-parent interactions in local communities and online forums. The American Vitiligo Research Foundation features testimonials from people of many ethnic backgrounds on their website, which highlights the varied experiences of teenagers and children while also supporting ongoing attempts to discover a cure [30]. It is crucial that healthcare professionals are aware of these groups so they may refer their patients to them. There are numerous additional organisations that operate as vitiligo support groups both domestically and overseas.

Another excellent option for people with chronic skin conditions like vitiligo is children's camps. Weeklong camps around the nation, Camp Wonder (37 for kids ages 6–16) and Camp Discovery (36 for kids ages 7–16), offer children the opportunity to participate in camp activities without having to worry about their skin ailment being stigmatised [31, 32]. The children get to enjoy free activities like swimming, fishing, rock climbing, horseback riding, and arts and crafts while getting professional dermatological and nurse care. For eligibility to be granted for these camps, the skin problem does not have to be clinically severe. In addition to feeling alone and upset due to their illness, patients with even modest clinical results may gain from the camp experience.

Over 80% of dermatological patients are estimated to utilise social media to learn about their illnesses. Social media can be used by vitiligo patients as a resource for support and a better understanding of the disease [33].

10.10 Conclusion

In conclusion, the management of vitiligo extends beyond medical treatments to encompass crucial psychological and ancillary support. Patients often experience significant emotional distress and social challenges due to the visible nature of the condition. Effective psychological interventions, such as cognitive-behavioural therapy and support groups, play a pivotal role in improving mental well-being and enhancing coping mechanisms. Ancillary support through educational resources, camouflage techniques, and advocacy further empowers individuals with vitiligo to manage their condition with confidence. By integrating comprehensive care that addresses both medical and psychosocial aspects, healthcare providers can significantly enhance the quality of life for patients living with vitiligo.

References

1. Bin Saif GA, Al-Balbeesiu AO, Binshabaib R, Alsaad D, Kwatra SG, Alzolibani AA, et al. Quality of life in family members of vitiligo patients: a questionnaire study in Saudi Arabia. Am J Clin Dermatol. 2013;14(6):489–95.
2. Salama AH, Alnemr L, Khan AR, Alfakeer H, Aleem Z, Ali-Alkhateeb M. Unveiling the unseen struggles: a comprehensive review of vitiligo's psychological, social, and quality of life impacts. Cureus. 2023;15(9):e45030.
3. Ezzedine K, Eleftheriadou V, Jones H, Bibeau K, Kuo FI, Sturm D, et al. Psychosocial effects of vitiligo: a systematic literature review. Am J Clin Dermatol. 2021;22(6):757–74.
4. Augustin M, Gewiss C, Ben-Anaya N, Böhm M. Quality of life, disease burden and healthcare need of patients with vitiligo. Dermatologie (Heidelb). 2024;75(5):404–11.
5. Parsad D, Dogra S, Kanwar AJ. Quality of life in patients with vitiligo. Health Qual Life Outcomes. 2003;1:58.
6. Liu J, Tang R, Xiao Y, Luo M, Shi Y, Deng Q, et al. Meta-analytic review of high anxiety comorbidity among patients with vitiligo. Biomed Res Int. 2021;2021:6663646.
7. Mattoo SK, Handa S, Kaur I, Gupta N, Malhotra R. Psychiatric morbidity in vitiligo: prevalence and correlates in India. J Eur Acad Dermatol Venereol. 2002;16(6):573–8.
8. Wang G, Qiu D, Yang H, Liu W. The prevalence and odds of depression in patients with vitiligo: a meta-analysis. J Eur Acad Dermatol Venereol. 2018;32(8):1343–51.

9. Anaba EL, Oaku RI. Prospective cross-sectional study of quality of life of vitiligo patients using a vitiligo specific quality of life instrument. West Afr J Med. 2020;37(7):745–9.
10. Alharbi MA. Identifying patients at higher risk of depression among patients with vitiligo at outpatient setting. Mater Sociomed. 2020;32(2):108–11.
11. Thompson AR, Clarke SA, Newell RJ, Gawkrodger DJ. Vitiligo linked to stigmatization in British South Asian women: a qualitative study of the experiences of living with vitiligo. Br J Dermatol. 2010;163(3):481–6.
12. Kussainova A, Kassym L, Akhmetova A, Glushkova N, Sabirov U, Adilgozhina S, et al. Vitiligo and anxiety: a systematic review and meta-analysis. PLoS One. 2020;15(11):e0241445.
13. Lai YC, Yew YW, Kennedy C, Schwartz RA. Vitiligo and depression: a systematic review and meta-analysis of observational studies. Br J Dermatol. 2017;177(3):708–18.
14. Krüger C, Schallreuter KU. Stigmatisation, avoidance behaviour and difficulties in coping are common among adult patients with vitiligo. Acta Derm Venereol. 2015;95(5):553–8.
15. Shourick J, Ahmed M, Seneschal J, Passeron T, Andreux N, Qureshi A, et al. Development of a shared decision-making tool in vitiligo: an international study. Br J Dermatol. 2021;185(4):787–96.
16. Mishra N, Rastogi MK, Gahalaut P, Agrawal S. Dermatology specific quality of life in vitiligo patients and its relation with various variables: a hospital based cross-sectional study. J Clin Diagn Res. 2014;8(6):Yc01–3.
17. Taïeb A, Meurant JM. Should we prioritize psychological interventions in the management of vitiligo? J Eur Acad Dermatol Venereol. 2018;32(12):2053–4.
18. AlGhamdi KM. Beliefs and perceptions of Arab vitiligo patients regarding their condition. Int J Dermatol. 2010;49(10):1141–5.
19. Mielck A, Reitmeir P, Vogelmann M, Leidl R. Impact of educational level on health-related quality of life (HRQL): results from Germany based on the EuroQol 5D (EQ-5D). Eur J Pub Health. 2013;23(1):45–9.
20. Elbuluk N, Ezzedine K. Quality of life, burden of disease, co-morbidities, and systemic effects in vitiligo patients. Dermatol Clin. 2017;35(2):117–28.
21. Tedeschi A, Dall'Oglio F, Micali G, Schwartz RA, Janniger CK. Corrective camouflage in pediatric dermatology. Cutis. 2007;79(2):110–2.
22. Hsu S. Camouflaging vitiligo with dihydroxyacetone. Dermatol Online J. 2008;14(8):23.
23. Rajatanavin N, Suwanachote S, Kulkollakarn S. Dihydroxyacetone: a safe camouflaging option in vitiligo. Int J Dermatol. 2008;47(4):402–6.
24. DeMaso DR, Walter HJ. Chapter 21: Psychological treatment of children and adolescents. In: Kliegman R, editor. Nelson textbook of pediatrics. Philadelphia: Elsevier, Inc.; 2016. p. 127–135.e1.
25. Bilgiç O, Bilgiç A, Akiş HK, Eskioğlu F, Kiliç EZ. Depression, anxiety and health-related quality of life in children and adolescents with vitiligo. Clin Exp Dermatol. 2011;36(4):360–5.
26. Abernethy RS, Schlozman SC. Chapter 10: An overview of the psychotherapies. In: Stern TA, ed. Massachusetts general hospital comprehensive clinical psychiatry. Boston: Elsevier, Inc. 2016: 102–110.e3.
27. Shah R, Hunt J, Webb TL, Thompson AR. Starting to develop self-help for social anxiety associated with vitiligo: using clinical significance to measure the potential effectiveness of enhanced psychological self-help. Br J Dermatol. 2014;171(2):332–7.
28. Goh C, Lane AT, Bruckner AL. Support groups for children and their families in pediatric dermatology. Pediatr Dermatol. 2007;24(3):302–5.
29. Vitiligo Support International Inc. (online). Available at https://www.vitiligosupport.org/. Accessed 24 June 2024.
30. American Vitiligo Research Foundation Inc: AVRF (online). Available at http://www.avrf.org/. Accessed 24 June 2024.

31. American Academy of Dermatology (AAD). Camp discovery 2017 (online). Available at http://www.campdiscovery.org/. Accessed June 2024.
32. Children's Skin Disease Foundation (CSDF). Camp wonder (online). Available at https://www.csdf.org/campwonder.aspx Accessed 24 June 2024.
33. Social media platforms as a resource for vitiligo support. J Drugs Dermatol. 2022;21(10):1135–6.

Part III
Medical Therapy

Chapter 11
Topical Medications in Vitiligo

Shyamrup Banerjee, Sambit Chatterjee, and Anupam Das

Abstract Vitiligo is an acquired, chronic depigmenting disorder characterized by the gradual loss of functional melanocytes in the epidermis, leading to well-demarcated amelanotic macules and patches. Its onset may occur at any age, with an average age of 30 years, and is influenced by complex interactions between genetic susceptibility, intrinsic melanocyte defects, oxidative stress, and autoimmune responses. The disease displays considerable clinical heterogeneity, with segmental, non-segmental, mixed, and rare variants such as follicular, trichrome, and vitiligo ponctué presentations. Histopathologically, lesions typically show an absence of melanocytes, with occasional lichenoid inflammation at the margins. Beyond cutaneous changes, vitiligo has a strong association with autoimmune comorbidities, including thyroid disorders, alopecia areata, and type 1 diabetes mellitus, alongside significant psychosocial implications.

Current topical therapies form the cornerstone of management, with corticosteroids, calcineurin inhibitors, and vitamin D analogs widely employed either as monotherapy or in combination with phototherapy. Psoralen-based photochemotherapy, phenylalanine, and newer approaches such as topical methotrexate, mycophenolate mofetil, JAK inhibitors (e.g., ruxolitinib), and growth factor-based treatments have expanded the therapeutic armamentarium. Adjunctive strategies like antioxidants, prostaglandin analogs, piperine, and camouflage play supportive roles. This review consolidates the pathogenesis, clinical spectrum, histopathology, comorbidities, and therapeutic advances in vitiligo, emphasizing the need for a holistic, individualized approach to management to address both physical and psychosocial impacts.

Keywords Vitiligo · Depigmentation · Topical therapies · JAK inhibitors

---

S. Banerjee · S. Chatterjee · A. Das (✉)
Department of Dermatology, KPC Medical College and Hospital, Kolkata, India

R. Sarkar, V. Narayan R (eds.), *A Concise Guide to The Management of Vitiligo*, https://doi.org/10.1007/978-981-95-3857-7_11

11.1 Manuscript

Vitiligo is an acquired, chronic, depigmented disorder in which melanocytes that determine colour of the skin, hair, and eyes are slowly lost [1–3]. It may appear any time, from shortly after birth to late adulthood, with an average age of 30 years at onset [4].

The pathogenesis of vitiligo involves both genetic and non-genetic factors in processes leading to loss of epidermal melanocytes; with evidence of significant genetic heterogeneity, as observed in different ethnic populations. Intrinsic abnormalities of melanocytes, in a background of genetic susceptibility, render them more vulnerable to oxidative stress and consequent damage [5].

Vitiligo commonly presents as totally amelanotic discrete round to oval irregular or linear macules or patches surrounded by normal skin, usually with convex borders, though lesions tend to be more ill-defined and hypomelanotic at their onset or when actively spreading. They may also present with a hyperpigmented border occasionally [6–8].

Vitiligo lesions enlarge centrifugally with time, either at slow or rapid rates. Lesions may develop anywhere on the body; frequently localizing to sites which are relatively hyperpigmented (face nipples axillae umbilicus inguinal anogenital) as well as areas subjected to repeated trauma (isomorphic Koebner phenomenon) pressure or friction [9].

Histologically, there seems to be complete absence of melanocytes, usually, without inflammatory infiltrate, but lichenoid or spongiotic inflammation may be detected at the edge of vitiligo lesions. This explains the scaling or hyperpigmentation sometimes observed around lesions of vitiligo.

11.1.1 Clinical Classification and Variants

"Vitiligo" was recommended to be used as the umbrella term for all non-segmental forms of the ailment, while mixed vitiligo represented co-existence of segmental and non-segmental vitiligo (by The 2012 Vitiligo Global Issues Consensus Conference) [10].

Localized:

- Segmental: Involves one or more body segments usually, with roughly quadrilateral shapes, not crossing the midline (more common in children than in adults).
- Focal: An undetermined/unclassified form in which depigmented macules are localized to one area but not clearly in a segmental distribution.
- Mucosal: Only the mucous membranes are involved.
- Generalized: Widespread vitiliginous lesions all across the body.
- Vulgaris: Scattered patches that are widely distributed (m.c. clinical type in children).
- Acrofacial: Distal extremities and face.

- Universal: Complete or, more commonly, nearly complete depigmentation.

11.1.2 Variants:

Follicular vitiligo presents with leukotrichia in the absence of depigmentation of the surrounding epidermis [11].

Vitiligo ponctué, an unusual clinical presentation of vitiligo, is characterized by multiple, small, discrete amelanotic macules sometimes superimposed upon a hyperpigmented macule.

Trichrome vitiligo is characterized by a hypopigmented zone between the normal and depigmented skin.

Hypochromic vitiligo presents with persistent hypopigmented macules in a seborrheic distribution, often coalescing together [12].

The onset of vitiligo, usually insidious, is followed by an unpredictable course, usually one of slow spread, as in case of generalized variants, but it may stabilize for a long period of time. In contrast, segmental vitiligo usually reaches its full extent within 1–2 years and remains restricted to the initial segmental area.

Generalized vitiligo is associated with an increased risk of developing autoimmune thyroid disease [13–15], alopecia areata, pernicious anaemia, type 1 diabetes mellitus, myasthenia gravis, and several connective tissue diseases—lupus erythematosus (discoid and systemic), Sjögren's syndrome, and rheumatoid arthritis [13, 16, 17]. Epidemiologic studies have also linked vitiligo with psoriasis, atopic diseases, inflammatory bowel disease, and metabolic syndrome [13, 18, 19]. Psychosocial conditions such as depression, anxiety, and adjustment disorders [20]. Patients with the autosomal recessive autoimmune polyenoic-cryopathy-candidiasis-ectodermal dystrophy (APECED) syndrome often develop vitiligo [21].

Figure 11.1 represents the pathogenesis of vitiligo.

11.2 Topical Corticosteroids (TCS)

Corticosteroids, at the cellular level, subserve their effects via binding to and activating GCR (glycoprotein-coupled-receptors) as follows:

1. The CS diffuses into the target cell and binds to the GCR (cytoplasmic) [22].
2. The CS-GCR complex undergoes necessary conformational changes [23].
3. The resulting active complex traverses the nuclear envelope and directly or indirectly binds to deoxyribonucleic acid [24, 25].
4. Gene regulation and transcription of various specific messenger ribonucleic acid (mRNA) occur [26].

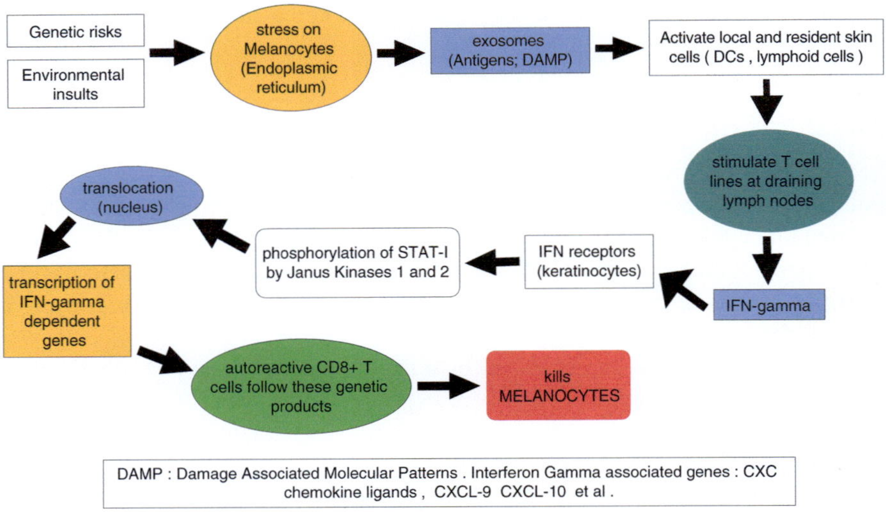

Fig. 11.1 Diagrammatic representation of vitiligopathogenesis

Thus, topical corticosteroids, likewise:

- Stabilize cell and lysosomal membranes thus preventing release of lysosomal contents and phospholipid precursors for synthesis of prostaglandins and platelet-activating factors (PAF).
- Induce anti-inflammatory proteins, lipocortins, vasocortin, and vasoregulin.

Lipocortins inhibit phospholipase A2 and block release of arachidonic acid and PAF from cell membranes; preventing the formation of potent inflammatory mediators (prostaglandins, leukotrienes, 12-hydroxyeicosatetraen-oic acid (12-HETE), and 15-HETE).

Additionally, they reduce production of interleukin-1 (both IL-1a and IL-1ß), interferon-y, tumour necrosis factor, IL-2, and granulocyte-monocyte colony-stimulating factor as well as have anti-inflammatory actions on specific cells (polymorphonuclear leukocytes monocytes lymphocytes Langerhans cells) [27].

Thus, within the given context, topical steroids are the main drugs used for the management of vitiligo, reducing the macrophages and T lymphocytes in the vitiligo patches as well as reduction in complement mediated destruction of the melanocytes. In patients with limited involvement, once-daily application of potent corticosteroids is advised for 3 months. Most studies done so far have confirmed the efficacy of topical steroids [28–31]. Efficacy is higher in children. When comparing the efficacy with other topical agents, results are similar when it comes to calcineurin inhibitors. Application of topical steroids can have some unwanted side effects like atrophy, telangiectasia, hypertrichosis, acneiform eruption, as well as striae. These side effects are more commonly seen with higher potency topical corticosteroids.

11.3 Topical Calcineurin Inhibitors (TCI)

Calcineurin after activation leads to formation of IL-2 and TNF-alpha. In vitiligo patches, the levels of these cytokines is elevated [32–34].

Tacrolimus, a common TCI, binds to the cellular protein FK506-binding protein (FKBP), a rotamase enzyme that is involved in protein folding. This complex then binds to the enzyme calcineurin, blocking its ability to dephosphorylate the transcription factor nuclear factor of activated T cells (NFAT-1). This in turn prevents transcription of the gene encoding the cytokine interleukin (IL)-2, blocking T cell activation and proliferation, and further cytokine production [35].

The mechanism of Pimecrolimus is the same as that of Tacrolimus. It binds to FKBP, leading to inhibition of calcineurin, subsequently preventing activation of NFAT-1. This blocks transcription of the gene encoding IL-2 and blocks T cell activation and further cytokine production [35].

Additionally, Pimecrolimus may act by other mechanisms, possibly by reducing NFAT-2 activity in follicular kertinocytes [36].

Thus, TCIs, by increasing proliferation of melanoblasts and melanocytes, are very useful in the treatment of vitiligo. Twice daily application is needed and can be given for a duration of 12 months. The onset of action is slightly faster than TCS but the repigmentation is less. The repigmentation rates increase when NB-UVB is combined with TCI. Combination of 308 nm excimer laser also has a high response rate [37–40].

Additional double-blind studies showed that 0.1% ointment plus narrowband UVB (NB-UVB) was equal to placebo plus NB-UVB and that twice-daily application was optimal for facial lesions.

Single-blind studies have shown a combination of 308 nm excimer laser plus pimecrolimus 1% cream to be superior to excimer laser only for facial lesions [41].

11.4 Topical Vitamin D 3 Analogues

Vitamin D in the form of 1,25 (OH)2-D acts mainly via the VDR to regulate cell proliferation, differentiation, and immune function, as well as calcium and phosphorus metabolism.

The VDR protein belongs to the nuclear receptor gene family. When the VDR is activated by its ligand 1,25 (OH)2D, the drug-receptor complex, in association with the retinoid X receptor-a (RXR-a) binds to specific deoxyribonucleic acid (DNA)-binding sites called vitamin D response elements, with subsequent induction or repression of the gene that contains these elements.

Thus Vitamin D modulates epidermal differentiation, promoting the formation of the cornified envelope by increasing gene expression and protein levels of involucrin, loricrin, filaggrin, and transglutaminase [42, 43].

It also inhibits production of interleukin (IL)-2, IL-6, and interferon (IFN)-y by T-helper (Th) 1 cells, and IL-17 by Th17 cells, blocks transcription of granulocyte macrophage colony stimulating factor (GM-CSF) messenger ribonucleic acid (mRNA), and inhibits cytotoxic T cell and natural killer cell activity. However, vitamin D increases the activity of T regulatory cells and the production of IL-4 by Th2 cells [44].

Thus, in the given context, Calcipotriene with its immunomodulatory as well as proliferative effect on melanocytes [45–48]. It is a good add on therapy when combined with topical steroids. There are some reports of repigmentation in children even when used as a monotherapy. Combination with NBUVB, however, is not effective.

11.5 Photochemotherapy

11.5.1 Psoralens

Photochemical reactions tend to be chiefly of two types (within the given context of the therapeutic under discussion). Type I (direct) photochemical reactions result in photoaddition of the compound to pyrimidines in deoxyribonucleic acid (DNA), forming monofunctional adducts and cross-linking of adjacent strands of DNA (bifunctional adducts) and conjugation of proteins. Type II (indirect) photochemical reactions result in the production of reactive oxygen species and free radicals that cause damage to cell membranes and cytoplasmic constituents.

Ground state Psoralen molecules are activated to the excited singlet state by absorption of photons in the UVA waveband, with peak absorption between 320 and 330 nm [49]. The singlet state undergoes decay to the triplet state, and given that this is a relatively long-lived state, it is responsible for most photochemical effects.

The aim of treatment is to consistently produce a high level of drug in the target organ (skin) only at the time of exposure to UV radiation.

Stimulation of melanocytes also causes selective immunosuppression [50–52].

Phototherapy with 8-methoxypsoralen (8-MOP) can be used in patients with lesions that cover less than 5% BSA. It can safely be used in children less than 12 years of age, however, systemic PUVA is contraindicated. Topical application of Psoralens can lead to pruritus, edema, erythema, blister formation, and skin necrosis. Treatment with these agents, require strict monitoring [53–55]. 8-MOP 0.001% is to be applied one to three times per week for 30 min. The skin is after this exposed UVA radation at 0.25–0.5 J/cm2. The exposure time is slowly increased by 15–30 s until a maximum dosage and exposure time is achieved which will produce erythema but no burning [56]. After the procedure, it is important to avoid adverse effects and patients should wash away the extra 8-MOP with soap. In addition, sunscreen should be applied [57–59].

11.5.2 Khellin

Khellin is a furanochrome extract obtained from the plant Amnivisnaga. KUVA is khellin application followed by exposure to UVA [59–61]. This stimulates melanogenesis as well as melanocyte proliferation.

11.5.3 Phenylalanine

Phenylalanine is an essential amino acid which initiates melanogenesis and can be used as a photosensitizer topically or artificial UVA light phototherapy in treating vitiligo [62, 63].

11.5.4 Topical Depigmeting Agents

Topical agents such as Hydroquinone and menobenzone cause melanocyte death [64–66]. These agents are approved for vitiligo and should be used only if conventional treatment options have failed and there are extensive lesions. Monobenzyl ether of Hydroquinone, causes irreversible depigmentation. It should be applied twice daily for 1–4 months, following which, depigmentation is seen. Some of the side effects include erythema, burning, and itching [67].

11.5.5 Comparison of Various Topical Therapies

Clobetasol has been found to be superior to pimecrolimus. Combination of clobetasol along with vitamin d analogues like calcipotriol has been found to show good results [68].

11.6 Newer Drugs

11.6.1 Antioxidants

Recent studies in the pathogenesis of vitiligo have shown that reactive oxygen species have a role in the inhibition of melanogenesis. Side effects that can be seen due to the use of superoxide dismutase are transient erythema, pruritus, and peeling [69–71].

11.6.2 Topical 5-Fluorouracil (5 FU)

It is an anti-mitotic agent that helps in vitiligo by inhibiting the immune cells that attack melanocytes. It can stimulate melanocyte reservoirin hair follicles as well as help melanocytes survive in the affected skin [72]. Several studies have shown success in combining mechanical dermabrasion along with topical 5-FU.

11.6.3 Piperine

Piperine along with its analogues stimulates melanocyte replication and are useful in treating conditions where depigmentation is present [73].

11.6.4 Prostaglandin E2 Analogs

PGE2 has got growth stimulatory effects and can regulate the proliferation and maturation of melanocytes. Studies have confirmed its efficacy [74, 75]. Side effects can rarely be seen and includes transient burning sensation of the lips.

11.6.5 Capsaicin and Curcumin

Treatment with antioxidants stops caspase induced apoptosis and increases the antioxidant reserve of the body, decreasing the ROS generation. Topical capsaicin can help in preventing the progress of vitiligo; however, more studies are required to confirm its efficacy [76–78].

11.6.6 Camouflage

Considering the fact that there is a lot of psychosocial trauma associated with vitiligo, camouflage plays a significant role in its management. Dihydroxyacetone (DHA) is a commonly used agent in camouflaging [79–81].

11.6.7 Basic Fibroblast Growth Related Deca-Peptide

Use of basic fibroblast growth factor is based on the theory that decrease in growth factors is responsible for melanocyte death in vitiligo. A randomized controlled trial assessing repigmentation of stable vitiligo lesions has confirmed that deca-peptide along with tacrolimus 0.1% is superior to tacrolimus used as a monotherapy [82–84].

11.6.8 Topical Methotrexate

MTX, within general context, at the cellular level, competitively and reversibly binds to DHFR, which prevents the conversion of dihydrofolate to tetrahydrofolate. Tetrahydrofolate is necessary for the production of 1-carbon units (as a co-factor), which are essential for synthesis of thymidylate and purine nucleotides needed for DNA and RNA synthesis.

Henceforth, MTX inhibits cell division, being specific for the S phase of the normal cell cycle. The effect of MTX on the proliferation of lymphoid cells is greater than its effect on human keratinocytes [85]. It is most likely that MTX acts via an immunosuppressive mechanism, rather than as an antiproliferative agent directed against the keratinocyte. It also blocks migration of activated T cells into certain tissues [86].

Thus, MTX not only inhibits DNA synthesis in immunologically competent cells but also suppresses primary and secondary antibody responses [87–89].

Topical methotrexate has been used successfully in psoriasis. A study by Abdelmaksoud et al. reported repigmentation. Twice daily application of 1% methotrexate for 12 weeks resulted in significant improvement. There were no major local of systemic side effects [90].

11.6.9 Topical Mycophenolate Mofetil

Topical MMF may have a modest effect in treating vitiligo. A pilot study enrolled 30 patients with limited vitiligo and found that after 3 months, 11 patients 36.6% showed repigmentation. No major side effects were observed [91].

11.6.10 Topical JAK Inhibitors

JAK are a family of nonreceptor tyrosine kinases which initiate a variety of intracellular effects in response to various cytokines. There are four members in the JAK family: JAK1, JAK2, JAK3, and Tyk2 can dimerize in different combinations within intracytoplasmic end of cytokine receptors and selectively respond to certain extracellular signals. When JAK activate STAT (signal transducer and activator of transcription) pathways, it results in the production of multiple proinflammatory cytokines including IFN-y, IL-12, and IL-23, and the maturation of dendritic cells [92, 93]. Inhibition of JAK signalling thus, has an overall anti-inflammatory effect, with decreased expression of proinflammatory cytokines [94].

Ruxolitinib 1.5% cream, a JAK 1 and 2 inhibitor has been FDA approved has been FDA approved for the treatment of nonsegmental vitiligo in adults and children aged 12 years and older. Pilot studies done with Tofactinib (Jak 1 and 3 inhibitor) have shown promising results [95].

Table 11.1 summarized the various topical medications used in vitiligo.

Table 11.1 Topical medications used in the treatment of vitiligo

Drug/classification	Mechanism of action	Common examples (where applicable)	Use case
Topical corticosteroids	Antiproliferative Anti-inflammatory Immunosuppressive (T cells/macrophages and dendritic cells)	Clobetasol 0.05% (I) Betamethasone (II) Fluticasone (IV) Hydrocortisone (V)	Monotherapy or in combination
Topical Calcineurin inhibitors	Block Calcineurin mediated transcription of genes encoding cytokines involved in T lymphocytic activity	Tacrolimus (0.1%) Pimecrolinus (1%)	Monotherapy or in combination
Topical vitamin D Analouges	Modulates epidermal differentiation, melanocyte proliferation inhibits pro-inflammatory cytokines, cytotoxic T cells	Calcipotriol Tacalcitol	Mostly in combination
Topical JAK inhibitors	Decreased expression of pro-inflammatory cytokines (anti-inflammatory-effect)	Ruxolitinib cream (1.5%)	Monotherapy or in combination
Topical methotrexate	Inhibits cell division, DNA synthesis of lymphoid cells (T cells) Inhibits T cell migration Suppresses antibody response	Methotrexate gel (1%)	
Topical 5 FU	Anti-mitotic activity on immune cells		May be used in combination with dermabrasion
Photochemotherapy	High level of drug within the target organ (skin) at the instance of UV exposure stimulates melanocytes	Psoralin Khellin Phenylalanine	Monotherapy or in combination

Pigmentary disorders tend to be more perceptible, and thus more important, in populations with darker constitutive pigmentation. The preference for unblemished skin is exceedingly important in cultures in which altered pigmentation may be confused with infectious diseases such as Hansen disease or associated with superstitions. Not only do persons with such dermatoses face the physical consequences of such ailments, but also a variety of social injustices. Thus, management of such ailments, with such far reaching consequences, which extend beyond the mere debility conferred upon by the underlying pathology or otherwise, becomes absolutely imperative under the current socio—cultural times, and such dermatoses are thus, becoming, an ailment of increasing concern, both from the perspective of the individuals suffering as well as their physicians/dermatologists, warranting a holistic approach, when managing such cases.

References

1. Felsten LM, Alikhan A, Petronic-Rosic V. Vitiligo: a comprehensive overview Part II: treatment options and approach to treatment. J Am Acad Dermatol. 2011;65(3):493–514.
2. Birlea SA, Costin GE, Norris DA. Cellular and molecular mechanisms involved in the action of vitamin D analogs targeting vitiligo depigmentation. Curr Drug Targets. 2008;9(4):345–59.
3. Wu CS, Lan CC, Wang LF, Chen GS, Wu CS, Yu HS. Effects of psoralen plus ultraviolet A irradiation on cultured epidermal cells in vitro and patients with vitiligo in vivo. Br J Dermatol. 2007;156:122–9.
4. Jin Y, Santorico SA, Spritz RA. Pediatric to adult shift in vitiligo onset suggests altered environmental triggering. J Invest Dermatol. 2020;140:241–3. €4
5. Regazzetti C, Joly F, Marty C, et al. Transcriptional analysis of vitiligo skin reveals the alteration of WNT pathway: a promising target for repigmenting vitiligo patients. J Invest Dermatol. 2015;135:3105–14.
6. Taïeb A, Picardo M. Clinical practice vitiligo. N Engl Med. 2009;360:160–9.
7. Ezzedine K, Eleftheriadou V, Whitton M, van Geel N. Vitiligo. Lancet. 2015;386:74–84.
8. Taieb A, Picardo M. The definition and assessment of vitiligo: a consensus report of the vitiligo European task force. Pigment Cell Res. 2007;20:27–35.
9. Lacovelli P, Filoni A, Martorina F, et al. Palmoplantar vitiligo: an overlooked entity published correction appears in. J Eur Acad Dermatol Venereol. 2020;34:904; J Eur Acad Dermatol Venereol 2019;33:300–3.
10. Ezzedine K, Lim HW, Suzuki T, et al. Vitiligo global issue consensus conference panelists revised classification/nomenclature of vitiligo and related issues: the vitiligo global issues consensus conference. Pigment Cell Melanoma Res. 2012;25:1-E13.
11. Gan EY, Cario-André M, Pain C, et al. Follicular vitiligo: a report of 8 cases. J Am Acad Dermatol. 2016;74:1178–84.
12. Ezzedine K, Mahe A, van Geel N, et al. Hypochromic vitiligo: delineation of a new entity. Br J Dermatol. 2015;172:716–21.
13. Lee JH, Ju HJ, Seo JM, et al. Comorbidities in patients with vitiligo: a systematic review and meta-analysis. J Invest Dermatol 2023;143:777-789 e6; Gill L, Zarbo A, Isedeh P, et al. Comorbid autoimmune diseases in patients with vitiligo: a cross-sectional study. J Am Acad Dermatol 2016;74:295–302.
14. Vrijman C, Kroon MW, Limpens J, et al. The prevalence of thyroid disease in patients with vitiligo: a systematic review Br J Dermatol. 2012;167:1224–35.

15. Bae JM, Lee JH, Yun JS, Han B, Han TY. Vitiligo and overt thyroid diseases: a nationwide population-based study in Korea. J Am Acad Dermatol. 2017;76:871–8.
16. Zhang XJ, Chen JJ, Liu JB. The genetic concept of vitiligo. J Dermatol Sci. 2005;39:137–46.
17. Sheth VM, Guo Y, Qureshi AA. Comorbidities associated with vitiligo: a ten-year retrospective study. Dermatology. 2013;227:311–5.
18. Chen YT, Chen Y, Hwang CY, et al. Comorbidity profiles in association with vitiligo: a nationwide population-based study in Taiwan. J Eur Acad Dermatol Venereol 2015;29:1362–1369.
19. Silverberg JI, Silverberg NB. Association between vitiligo and atopic disorders: a pilot study. JAMA Dermatol. 2013;149:983–6.
20. Ezzedine K, Eleftheriadou V, Jones H, et al. Psychosocial effects of vitiligo: a systematic literature review. Am J Clin Dermatol. 2021;22:757–74.
21. Zhu ML, Nagavalli A, Su MA. Aire deficiency promotes TRP-1-specific immune rejection of melanoma. Cancer Res. 2013;73:2104–16.
22. Catt K.J, Dufau M.L. Hormone action: control of target cell function by peptide, thyroid and steroid hormones. In: Felig P, Baxter JD, Broadus AE, et al., editors. Endocrinology and metabolism. New York: McGraw-Hill; 1981. p. 61–105; Thompson EB. The structure of the human glucocorticoid receptor and its gene. J Steroid Biochem. 1987;27(1–3):105–8.
23. Lan NC, Karin M, Nguyen T, et al. Mechanisms of glucocorticoid hormone action. J Steroid Biochem. 1984;20(1):77–88.
24. Spindler SR, Mellon SH, Baxter JD. Growth hormone gene transcription is regulated by thyroid. J Biol Chem. 1982;257(19):11627–32.
25. Evans RM, Birnberg NC, Rosenfeld MG. Glucocorticoid and thyroid hormones transcriptionally regulate growth hormone gene expression. Proc Natl Acad Sci USA. 1982;79(24):7659–63.
26. Modified from, Yohn JJ, Weston WL. Topical glucocorticosteroids. Curr Probl Dermatol. 1990;2:38–63.
27. Falabella R, Barona MI. Update on skin repigmentation therapies in vitiligo. Pigment Cell Melanoma Res. 2008;22:42–65.
28. Shenoi SD, Prabhu S. Photochemotherapy (PUVA) in psoriasis and vitiligo. Ind J Dermatol Venereol Leprol. 2014;80:497–504.
29. Van doonBoorn JG, Melief CJ, Luiten RM. Monobenzone induced depigmentation: from enzymatic blockade to autoimmunity. Pigment Cell Melanoma Res. 2011;24:673–9.
30. Gauthier Y, Anbar T, Lepreux S, Cario-André M, Benzekri L. Possible mechanisms by which topical 5fluorouracil and dermabrasion could induce pigment spread in vitiligo skin: an experimental study. ISRN Dermatol. 2013;2013:852497.
31. Faas L, Venkatasamy R, Hider RC, Young AR, Soumyanath A. In vivo evaluation of piperine-and synthetic analogues asn potential treatments for vitiligo using a sparsely pigmented mouse model. Br J Dermatol. 2008;158:941–50.
32. Lan CC, Chen GS, Chiou MH, Wu CS, Chang CH, Yu HS. FK506 promotes melanocyte and melanoblast growth and creates a favourablemilieu for cell migration via keratinocytes: possible mechanisms of how tacrolimus ointment induces repigmentation in patients with vitiligo. Br J Dermatol. 2005;153:498–505.
33. Hartmann A, Brocker EB, Hamm H. Repigmentation of pretibial vitiligo with calcineurin inhibitors under occlusion. J Deutschen Dermatologischen Gesellschaft. 2008;6:383–5.
34. Silverberg NB, Lin P, Travis L, Farley-Li J, Mancini AJ, Wagner AM, et al. Tacrolimus ointment promotes repigmentation of vitiligo in children: a review of 57 cases. J Am AcadDermatol. 2004;51:760–6.
35. Nghiem P, Pearson G, Langley RG. Tacrolimus and pimecrolus: from clever prokaryotes to inhibiting calcinuerin and treating atopic dermatitis. J Am Acad Dermatol. 2002;46:228–41.
36. Fiorentino DF, Chen RO, Stewart DB, Brown KK, Sundram UN. The direct cellular target of topically applied pimecrolimus may not be infiltrating lymphocytes. Br J Dermatol. 2011;164(5):996–1003.

37. Kwinter J, Pelletier J, Khambalia A, Pope E. High-potency steroid use in children with vitiligo: a retrospective study. J Am AcadDermatol. 2007;56:236–41.
38. Lepe V, Moncada B, Castanedo-Cazares JP, Torres-Alvarez MB, Ortiz CA, Torres-Rubalcava AB. A double-blind randomized trial of 0.1% tacrolimus vs 0.05% clobetasol for the treatment of childhood vitiligo. Arch Dermatol. 2003;139:581–5.
39. Coskun B, Saral Y, Turgut D. Topical 0.05% clobetasol propionate versus 1% pimecrolimus ointment in vitiligo. Eur J Dermatol. 2005;15:88–91.
40. Westerhof W, Nieuweboer-Krobotova L, Mulder PG, Glazenburg EJ. Left-right comparison study of the combination of fluticasone propionate and UV-A vs. either fluticasone propionate or UV-A alone for the long-term treatment of vitiligo. Arch Dermatol. 1999;135:1061–6.
41. Esfandiarpour I, Ekhlasi A, Farajzadeh S, Shamsa-dini S. The efficacy of pimecrolimus 1% cream plus narrow-band ultraviolet B in the treatment of vitiligo: a double-blind, placebo-controlled clinical trial, J Dermatolog Treat. 2009;20(1):14–8.
42. Khammissa RAG, Fourie J, Motswaledi MH, Bally-ram R, Lemmer J, Feller L. The biological activities of vitamin D and its receptor in relation to calcium and bone homeostasis, cancer, immune and cardiovascular systems, skin biology, and oral health. Biomed Res Int. 2018;2018:9276380.
43. Bikle DD, Ng D, Tu CL, Oda Y, Xie Z. Calcium- and vitamin D-regulated keratinocyte differentiation. Mol Cell Endocrinol. 2001;177(1–2):161–71.
44. van de Kerkhof PC. An update on vitamin D3 analogues in the treatment of psoriasis. Skin Pharmacol Appl Ski Physiol. 1998;11:2–10.
45. Grimes PE, Morris R, Avaniss-Aghajani E, Soriano T, Meraz M, Metzger A. Topical tacrolimus therapy for vitiligo: therapeutic responses and skin messenger RNA expression of proinflammatory cytokines. J Am AcadDermatol. 2004;51:52–61.
46. Hartmann A, Brocker EB, Hamm H. Occlusive treatment enhances efficacy of tacrolimus 0.1% ointment in adult patients with vitiligo: results of a placebo-controlled 12-month prospective study. Acta Derm Venereol. 2008;88:474–9.
47. Fai D, Cassano N, Vena GA. Narrow-band UVB phototherapy combined with tacrolimus ointment in vitiligo: a review of 110 patients. J Eur Acad Dermatol Venereol. 2007;21:916–20.
48. Nordal E, Guleng G, Ro¨nnevig J. Treatment of vitiligo with narrowband-UVB (TL01) combined with tacrolimus ointment (0.1%) vs. placebo ointment, a randomized right/left double-blindcomparative study. J Eur Acad Dermatol Venereol. 2011;25:1440–3.
49. Cripps DJ, Lowe NJ, Lerner AB. Action spectra of topical psoralens: a re-evaluation. Br J Dermatol. 1982;107:77–82.
50. Epstein JH, Fukuyama K. Effects of 8-methoxyp-soralen-induced phototoxic effects of mammalian epidermal macromolecule synthesis in vivo. Photochem Photobiol. 1975;24:325–30.
51. Fritsch PO, Gschnait F, Kaaserer G, et al. PUVA suppresses the proliferative stimulus produced by stripping on hairless mice. J Invest Dermatol. 1979;73(2):188–90.
52. Anbar TS, El-Sawy AE, Attia SK, et al. Effect of PUVA therapy on melanocytes and keratinocytes in non-segmental vitiligo: histopatho-logical, immuno-histochemical and ultrastructural study. Photodermatol Photoimmunol Photomed. 2012;28(1):17–25.
53. Passeron T, Ostovari N, Zakaria W, Fontas E, Larrouy JC, Lacour JP, et al. Topical tacrolimus and the 308-nm excimer laser: a synergistic combination for the treatment of vitiligo. Arch Dermatol. 2004;140:1065–9.
54. Korobko IV. Review of current clinical studies of vitiligo treatments. Dermatol Ther. 2012;25(S1):S17–27.
55. Kathuria S, Khaitan BK, Ramam M, Sharma VK. Segmental vitiligo: a randomized controlled trial to evaluate efficacy and safety of 0.1% tacrolimus ointment vs 0.05% fluticasone propionate cream. Ind J Dermatol Venereol Leprol. 2012;78:68–73.
56. Juan D, Qianxi X, Zhou C, Jianzhong Z. Clinical efficacy and safety of tacrolimus ointment in patients with vitiligo. J Dermatol. 2011;38:1092–4.

57. Ho N, Pope E, Weinstein M, Greenberg S, Webster C, Krafchik BR. A double-blind, randomized, placebocontrolled trial of topical tacrolimus 0.1% vs. clobetasol propionate 0.05% in childhood vitiligo. Br J Dermatol. 2011;165:626–32.
58. Lee DY, Kim CR, Lee JH, Yang JM. Recent onset vitiligo treated with systemic corticosteroid and topical tacrolimus: need for early treatment in vitiligo. J Dermatol. 2010;37:1057–9.
59. Xu AE, Zhang DM, Wei XD, Huang B, Lu LJ. Efficacy and safety of tarcrolimus cream 0.1% in the treatment of vitiligo. Int J Dermatol. 2009;48:86–90.
60. Mehrabi D, Pandya AG. A randomized, placebo-controlled, double-blind trial comparing narrowband UV-B plus 0.1% tacrolimus ointment with narrowband UV-B plus placebo in the treatment of generalized vitiligo. Arch Dermatol. 2006;142:927–9.
61. De D, Kanwar AJ. Tacrolimus-induced hyperpigmentation in a patch of vitiligo. Skinmed. 2008;7:93–4.
62. Bakos L, Bakos RM. Focal acne during topical tacrolimus therapy for vitiligo. Arch Dermatol. 2007;143:1223–4.
63. US Food and Drug Administration Web site. Available from: www.fda.gov. Accessed 1 Oct 2015.
64. Wong R, Lin AN. Efficacy of topical calcineurin inhibitors in vitiligo. Int J Dermatol. 2013;52(4):491–6.
65. Parsad D, Saini R, Nagpal R. Calcipotriol in vitiligo: a preliminary study. Pediatr Dermatol. 1999;16:317–20.
66. Gargoom AM, Duweb GA, Elzorghany AH, Benghazil M, Bugrein OO. Calcipotriol in the treatment of childhood vitiligo. Int J Clin Pharmacol Res. 2004;24:11–4.
67. Kumaran MS, Kaur I, Kumar B. Effect of topical calcipotriol, betamethasone dipropionate and their combination in the treatment of localized vitiligo. J Eur Acad Dermatol Venereol. 2006;20:269–73.
68. Travis LB, Silverberg NB. Calcipotriene and corticosteroid combination therapy for vitiligo. Pediatr Dermatol. 2004;21:495–8.
69. Newman MD, Silverberg NB. Once-daily application of calcipotriene 0.005%-betamethasone dipropionate 0.064% ointment for repigmentation of facial vitiligo. Cutis. 2011;88:256–9.
70. Arca E, Tastan HB, Erbil AH, Sezer E, Koc E, Kurumlu Z. Narrow-band ultraviolet B as monotherapy and in combination with topical calcipotriol in the treatment of vitiligo. J Dermatol. 2006;33:338–43.
71. Hartmann A, Lurz C, Hamm H, Brocker EB, Hofmann UB. Narrow-band UVB311 nm vs. broad-band UVB therapy in combination with topical calcipotriol vs. placebo in vitiligo. Int J Dermatol. 2005;44:736–42.
72. Ada S, Sahin S, Boztepe G, Karaduman A, Kolemen F. No additional effect of topical calcipotriol on narrow-band UVB phototherapy in patients with generalized vitiligo. Photodermatol Photoimmunol Photomed. 2005;21:79–83.
73. Ortel B, Petronic-Rosic V, Calzavara-Pinton P. Phototherapeutic options for vitiligo. In: Krutmann J, Honigsmann H, Elmets CA, Bergstresser PR, editors. Dermatological phototherapy and photodiagnostic methods. Heidelberg: Springer; 2009. p. 151–83.
74. Orecchia G, Perfetti L. Photochemotherapy with topical khellin and sunlight in vitiligo. Dermatol. 1992;184:120–3.
75. Saraceno R, Nistico SP, Capriotti E, Chimenti S. Monochromatic excimer light 308 nm in monotherapy and combined with topical khellin4% in the treatment of vitiligo: a controlled study. Dermatol Ther. 2009;22:391–4.
76. Greiner D, Ochsendorf FR, Milbradt R. Vitiligo therapy with phenylalanine/UV A. Catamnesticstudies after five years [in German]. Hautarzt. 1994;45:460–3.
77. Lotti T, Buggiani G, Troiano M, Assad GB, Delescluse J, De Giorgi V, et al. Targeted and combination treatments for vitiligo. Comparative evaluation of different current modalities in 458 subjects. Dermatol Ther. 2008;21(S1):S20–6.
78. Camacho F, Mazuecos J. Treatment of vitiligo with oral and topical phenylalanine: 6 years of experience. Arch Dermatol. 1999;135:216–7.

79. Antoniou C, Schulpis H, Michas T, Katsambas A, Frajis N, Tsagaraki S, et al. Vitiligo therapy with oral and topical phenylalanine with UVA exposure. Int J Dermatol. 1989;28:545–7.
80. Hariharan V, Klarquist J, Reust MJ, KoshofferA, McKee MD, Boissy RE, et al. Monobenzylether of hydroquinone and 4-tertiary butyl phenol activate markedly different physiological responses in melanocytes: relevance to skin depigmentation. J Invest Dermatol. 2010;130:211–20.
81. Njoo MD, Vodegel RM, Westerhof W. Depigmentation therapy in vitiligo universalis with topical 4-methoxyphenol and the Qswitchedruby laser. J Am Acad Dermatol. 2000;42:760–9.
82. Kasraee B, Fallahi MR, Ardekani GS Ebrahimi S, Doroudchi G, Omrani GR, et. al. Retinoic acid synergistically enhances the melanocytotoxicand depigmenting effects of monobenzylether of hydroquinone in black Guinea pig skin. Exp Dermatol 2006;15:509–514.
83. Eryilmaz A, Seckin D, Baba M. Pimecrolimus: a new choice in the treatment of vitiligo? J Eur Acad Dermatol Venereol. 2009;23:1327–49.
84. Dawid M, Veensalu M, Grassberger M, Wolff K. Efficacy and safety of pimecrolimus cream 1% in adult patients with vitiligo: results of a randomized, double-blind, vehicle-controlled study. J Dtsch Dermatol Ges. 2006;4:942–6.
85. Jeffes EW 3rd, JL MC, Pittelkow MR, et al. Methotrexate therapy of psoriasis. Differential sensitivity of proliferating lymphoid and epithelial cells to the cytotoxic and growth-inhibitory effects of methotrexate. J Invest Dermatol. 1995;104(2):183–8.
86. Sigmundsdottir H, Johnston A, Gudjonsson JE, Bjarnason B, Valdimarsson H. Methotrexate markedly reduces the expression of vascular E-selectin, cutaneous lymphocyte-associated antigen and the numbers of mononuclear leucocytes in psoriatic skin. Exp Dermatol. 2004;13(7):426–34.
87. Hersh EM, Carbone PP, Wong VG, Freireich EJ. Inhibition of primary immune response in man by antimetabolites. Cancer Res. 1965;25(7):1997–2001.
88. Mitchell MS, Wade ME, DeConti RC, Bertino JR, Calabresi P. Immune suppressive effects of cytosine arabinoside and methotrexate in man. Ann Intern Med. 1969;70(3):535–47.
89. Chan ES, Cronstein BN. Molecular action of metho treate in inflammatory diseases. Arthritis Res. 2002;4(4):266–73.
90. Radakovic S, Breier-Maly J, Konschitzky R, et al. Response of vitiligo to once vs. twice-daily topical tacrolimus: a controlled prospective, randomized, observer-blinded trial. J Eur Acad Dermatol Venereol. 2009;23:951–3.
91. Esfandiarpour I, Ekhlasi A, Farajzadeh S, Shamsadini S. The efficacy of pimecrolimus 1% cream plus narrow-band ultraviolet B in the treatment of vitiligo: a double-blind, placebo-controlled clinical trial. J Dermatolog Treat. 2009;20:14–8.
92. Azevedo A, Torres T. Tofacitinib: a new oral therapy for psoriasis. Clin Drug Investig. 2018;38(2):101–12.
93. Ghoreschi K, Laurence A, O'Shea JJ. Janus kinases in immune cell signaling. Immunol Rev. 2009;228(1):273–87.
94. Hald A, Andrés RM, Salskov-Iversen ML, Kjellerup RB, Iversen L, Johansen C. STAT1 expression and activation is increased in lesional psoriatic skin. Br J Dermatol. 2013;168(2):302–10.
95. Joshipura D, Alomram A, Zancanaro P, Rosmarin D. Treatment of vitiligo with the topical Janus kinase inhibitor ruxolitinib: a 32-week open-label extension study with optical narrow-band UVB. J Am Acad Dermatol Ther. 2020;33(1):e13175.

Chapter 12
Systemic Immunomodulatory and Immunosuppressive Therapies

Rashmi Sarkar and Amit Kumar Meena

Abstract Vitiligo is an autoimmune disease characterized by the presence of depigmented macules over the body. It may have a significant effect on the quality of life and may cause psychological distress to the patient, especially in skin of color. The treatment of vitiligo is aimed at halting the progression of the disease, repigmentation of depigmented patches, and prevention of recurrence. Various treatment modalities used in the management of vitiligo include topical agents, systemic therapies, and phototherapy. These therapies may be used alone or in combination depending on various factors like body surface area involved, age, sites involved, progression of the disease, presence of comorbidities, availability of the treatment, etc. Systemic immunomodulatory and immunosuppressive agents are used in patients with slowly or rapidly progressive disease and patients with extensive body surface area involvement. These immunosuppressive and immunomodulatory agents include corticosteroids, azathioprine, methotrexate, cyclosporine, mycophenolate mofetil, cyclophosphamide, zinc, levamisole, and minocycline. Out of all these agents, systemic corticosteroids in the form of oral mini pulse are most commonly used. Azathioprine and methotrexate may be used when corticosteroids are contraindicated. The definitive role of zinc, levamisole and cyclophosphamide in vitiligo is yet to be proven.

Keywords Azathioprine · Corticosteroids · Immunosuppressive agents · Levamisole · Methotrexate · Minocycline · Oral mini pulse

12.1 Introduction

Vitiligo is a depigmentary disorder characterized by the presence of depigmented macules and patches over the body. These patches of depigmentation occur as a result of autoimmune destruction of melanocytes in the involved area. It affects

R. Sarkar (✉) · A. K. Meena
Department of Dermatology and STD, Lady Hardinge Medical College, New Delhi, Delhi, India

R. Sarkar, V. Narayan R (eds.), *A Concise Guide to The Management of Vitiligo*,
https://doi.org/10.1007/978-981-95-3857-7_12

people of all races and has no gender predilection. The prevalence of vitiligo ranges from 0.5% to 2% of the world population [1]. It may have a significant effect on the quality of life and may cause psychological distress to the patient, especially in skin of color. Treatment is aimed at achieving three targets—halting the progression of disease, repigmentation of depigmented patches, and prevention of recurrence.

12.2 Treatment Modalities in Vitiligo

Various treatment modalities used in the management of vitiligo include:

12.2.1 Topical Therapy

(a) Topical corticosteroids—clobetasol propionate, mometasone furoate, fluticasone propionate
(b) Calcineurin inhibitors—Tacrolimus, pimecrolimus
(c) Vitamin D analogues—calcipotriol, calcitriol

12.2.2 Systemic Therapy

Immunosuppressive and immunomodulatory agents:

(a) Corticosteroids
(b) Azathioprine
(c) Methotrexate
(d) Cyclosporine
(e) Mycophenolate mofetil
(f) Cyclophosphamide
(g) Zinc
(h) Levamisole
(i) Minocycline
(j) Apremilast

12.2.3 Phototherapy

(a) Narrow band ultraviolet B, broad band ultraviolet B, Ultraviolet A

12.3 Rationale of Using Systemic Immunomodulatory and Immunosuppressive Therapies

Although exact etiopathogenesis of vitiligo is still to be elucidated, there are many theories regarding this. The various theories regarding its pathogenesis include autoimmune theory, oxidative stress, viral theory, neural theory, zinc-alpha-2-glycoprotein deficiency, and melanocytorrhagy theory.

Autoimmune hypothesis is one of the most accepted theories proposed in the pathogenesis of vitiligo. In vitiligo, there is abnormality in both the innate and adaptive immune systems, which leads to destruction of melanocytes. There is destruction of melanocytes by the antibody-mediated autoreactive CD8+ T cells through the interferon gamma-mediated signaling [2]. Recurrence of vitiligo is mainly due to the presence of memory T cells which remain in the lesion. Apart from this, there is imbalance between the Th1 and Th2 cytokines [3].

Hence, by modulating the immune response, activity of the vitiligo can be halted and repigmentation may be induced in the depigmented patches of vitiligo.

12.4 Systemic Immunomodulatory and Immunosuppressive Therapies

The various immunomodulatory and immunosuppressive therapies used in vitiligo are mentioned in Table 12.1 along with their adverse effects and monitoring guidelines.

Indication Patients with progressive disease and extensive body surface area involvement.

12.4.1 Corticosteroids

Mechanism of Action Corticosteroids have broad-spectrum immunosuppressive activity, both on the innate as well as adaptive immune system. They act by binding to a cytoplasmic receptor which regulates gene transcription of the inflammatory pathways and cause production of anti-inflammatory proteins. This leads to inhibition of autoantibody formation, inhibits T cell activity, and also causes apoptosis of cytotoxic T cells. Corticosteroids also lead to reduced levels of serum melanocyte autoantibodies and antibody titers to melanocyte surface antigens [2].

Corticosteroids are used in the form of daily oral corticosteroids, oral mini pulse, or intravenous form. Out of these, OMP is the most commonly used form of corticosteroid in vitiligo. It refers to use of supra-pharmacologic doses in an intermittent manner to increase the therapeutic effect and at the same time decrease the side

Table 12.1 Adverse effects and monitoring guidelines of systemic immunomodulatory and immunosuppressive therapies used in vitiligo

Drug	Adverse effects	Monitoring
Corticosteroids	HPA axis suppression, hypertension, hyperglycemia, osteoporosis, increased risk of infection, weight gain, acneiform eruption, menstrual disturbance, hypertrichosis, cataract, glaucoma	Baseline monitoring: Screening for tuberculosis, hepatitis B, hepatitis C, human immunodeficiency virus, fasting blood sugar, lipid profile, serum potassium levels and bone densitometry Serum potassium levels, fasting glucose and triglycerides should be repeated at 1 month and then every 3–4 monthly
Azathioprine	Bone marrow suppression, hepatotoxicity, gastric irritation, increased risk of infection and nonmelanoma skin cancer in transplant patients	Baseline monitoring: complete blood count, liver function test, kidney function test, thiopurine methyltransferase assay, urine analysis, screening for tuberculosis, hepatitis B, hepatitis C, human immunodeficiency virus Complete blood count and liver function test should be done biweekly for the first 2 months then every 2–3 monthly
Methotrexate	Bone marrow suppression, hepatotoxicity, increased risk of infection, gastrointestinal disturbance	Baseline: complete blood count, liver function test, hepatitis B, hepatitis C, human immunodeficiency virus, screening for tuberculosis Complete blood count and liver function test after 5–6 days of test dose. Then every 1–2 weeks for initial 2–4 weeks then every 3–4 monthly
Cyclosporine	Hypertension, nephrotoxicity, deranged lipid profile, hyperkalemia, hyperuricemia, hypomagnesemia, tremor, paresthesia, nausea, diarrhea	Baseline: Complete blood count, liver function test, kidney function test, fasting lipid profile, serum magnesium, potassium and uric acid Complete blood count, liver function test, kidney function test, lipid profile, serum magnesium, potassium, uric acid levels should be done every 2 weekly for the first 1–2 months, then every monthly

(continued)

Table 12.1 (continued)

Drug	Adverse effects	Monitoring
Mycophenolate mofetil	Increased risk of infection, nausea, diarrhea, abdominal cramps, dose dependent neutropenia, anemia, thrombocytopenia, lymphoproliferative disorders, nonmelanoma skin cancer	Baseline: complete blood count, liver function test, kidney function test, hepatitis B, hepatitis C, human immunodeficiency virus, screening for tuberculosis, serum or urine β-human chorionic gonadotropin Complete blood count, liver function test and kidney function should be repeated every 2–4 weeks following dose escalation and every 2–3 months once dose is stable. Serum or urine β-human chorionic gonadotropin test should be repeated monthly
Cyclophosphamide	Nausea, vomiting, bone marrow suppression, hemorrhagic cystitis, gonadal toxicity (amenorrhea, azoospermia, ovarian failure), anagen effluvium, pigmentation of skin and nails	Baseline: Complete blood count, liver function test, kidney function test, urinalysis, serum pregnancy test Complete blood count and urinalysis should be performed weekly for 2–3 months, then biweekly after 2–3 months and then monthly with stable dose. Liver function test and kidney function test should be performed monthly and then after 3–6 months
Zinc	Nausea, vomiting, diarrhea	No routine lab monitoring is required
Levamisole	Nausea, abdominal cramps, flu-like syndrome, arthralgia, agranulocytosis, psychosis, lichenoid eruptions	No routine lab monitoring is required
Minocycline	Nausea, abdominal discomfort, pill esophagitis, hyperpigmentation of skin, teeth, nail bed and mucous membrane, photosensitivity, hypersensitivity reactions like urticaria, fixed drug eruption, lupus like syndrome, autoimmune hepatitis, pseudotumor cerebri	No baseline monitoring is required. However, in the long term, periodic laboratory evaluation of organ systems, including hematopoietic, renal and hepatic functions should be done
Apremilast	Diarrhea, abdominal pain, suicidal ideation, hypersensitivity to apremilast	No routine lab monitoring is required

effects of daily corticosteroids. In a study by Pasricha et al. [4], 5 mg of betamethasone/dexamethasone was given on two consecutive days per week. In this study, 36 patients with active vitiligo were recruited. Within 1–3 months of treatment with OMP, progression of the disease was arrested in 89% of the patients.

Kim et al. [5], in their study, recruited 81 patients with active vitiligo and treated them with oral prednisolone at 0.3 mg/kg body weight. At the end of 4 months, stabilization of vitiligo and repigmentation were observed in 87.7% and 70.4% of the patients respectively. In a recent study, 500 mg of intravenous methylprednisolone was given on three consecutive days which leads to arrest of disease progression in 56% of the patients [6].

For treatment of active vitiligo, corticosteroids are usually given for a period of at least 3–6 months.

12.4.2 *Azathioprine*

Mechanism of Action It is a purine analogue that acts by suppressing DNA and RNA synthesis. This leads to inhibition of B cell and T cell proliferation and function.

In a study by Madarkar et al. [7], oral azathioprine (100 mg) was compared with betamethasone OMP (5 mg on two consecutive days per week) for a period of 6 months. Both drugs were found to be equally effective at the end of 6 months.

In a study by Radmanesh et al. [8], 60 patients were recruited and were randomized into two groups. Group 1 received azathioprine 0.6–0.75 mg/kg/day in combination with oral psoralen plus ultraviolet A (PUVA) while group 2 received PUVA alone. Patients in group 1 developed earlier repigmentation (five PUVA sessions) as compared to group 2 (eight PUVA sessions). Similarly, repigmentation was also seen in a greater percentage of patients in group 1 (58.4%) as compared to group 2 (24.8%).

In patients with progressive vitiligo, a randomized study was done in which group A received OMP (betamethasone 5 mg on two consecutive days per week) and group B received azathioprine 50 mg twice daily. A greater percentage of patients in group A achieved halting of the disease progression at 2 and 4 months. However, at the end of 6 months the difference was not significant in both groups [9].

Azathioprine may be used in patients with progressive vitiligo when steroids are contraindicated. However, regular blood monitoring should be done to monitor for any adverse effects.

12.4.3 *Methotrexate*

Mechanism of Action Methotrexate is a folic acid antagonist and acts as an immunomodulatory, anti-inflammatory and anti-proliferative agent. In vitiligo, it increases the levels of anti-inflammatory cytokines (IL-4, 10) and decreases levels of inflammatory cytokines (IL-1, 2, 6, IFN-γ). It also decreases levels of TNF-α by inhibiting T cells [10].

There is limited data on the use of methotrexate in vitiligo. Singh et al. [11], in a prospective randomized comparative study, compared low-dose oral methotrexate (10 mg/week) with oral mini pulse (dexamethasone 2.5 mg on two consecutive days per week). At the end of the study, both groups had similar reduction in the vitiligo disease activity (VIDA) score. During the treatment period, disease stabilization was achieved in 76% and 72% of the patients in the methotrexate and OMP groups, respectively, which was not statistically significant.

In a study from Egypt, 42 patients with vitiligo were recruited to assess the efficacy and safety of oral methotrexate and dexamethasone oral mini pulse for a period of 3 months. Group A received 15 mg of methotrexate divided into three doses with a 12 hourly weekly interval. Group B received 5 mg of dexamethasone on two consecutive days per week and group C received a combination of both. This study reported a significant decrease in vitiligo extension in group C as compared to the other two groups [12].

A pilot study from Saudi Arabia on six vitiligo patients reported no improvement with 25 mg weekly methotrexate for 6 months [13].

Methotrexate may be used in rapidly progressive vitiligo patients when corticosteroids are contraindicated.

12.4.4 Cyclosporine

Mechanism of Action It binds to cyclophilin and inhibits calcineurin, which activates nuclear factor of activated T cells, a transcription factor that is required for interleukin-2 (IL-2) regulation. This IL-2 is an important cytokine that is required for T cell pathway activation [14]. In vitiligo, it acts by decreasing macrophages, T lymphocytes and Langerhans cells in the skin [10].

Taneja et al. [15] conducted an open-label study on 18 patients with progressive vitiligo. All patients were treated with 3 mg/kg/day of cyclosporine for a period of 12 weeks. At the end of 3 months, 61% of patients reported arrest of disease progression which was assessed using Vitiligo Area Scoring Index (VASI).

Metha et al. [16], compared oral cyclosporine (3 mg/kg/day) with dexamethasone oral mini pulse (2.5 mg on two consecutive days per week) in active vitiligo patients. Both treatments were given for a period of 4 months and patients were followed up for another 2 months after stopping treatment. There was no significant difference in arrest of disease progression assessed by change of Vitiligo Disease Activity Index from 4+ to 3+ at 6 months. However, the mean time to arrest disease progression was significantly lower in the cyclosporine group as compared to the OMP group.

There are only a few studies on the efficacy of cyclosporine in vitiligo. At present, more well-controlled prospective studies are required for establishing the efficacy of cyclosporine in vitiligo.

12.4.5 *Mycophenolate Mofetil*

Mechanism of Action It acts by inhibiting inosine-5′-monophosphate dehydrogenase, an enzyme required for de novo synthesis of guanine nucleotides and subsequently DNA synthesis. It specifically affects B and T lymphocytes as they are dependent on de novo purine synthesis [17].

In a randomized, investigator-blinded study from India, 50 vitiligo patients with vitiligo disease activity score of four were recruited and were randomized into two groups. Group A received dexamethasone OMP (2.5 mg on two consecutive days per week) and group B received mycophenolate mofetil (up to 2 gm) for 180 days followed by 90 days drug-free period. Disease stabilization of vitiligo was assessed using vitiligo disease activity index 2+ and no significant difference was observed between both groups in disease stabilization [18].

12.4.6 *Cyclophosphamide*

Mechanism of action It exerts its effects mainly by causing alkylation of deoxyribonucleic acid (DNA). Apart from its anti-neoplastic and anti-mitotic effects, it also has immunosuppressive effects particularly on T cells.

The data regarding use of cyclophosphamide in vitiligo is very limited. In a study, 50 mg of cyclophosphamide was given twice daily in 33 cases. Out of these, 29 cases showed good repigmentation. However, the side effects observed with cyclophosphamide were very severe [19].

12.4.7 *Zinc*

Mechanism of Action It acts as a metal co-factor for superoxide dismutase, an enzyme responsible for the elimination of free radicals. It has anti-oxidant and immunomodulatory properties and also alters melanin production in melanocytes [20].

In a study by Yaghoobi et al. [21], topical steroid was compared with oral zinc in combination with topical corticosteroid, the mean response rate was found to be higher in the combination group as compared to the steroid group alone. However, the difference was not statistically significant between both the groups.

12.4.8 Levamisole

Mechanism of Action It is an anti-helminthic drug and is used in vitiligo as it has immunomodulatory properties.

In a study by Pasricha et al., levamisole was used in patients with limited and slowly spreading vitiligo at a dose of 150 mg on two consecutive days per week for a duration ranging from 4 to 48 months. Out of the total 36 patients with active disease, 34 (94%) of the patients reported halting of the disease [22]. However, in another study levamisole was compared with placebo in patients with limited and slowly progressive vitiligo. The mean number of new lesions developed during the study period of 6 months was similar in both groups [23].

12.4.9 Minocycline

Mechanism of Action Minocycline has anti-inflammatory, immunomodulatory, free-radical scavenging agent properties, and also has anti-apoptotic properties. In vitro studies have shown that minocycline protects melanocytes against hydrogen peroxide-induced death [24].

In a preliminary study, 32 patients with slowly progressive vitiligo were treated with 100 mg minocycline daily. It was effective in halting the disease progression in 90.62% of the patients [25]. In a randomized controlled study, oral minocycline (100 mg once daily) was compared with dexamethasone oral mini pulse (2.5 mg on two consecutive days per week) for 6 months. Patients in both groups reported significant reduction in the vitiligo severity scores. However, there was no difference in arresting the activity of disease in both the groups [26].

12.4.10 Apremilast

Mechanism of Action It is a phosphodiesterase 4 inhibitor and increases intracellular cyclic adenosine monophosphate (cAMP). This increase in cAMP results in an increase in anti-inflammatory cytokines like IL-10 and a decrease in pro-inflammatory cytokines like IL-17, IL-23, TNF-α, IFN-γ) [27].

In a case series of 13 patients with rapidly progressive non-segmental vitiligo, apremilast 30 mg was given twice daily for 3 months after initial titration. On exposed parts of the body, they also applied tacrolimus 0.1% twice daily. All patients reported stabilization and partial repigmentation was noticed in 61.5% of the patients [28].

12.5 Conclusion

In patients with slowly progressive and rapidly progressive vitiligo, systemic immunosuppressive and immunomodulatory agents are required to halt the progression of the disease. Of all these agents, systemic corticosteroids in the form of oral mini pulse are most commonly used. Azathioprine and methotrexate may be used when corticosteroids are contraindicated. The role of zinc, levamisole, and cyclophosphamide in vitiligo is yet to be proven.

References

1. Krüger C, Schallreuter KU. A review of the worldwide prevalence of vitiligo in children/adolescents and adults. Int J Dermatol. 2012;51(10):1206–12.
2. Ju HJ, Bae JM. Bridging molecular mechanism and clinical practice in vitiligo treatment: an updated review. Dermatology. 2024;240(3):474–86.
3. Chang WL, Lee WR, Kuo YC, Huang YH. Vitiligo: an autoimmune skin disease and its immunomodulatory therapeutic intervention. Front Cell Dev Biol. 2021;9:797026.
4. Pasricha JS, Khaitan BK. Oral mini-pulse therapy with betamethasone in vitiligo patients having extensive or fast-spreading disease. Int J Dermatol. 1993;32(10):753–7.
5. Kim SM, Lee HS, Hann SK. The efficacy of low-dose oral corticosteroids in the treatment of vitiligo patients. Int J Dermatol. 1999;38(7):546–50.
6. Wada-Irimada M, Tsuchiyama K, Sasaki R, Hatchome N, Watabe A, Kimura Y, et al. Efficacy and safety of i.v. methylprednisolone pulse therapy for vitiligo: a retrospective study of 58 therapy experiences for 33 vitiligo patients. J Dermatol. 2021;48(7):1090–3.
7. Madarkar M, Ankad BS, Manjula R. Comparative study of safety and efficacy of Oral betamethasone pulse therapy and azathioprine in vitiligo. Clin Dermatol Rev. 2019;3(2):121.
8. Radmanesh M, Saedi K. The efficacy of combined PUVA and low-dose azathioprine for early and enhanced repigmentation in vitiligo patients. J Dermatol Treat. 2006;17(3):151–3.
9. Patra S, Khaitan BK, Sharma VK, Khanna N. A randomized comparative study of the effect of betamethasone oral mini-pulse therapy versus oral azathioprine in progressive nonsegmental vitiligo. J Am Acad Dermatol. 2021;85(3):728–9.
10. Fatima S, Abbas T, Refat MA, Harris JE, Lim HW, Hamzavi IH, et al. Systemic therapies in vitiligo: a review. Int J Dermatol. 2023;62(3):279–89.
11. Singh H, Kumaran MS, Bains A, Parsad D. A randomized comparative study of oral corticosteroid minipulse and low-dose oral methotrexate in the treatment of unstable vitiligo. Dermatol Basel Switz. 2015;231(3):286–90.
12. ElGhareeb MI, Metwalli M, AbdelMoneim N. Combination of oral methotrexate and oral mini-pulse dexamethasone vs either agent alone in vitiligo treatment with follow up by dermoscope. Dermatol Ther. 2020;33(4):e13586.
13. AlGhamdi K, Khurrum H. Methotrexate for the treatment of generalized vitiligo. Saudi Pharm J SPJ. 2013;21(4):423–4.
14. Amor KT, Ryan C, Menter A. The use of cyclosporine in dermatology: part I. J Am Acad Dermatol. 2010;63(6):925–46.
15. Taneja A, Kumari A, Vyas K, Khare AK, Gupta LK, Mittal AK. Cyclosporine in treatment of progressive vitiligo: an open-label, single-arm interventional study. Indian J Dermatol Venereol Leprol. 2019;85:528.

16. Mehta H, Kumar S, Parsad D, Bishnoi A, Vinay K, Kumaran MS. Oral cyclosporine is effective in stabilizing active vitiligo: results of a randomized controlled trial. Dermatol Ther. 2021;34(5):e15033.
17. Orvis AK, Wesson SK, Breza TS, Church AA, Mitchell CL, Watkins SW. Mycophenolate mofetil in dermatology. J Am Acad Dermatol. 2009;60(2):183–99.
18. Bishnoi A, Vinay K, Kumaran MS, Parsad D. Oral mycophenolate mofetil as a stabilizing treatment for progressive non-segmental vitiligo: results from a prospective, randomized, investigator-blinded pilot study. Arch Dermatol Res. 2021;313(5):357–65.
19. Gokhale BB. Cyclophosphamide and vitiligo. Int J Dermatol. 1979;18(1):92.
20. Bagherani N, Yaghoobi R, Omidian M. Hypothesis: zinc can be effective in treatment of vitiligo. Indian J Dermatol. 2011;56(5):480–4.
21. Yaghoobi R, Omidian M, Bagherani N. Original article title: "Comparison of therapeutic efficacy of topical corticosteroid and oral zinc sulfate-topical corticosteroid combination in the treatment of vitiligo patients: a clinical trial.". BMC Dermatol. 2011;11:7.
22. Pasricha J s, Khera V. Effect of prolonged treatment with levamisole on vitiligo with limited and slow-spreading disease. Int J Dermatol. 1994;33(8):584–7.
23. Agarwal S, Ramam M, Sharma VK, Khandpur S, Pal H, Pandey RM. A randomized placebo-controlled double-blind study of levamisole in the treatment of limited and slowly spreading vitiligo. Br J Dermatol. 2005;153(1):163–6.
24. Song X, Xu A, Pan W, Wallin B, Kivlin R, Lu S, et al. Minocycline protects melanocytes against H2O2-induced cell death via JNK and p38 MAPK pathways. Int J Mol Med. 2008;22(1):9–16.
25. Parsad D, Kanwar A. Oral minocycline in the treatment of vitiligo–a preliminary study. Dermatol Ther. 2010;23(3):305–7.
26. Singh A, Kanwar AJ, Parsad D, Mahajan R. Randomized controlled study to evaluate the effectiveness of dexamethasone oral minipulse therapy versus oral minocycline in patients with active vitiligo vulgaris. Indian J Dermatol Venereol Leprol. 2014;80(1):29–35.
27. Kubelis-López DE, Zapata-Salazar NA, Said-Fernández SL, Sánchez-Domínguez CN, Salinas-Santander MA, Martínez-Rodríguez HG, et al. Updates and new medical treatments for vitiligo (review). Exp Ther Med 2021;22(2):797.
28. Majid I, Imran S, Batool S. Apremilast is effective in controlling the progression of adult vitiligo: a case series. Dermatol Ther. 2019;32(4):e12923.

Chapter 13
Small Molecules and Biologic Therapies

Hitaishi Mehta and Kumari Sweta Leena Patra

Abstract Vitiligo is a multifaceted disorder with diverse etiological factors, including genetic predisposition, oxidative stress, autoimmune responses, and neurogenic influences. Recent research has focused on the interferon-gamma (IFN-γ) and CXCL9/10-CXCR3 axis, and the JAK/STAT pathway, highlighting their roles in melanin production inhibition, melanocyte apoptosis, and immune cell recruitment. Cytokines like IL-15, IL-17/23, and TNF-α and pathways such as the Wnt/β-catenin, regulatory T cells (Tregs), heat shock protein 70i (HSP70i), and microRNAs (miRNAs) have also been implicated in vitiligo pathogenesis. This chapter examines small molecules and biologics targeting these pathways, detailing their mechanisms, therapeutic outcomes, and clinical statuses. Apremilast, a phosphodiesterase-4 inhibitor, has shown mixed results in clinical studies. JAK inhibitors, particularly topical ruxolitinib and oral tofacitinib, have demonstrated promising repigmentation effects. WNT signaling agonists and miRNA-based therapies are emerging areas of interest. Enhancing Tregs through direct infusion or microbiota modulation shows potential in regulating immune responses. Afamelanotide, targeting MC1R, promotes repigmentation and reduces oxidative stress. Biologics targeting inflammatory mediators like TNF-α, IL-17/23, and IFN-γ-CXCL9/10-CXCR3 axis offer new therapeutic avenues. However, adverse effects, such as infection risk and cardiovascular concerns, necessitate thorough patient evaluation and monitoring. As research progresses, personalized and targeted therapies for vitiligo are becoming increasingly viable, offering hope for more effective and safer treatments.

Keywords Vitiligo · Melanocyte destruction · IFN-γ/CXCL9/10-CXCR3 axis · JAK/STAT pathway · Apremilast · JAK inhibitors · Wnt signaling · miRNA therapy · Regulatory T cells (Tregs) · Afamelanotide · TNF-α inhibitors · IL-17/23 inhibitors · PD-1/PD-L1 axis · Inflammatory mediators · Depigmentation treatment

---

H. Mehta (✉) · K. S. L. Patra
Department of Dermatology, Venereology and Leprology, Post Graduate Institute of Medical Education and Research, Chandigarh, India

R. Sarkar, V. Narayan R (eds.), *A Concise Guide to The Management of Vitiligo*,
https://doi.org/10.1007/978-981-95-3857-7_13

13.1 Introduction

Vitiligo is a complex disorder with a multifaceted etiology that remains to be fully deciphered. Various theories have been proposed to explain its causes, including genetic predisposition, oxidative stress, autoimmune responses, neurogenic influences, melanocytorrhagy, apoptosis, and other factors. Recent studies have highlighted the role of interferon-gamma (IFN-γ) and the chemokine ligand 9/10-chemokine receptor 3 (CXCL9/10-CXCR3) axis, which inhibit melanin production, induce melanocyte apoptosis, and recruit immune cells to the epidermis [1]. These processes are intricately linked to the Janus kinase/signal transducer and activator of transcription (JAK/STAT) pathway. Additionally, cytokines such as interleukin-15 (IL-15), IL-17/23, tumor necrosis factor-alpha (TNF-α), Wnt/β--catenin signaling pathway, regulatory T cells (Tregs), heat shock protein 70i (HSP70i), and various microRNAs (miRNAs) have been implicated in the pathogenesis of vitiligo [2]. This chapter delves into the role of small molecules and biologics that target these pathways, examining their mechanisms of action, therapeutic outcomes, and current clinical statuses in the treatment of vitiligo. Figure 13.1 shows several small molecules and biologics that have been utilized or are upcoming options for the management of vitiligo.

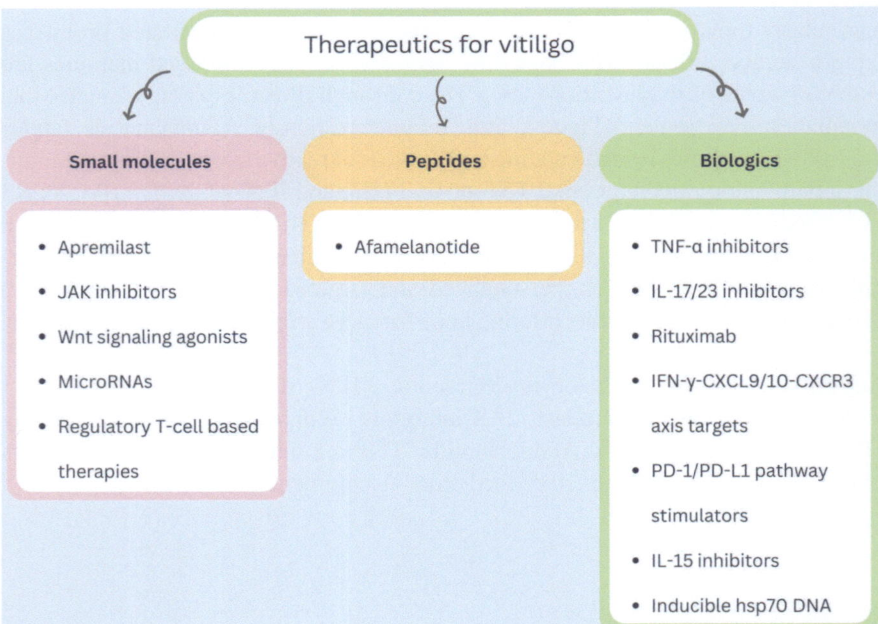

Fig. 13.1 Small molecules, peptides, and biologics for the management of vitiligo

13.2 Small Molecules

13.2.1 Apremilast

Apremilast, a phosphodiesterase-4 inhibitor, may promote repigmentation in vitiligo by activating the cAMP pathway, which enhances melanocyte proliferation and melanogenesis while simultaneously halting disease progression through its anti-inflammatory effects by reducing T helper 1, IL-17, CXCL9, and CXCL10 production. However, studies have produced conflicting results. In an Indian study recruiting 13 vitiligo patients, every patient showed disease stabilization after 3 months, with 8 patients (61.5%) experiencing repigmentation, and there was an average decrease of 7.11% in the Vitiligo Area Scoring Index (VASI) [3]. In contrast, a randomized controlled trial (RCT) involving 80 vitiligo patients with skin types I–III over a period of 52 weeks found that adding apremilast to narrowband UV-B (NB-UVB) therapy did not provide any additional benefit compared to NB-UVB therapy alone, as both groups experienced similar reductions in the VASI [4]. A split-body RCT of 28 patients with skin types IV-VI compared NB-UVB alone, apremilast alone, and a combination of the two [5]. The combination therapy expedited repigmentation more effectively than either treatment alone. Additionally, several case reports have documented arrest of disease progression and repigmentation with apremilast treatment [6].

13.2.2 JAK Inhibitors

The JAK family, comprising JAK1, JAK2, JAK3, and TYK2, plays a critical function in the JAK/STAT pathway, facilitating diverse cellular responses such as proliferative signaling, differentiation, migration, and apoptosis regulation. Among the JAK inhibitors currently available, topical ruxolitinib 1.5% is approved for use in patients aged 12 years and older for treating nonsegmental vitiligo (NSV) [7]. No oral JAK inhibitor has yet been approved for managing vitiligo. Nonetheless, the off-label use of various JAK inhibitors in vitiligo treatment has shown promise. Understanding the efficacy and safety profiles of these drugs is essential for assessing their risk-benefit balance.

13.2.2.1 Mechanism of Action

Oral JAK inhibitors target key cytokine pathways implicated in the pathogenesis of vitiligo by inhibiting the JAK signaling pathways. Additionally, these drugs activate Sonic Hedgehog and Wnt signaling, promoting repigmentation by stimulating the migration, multiplication, and differentiation of melanocytes [8].

JAK inhibitors act primarily on the IFN-γ/CXCL9/10 axis and IL-15, which are crucial in maintaining inflammation and immune responses in vitiligo. IL-15 produced by keratinocytes under oxidative stress interacts with its receptor on resident memory T cells (TRMs), leading to the production of IFN-γ and the recruitment of cytotoxic T cells and other immune cells to the skin. By inhibiting JAK1/JAK2 for IFN-γ signaling and JAK1/JAK3 for IL-15 signaling, oral JAK inhibitors reduce the activation and maintenance of these proinflammatory pathways [9]. This systemic inhibition helps mitigate the inflammatory environment and prevent melanocyte destruction, offering a promising therapeutic approach for vitiligo.

13.2.2.2 Clinical Use

Oral JAK inhibitors used in vitiligo management include first-generation nonselective inhibitors like baricitinib and tofacitinib and second-generation drugs such as upadacitinib and povorcitinib (selective JAK1 inhibitors), ritlecitinib (selective JAK3 inhibitor), and brepocitinib (TYK2 inhibitor) [10].

In a study on NSV, 15 patients received oral tofacitinib (5 mg bid) with topical therapies and NB-UVB treatment for 16 weeks. A control group of 19 patients received only topical therapies and NB-UVB phototherapy. By week 8, the combination therapy group showed significantly higher repigmentation rates compared to controls, continuing through week 16, where the combination therapy achieved near-complete repigmentation (VASI 1.50 ± 1.52) versus less improvement in the control group (VASI 12.68 ± 11.87), highlighting tofacitinib efficacy in enhancing repigmentation in NSV, with no serious adverse events [11].

Baricitinib, an inhibitor of JAK1/2, has demonstrated repigmentation in vitiligo patients in a few case reports [12]. A phase 2 clinical trial (NCT04822584) investigating the effects of a combination therapy of 4 mg/day baricitinib and NB-UVB demonstrated superiority over placebo and NB-UVB in terms of both repigmentation and improvement in quality-of-life measures [13].

A prospective case series compared the efficacy of tofacitinib, baricitinib, and upadacitinib in treating NSV. At month 6, the average reduction in VASI was 41.72% for tofacitinib, 35.15% for baricitinib, and 41.90% for upadacitinib [14]. All three treatments also significantly decreased serum CXCL10 levels [14].

Ritlecitinib (PF-06651600), a selective JAK3 and TEC kinase inhibitor, has been used in treating moderate-to-severe RA. Phase 2a study results reported the efficacy of ritlecitinib, with a percent decrease in facial VASI after 24 weeks being significantly higher in the 200/50 mg, 100/50 mg, and 50 mg groups compared to placebo ($p < 0.05$) [15]. A registered trial (NCT03715829) is being conducted comparing the efficacy of ritlecitinib and brepocitinib (an oral TYK2/JAK1 inhibitor) in vitiligo treatment, both with and without NB-UVB [16].

Table 13.1 summarizes the therapeutic outcomes and status of various oral JAK inhibitors in vitiligo [11, 15, 17–19].

Table 13.1 Current evidence on JAK inhibitor use in vitiligo

Drug	Mechanism of action	Therapeutic outcomes	Current status
Tofacitinib	JAK1/3 inhibitor	Combination therapy group receiving oral tofacitinib (5 mg bid) with topical corticosteroid (halometasone cream, tacrolimus 0.1% ointment, or pimecrolimus cream) and NB-UVB achieved near-complete repigmentation with a VASI of 1.50 ± 1.52, compared to the control group treated only with topical therapies and NB-UVB, which showed less improvement with a VASI of 12.68 ± 11.87, from baseline scores of 15.55 ± 13.40 and 18.14 ± 17.78, respectively [11]	Approved for other indications; additional studies needed for vitiligo
Ritlecitinib	JAK3/TEC inhibitor	Significant repigmentation compared to placebo in %CFB in F-VASI at week 24 (−21.2 vs. 2.1, $p < 0.001$). Consistent improvement through week 48 [15]	Phase 3 study ongoing
Upadacitinib	Selective JAK1 inhibitor	Average improvement in pigmentation: 51.4% in facial vitiligo and 16.8% in acral vitiligo. Primary endpoint achieved in % change from baseline in F-VASI at week 24 with improvements in 11 mg (−35.6%) and 22 mg (−34.0%) vs. placebo (−14.4%; $p \leq 0.01$ and $p \leq 0.05$, respectively) [17]	Phase 3 study ongoing
Povorcitinib	Selective JAK1 inhibitor	Statistically superior T-VASI change from baseline at week 24 compared to placebo: −19.1%, −17.8%, −15.7%, and + 2.3% for 15 mg, 45 mg, 75 mg, and placebo, respectively ($p < 0.01$). Higher F-VASI50 percentages at week 24 for 15, 45, and 75 mg (16.3%, 34.9%, and 23.8%) compared to placebo (7.0%). Improved repigmentation at week 52 [18]	Phase 2b completed
Baricitinib	JAK1/2 selective inhibitor	At week 36, %CFB for T-VASI and F-VASI scores were − 44.8% ($p = 0.0223$) and − 65.2% ($p = 0.0011$) in the baricitinib + NB-UVB group, and − 9.2% and + 4.2% in the placebo + NB-UVB group [19]	Phase 2b completed

%CFB percentage change from baseline, *F-VASI* Facial Vitiligo Area Scoring Indexm *JAK* Janus kinase, *NB-UVB* narrowband ultraviolet B, *T-VASI* Total Vitiligo Area Scoring Index, *VASI* Vitiligo Area Scoring Index

13.2.2.3 Adverse Effects and Cautions

Adverse effects are typically mild and include nasopharyngitis, upper respiratory and urinary tract infections, headache, and gastrointestinal adverse effects such as nausea and diarrhea. However, more severe adverse events can occur, warranting thorough patient evaluation and continuous monitoring.

Infection risk is notably heightened with JAK inhibitors, with the increased incidence of herpes zoster being particularly significant. In cases where herpes zoster develops, a JAK inhibitor should be temporarily discontinued until the infection is resolved and antiviral treatment is completed. Tuberculosis is another serious infection risk, with occurrences noted in both primary and reactivation cases. Screening for latent tuberculosis is essential prior to initiating therapy. Opportunistic infections such as invasive candidiasis, pneumocystis pneumonia, cytomegalovirus disease, and cryptococcosis have also been reported [20].

Cardiovascular concerns include dyslipidemia and a potential increase in major adverse cardiovascular events (MACE). Dyslipidemia manifests as elevated levels of total cholesterol, HDL, and LDL, typically appearing within 12 weeks of treatment initiation. While some studies have shown a potential link between JAK inhibitors and an elevated risk of MACEs, especially in patients with preexisting atherosclerotic disease, other studies have not consistently supported this association [21, 22]. Venous thromboembolic events, including pulmonary embolism, pose a dose-dependent increased risk, prompting the need for vigilance and possible adjustment of treatment in patients with a history of thromboembolic disorders.

Malignancy risks with JAK inhibitors are debated, with mixed findings from various studies. While some trials indicate an increased risk [21], particularly for lung cancer and lymphoma in patients with cardiovascular risk factors, observational studies have not consistently confirmed these results [21].

Hematologic adverse events include lymphopenia, neutropenia, and anemia. These conditions generally require temporary interruption of treatment and possible dose adjustments. Deranged liver enzymes and gastrointestinal perforations have also been observed, necessitating careful monitoring of liver function and gastrointestinal health, particularly in patients with a history of diverticulitis.

Table 13.2 provides an overview of the JAK inhibitors currently in use for vitiligo.

13.2.3 WNT Signaling and Its Agonists

Research has demonstrated that WNT/β-catenin signaling is crucial for the multiplication, migration, and differentiation of pigment cells in patients with vitiligo. Activation of the Wnt/β-catenin signaling pathway could potentially regulate immune responses, shielding melanocytes from oxidative stress, suppressing CD8+ cytotoxic T cells, and promoting regulatory T cell activation [23].

Injecting IWR-1, a Wnt response-1 inhibitor, intradermally, along with small interfering RNA (siRNA) targeting WNT, has demonstrated efficacy in decreasing the population of melanocytes within the epidermis [24]. Techniques like microinjury and certain phenanthridine-derived WNT-specific agonists have been shown to promote melanin production and repigmentation [25, 26].

Various compounds, including simvastatin and lithium chloride, which activate the Wnt/β-catenin signaling pathway, may have a potential role in vitiligo

Table 13.2 Overview of JAK inhibitors in use for vitiligo

Category	Details
Clinical evaluation	Screen for conditions like herpes infection, diverticulitis, gastrointestinal perforation, thrombosis, cardiovascular risk factors, malignancies, and smoking history
Baseline laboratory testing	Complete blood count (CBC) Liver function tests Lipid panel Chest X-ray Urine routine and microscopy Screening for latent tuberculosis (Mantoux test or interferon gamma release assay), hepatitis B (HBV surface antigen and core antibody), hepatitis C, and human immunodeficiency virus Test for pregnancy in females of reproductive age and provide reproductive health counseling
Follow-up monitoring (after 4–8 weeks, thereafter every 3 months)	Regular clinical assessments for complications and adverse effects Periodic laboratory testing to monitor CBC, liver function, and lipid levels Continuous monitoring for infections, particularly tuberculosis and hepatitis Ongoing reproductive health monitoring and counseling for females of reproductive age
Dosages (in adults)	Tofacitinib: 5–10 mg twice daily Baricitinib: 2 mg once a day; may increase up to 4 mg once a day if no response Upadacitinib: 15 mg once a day; may increase up to 30 mg once a day if no response Ritlecitinib: 50 mg once daily
Drug interactions	Should not be combined with strong immunosuppressants (azathioprine/cyclosporine) in view of the risk of additive immunosuppression JAK inhibitors are CYP3A4 substrates: CYP3A4 inducers and inhibitors may decrease and increase the serum concentrations, respectively
Vaccination	Vaccinations recommended prior to commencement of therapy, in view of the risk of herpes zoster reactivation and streptococcal pneumonia Live and attenuated vaccines should be avoided during treatment with JAK inhibitors
Use in special situations	Children: safety and efficacy not established, use with caution Elderly: higher risk of adverse events, close monitoring recommended Pregnancy: not recommended; potential risk to the fetus Lactation: not recommended; potential risk to the infant

treatment. However, while simvastatin has been investigated in phase II clinical trials, studies have generally not found a clear correlation between its oral intake and repigmentation [27].

13.2.4 MicroRNAs (miRNAs)

MicroRNAs (miRNAs) have a crucial part in vitiligo pathogenesis by modulating gene expression in melanocytes, making them promising therapeutic targets. Two primary strategies exist for miRNA-based therapy: gain of function and miRNA replacement. The gain-of-function approach involves inhibiting pathogenic miRNAs using antagonists like anti-miRNAs, locked nucleic acids (LNAs), or antagomiRs, which trap or degrade the miRNAs, preventing their function [28]. The miRNA replacement strategy involves reintroducing gene-suppressor miRNA mimics to modulate gene expression [29]. This emerging therapeutic approach holds great promise for treating vitiligo and potentially other skin pigmentation disorders.

13.2.5 Therapeutics Enhancing Regulatory T Cells (Tregs)

Tregs, a specialized subset of CD4+ T cells, play a critical role in inhibiting the activation and proliferation of autoreactive T cells. Vitiligo patients exhibit reduced Treg populations across lesional, nonlesional, and perilesional skin areas, indicating that augmenting Treg abundance and activity may hold promise as a therapeutic strategy.

- Direct infusion of purified Tregs, including polyclonally expanded, antigen specific, and engineered Tregs, shows promise. In a murine vitiligo model, transferring polyclonal Tregs has shown short-term effectiveness but may cause systemic immunosuppression [30].
- Hemin, an HO-1 agonist, enhances Treg function by upregulating IL-10. Modulating the microbiota, such as with neomycin, can delay depigmentation and promote Treg infiltration [31].
- Rapamycin, an inhibitor of PI3K-Akt-mTORC1 signaling, increases Treg abundance and halts depigmentation in h3TA2 mice, with effects lasting up to 6 weeks posttreatment. A phase 2 clinical trial (NCT05342519) is currently evaluating the efficacy of 0.1% topical rapamycin [32].
- Microbiota modulation with antibiotics like neomycin has been shown to delay vitiligo depigmentation and promote Treg infiltration in the skin in animal models, highlighting the potential for dietary or microbiome-targeted therapies in vitiligo management [33].

13.3 Afamelanotide

Afamelanotide, a synthetic α-melanocyte-stimulating hormone (MSH) analogue, targets the melanocortin 1 receptor (MC1R), promoting eumelanin transfer into melanosomes and exerting antioxidant and anti-inflammatory effects via MC1R on inflammatory cells. In clinical studies, afamelanotide administered as 16 mg subcutaneous implants every 28 days, in combination with NB-UVB, exhibited superior repigmentation compared to phototherapy alone in patients with nonsegmental vitiligo, notably showing efficacy in areas such as the face and upper extremities [34, 35]. Adverse events included erythema and nausea.

13.4 Biologics

Recent studies have elucidated the mechanisms underlying vitiligo pathogenesis and chronicity, emphasizing the critical involvement of cell-mediated immune responses and cytokine dysregulation in the depigmentation process. The aberrant immune reactions and disrupted cytokine profiles observed in vitiligo underscore the potential benefits of targeting inflammatory mediators like TNF-α, IL-12, IL-23, and IL-17 as promising therapeutic strategies.

13.4.1 TNF-α Inhibitors

TNF-α is postulated to contribute to vitiligo pathogenesis by promoting melanocyte apoptosis, triggering B-cell stimulation, enhancing autoantibody production, and suppressing melanin production. Elevated TNF-α expression in vitiligo-affected skin has been observed in recent research [36]. Infliximab, an anti-TNF-α monoclonal antibody, has shown efficacy in treating patients with ankylosing spondylitis and comorbid refractory vitiligo. Substantial improvement was observed after 6 months of treatment, administered intravenously at a dose of 5 mg/kg at weeks 0, 2, and 6, followed by maintenance doses every 8 weeks [37]. In another pilot study with six unstable vitiligo patients, etanercept, infliximab, or adalimumab was administered following psoriasis guidelines. No repigmentation was achieved although five patients saw no new lesions during treatment and the 6-month follow-up [38]. Another pilot trial with four patients treated with etanercept for 16 weeks achieved disease stabilization although follow-up data was not recorded [39]. In another study, two patients experiencing unstable refractory vitiligo demonstrated disease stabilization and repigmentation when treated with etanercept in addition to other therapies [40].

However, research indicates that TNF-α blockers, particularly infliximab and adalimumab, can potentially worsen preexisting vitiligo and trigger new-onset vitiligo when used to treat other autoimmune diseases [41]. The possible adverse effects of TNF-α inhibitors include injection site reactions, risk of infectious complications, potential development of autoimmune conditions, reactivation of latent tuberculosis, lymphoma, heart failure, demyelinating diseases, and liver toxicity. Overall, TNF-α inhibitors appear to exhibit some efficacy in halting the progression of active vitiligo; however, given the potential adverse effects and the possibility of exacerbating vitiligo, their use is best confined to treating vitiligo associated with autoimmune conditions where their use may be indicated.

13.4.2 IL-17/23 Inhibitors

Several clinical investigations have examined the efficacy of modulating the IL-17 and Th17 pathways as a therapeutic strategy for vitiligo. In a case study involving a patient with psoriasis, vitiligo, and alopecia areata previously unresponsive to etanercept, treatment with the IL-23 inhibitor ustekinumab was initiated [42]. Complete clearance of psoriatic lesions was observed, along with some improvement in vitiligo lesions, indicating a potential benefit of targeting the IL23 pathway. Conversely, another case report described the use of ixekizumab, an IL-17A inhibitor, in a patient with comorbid vitiligo and psoriasis. While psoriasis completely cleared, vitiligo lesions showed no response and disease progression continued [43]. In a small-scale trial with eight patients receiving secukinumab for active vitiligo, seven patients experienced continued progression of their condition [44]. Biomarker assessments revealed no significant changes over time, suggesting the limited efficacy of IL17 inhibition in treating active vitiligo. Additionally, an independent group of active nonsegmental vitiligo patients showed a change in the Th1/Th17.1/Th17 balance toward the Th1 axis, indicating that IL17 inhibition may offer little benefit in treating this disease [44]. These findings indicate a limited role of targeting the IL17 and Th17 pathways in vitiligo management.

13.4.3 Rituximab

Rituximab binds specifically to CD20, a transmembrane protein on B lymphocytes involved in activating CD8+ T cells and subsequent autoreactive responses. Studies indicate that antibodies against melanocyte-associated antigens can induce the apoptosis of cultured melanocytes in vitro, and increased antibody levels in patient serum may correlate with disease activity, underscoring the potential role of autoantibodies in vitiligo pathogenesis [45, 46]. In a clinical trial, five unstable vitiligo patients with generalized lesions received intravenous rituximab infusion, resulting in significant improvement in symptoms and histological findings for three of them [47].

13.4.4 Targeting IFN-γ-CXCL9/10-CXCR3 Axis

The IFN-γ-CXCL9/10-CXCR3 axis plays a crucial role in vitiligo pathogenesis by perpetuating an autoimmune response that leads to melanocyte destruction. In this cascade, CD8+ T cells encounter antigens presented by dendritic cells (DCs) and subsequently release significant quantities of IFN-γ. This cytokine triggers the activation of the JAK-STAT pathway in keratinocytes, which subsequently increases the transcription of the chemokines CXCL9 and CXCL10. These chemokines bind to the CXCR3 receptor on CD8+ T cells, attracting additional melanocyte-reactive T cells to the skin and thereby exacerbating melanocyte destruction. Studies have shown higher IFN-γ mRNA expression in nonlesional and perilesional skin, particularly in unstable vitiligo, correlating with disease activity [48]. Recent studies underscore the therapeutic promise of intervening with this pathway in vitiligo.

Anti-IFN-γ treatments, which have shown efficacy in other autoimmune conditions, have been tested in vitiligo-induced mice, where intraperitoneal injections of IFN-γ neutralizing antibodies resulted in significant repigmentation [49]. Similarly, four vitiligo patients who received intradermal perilesional injections experienced marginal repigmentation in the treated areas [50].

CXCL10 is critical for guiding T cell migration to specific sites, initiating immune cell infiltration early in the disease process, and contributes to the suppression of keratinocyte glycoprotein nonmetastatic melanoma protein B (GPNMB) [51]. A study illustrated that mice treated with CXCL10 neutralizing antibodies displayed substantial repigmentation within 4 weeks, continuing for an additional 4 weeks, suggesting that targeting CXCL10 could offer an effective therapeutic approach for vitiligo [1].

Additionally, CXCR3, found on skin lesions and autoreactive T cells, has been targeted in studies where vitiligo mice treated with CXCR3-depleting antibodies showed reversal of depigmentation and a reduction of CD8+ T cell numbers in the skin [52]. These findings underscore the potential of therapeutics targeting the IFN-γ-CXCL9/10-CXCR3 axis in managing vitiligo.

13.4.5 PD-1/PD-L1 Axis

The PD-1/PD-L1 pathway plays a critical function in regulating immune tolerance and preventing autoimmune responses; in vitiligo, dysfunction of this pathway leads to increased T cell-mediated destruction of melanocytes [53]. Modulating this axis presents a promising treatment approach to reestablish immune tolerance and prevent melanocyte destruction in vitiligo patients. Targeting PD-L1 through PD-L1 fusion protein therapy was shown to inhibit immune responses and reverse depigmentation in vitiligo by enriching Tregs in the skin, spleen, and circulation of Pmel-1 vitiligo mice [54].

13.4.6 Interleukin-15 Inhibitors

IL-15 plays a crucial role in the development and function of TRMs, which are implicated in the persistence of vitiligo. Targeting IL-15 or its receptor to deplete autoreactive TRM while sparing other T cell populations presents a promising therapeutic approach. Blocking IL-15 signaling by anti-CD122 antibody has shown potential in reducing the effector functions of TRM and promoting durable treatment effects in vitiligo [55]. A phase 2a trial (NCT04338581) is currently underway to assess this therapeutic strategy.

13.4.7 Inducible hsp70 (HSP70i) DNA

HSP70i plays a pivotal role in the pathogenesis of vitiligo, acting as a crucial damage-associated molecular pattern (DAMP) involved in cellular stress responses. In therapeutics, blocking HSP70i activity presents a promising avenue for reversing vitiligo development. Studies utilizing HSP70iQ435A-encoding DNA treatment (carrying a single amino acid alteration within the dendritic cell-activating region) have demonstrated remarkable repigmentation in animal models [56]. This treatment also prevents T cell accumulation and shift to an inflammatory phenotype in both mouse and human skin, highlighting its multifaceted therapeutic benefits in vitiligo management [57].

13.5 Conclusion

Treating vitiligo remains challenging, but ongoing research into precision treatments offers promising avenues. As therapeutic targets are better understood and validated, patients can receive more personalized care. Current treatment models for vitiligo are often nonspecific, ranging from systemic glucocorticoids and immunosuppressants for active vitiligo to topical corticosteroids, topical calcineurin inhibitors, NB-UVB, and surgical procedures for stable vitiligo. Novel targeted therapies, such as JAK inhibitors, have shown promise in the management of vitiligo, although risks of latent infection activation and various other adverse effects exist. Studies are currently exploring cytokines implicated in vitiligo pathogenesis, including IFN-γ, CXCR3, CXCL10, HSP70i, IL-15, IL-17/23, and TNF-α, with efforts to modulate their function both in vitro and in vivo. Additionally, studies on miRNA-based therapies and adoptive Treg cell therapeutics are ongoing, requiring further investigation for potential clinical applications.

References

1. Rashighi M, Agarwal P, Richmond JM, et al. CXCL10 is critical for the progression and maintenance of depigmentation in a mouse model of vitiligo. Sci Transl Med. 2014;6(223):223ra23.
2. Abdou AG, Maraee A, Yassien H, Sarhan M. Immunohistochemistry of Janus kinase 1 (JAK1) expression in vitiligo. J Pathol Transl Med. 2018;52(6):363–8.
3. Majid I, Imran S, Batool S. Apremilast is effective in controlling the progression of adult vitiligo: a case series. Dermatol Ther. 2019;32(4):e12923.
4. Khemis A, Fontas E, Moulin S, Montaudié H, Lacour JP, Passeron T. Apremilast in combination with narrowband UVB in the treatment of vitiligo: a 52-week monocentric prospective randomized placebo-controlled study. J Invest Dermatol. 2020;140(8):1533–1537.e2.
5. Kim HJ, Singer G, Abittan BJ, Chima MA, Kimmel G, Bares J, et al. Combination of apremilast and narrowband ultraviolet B light in the treatment of generalized vitiligo in skin phototypes IV to VI: a randomized split-body pilot study. J Am Acad Dermatol. 2021 Dec;85(6):1657–60.
6. Plachouri KM, Kyriakou G, Chourdakis V, Georgiou S, Grafanaki K. One stone, two birds: improvement of early-onset vitiligo under apremilast in a patient with plaque psoriasis. Dermatol Ther. 2019;32(5):e13064.
7. Sheikh A, Rafique W, Owais R, Malik F, Ali E. FDA approves Ruxolitinib (Opzelura) for vitiligo therapy: a breakthrough in the field of dermatology. Ann Med Surg (Lond). 2022;81:104499.
8. Diotallevi F, Gioacchini H, De Simoni E, Marani A, Candelora M, Paolinelli M, Molinelli E, Offidani A, Simonetti O. Vitiligo, from pathogenesis to therapeutic advances: state of the art. Int J Mol Sci. 2023;24(5):4910.
9. Morris R, Kershaw NJ, Babon JJ. The molecular details of cytokine signaling via the JAK/STAT pathway. Protein Sci. 2018;27(12):1984–2009.
10. Karagaiah P, Schwartz RA, Lotti T, Wollina U, Grabbe S, Goldust M. Biologic and targeted therapeutics in vitiligo. J Cosmet Dermatol. 2023;22(1):64–73.
11. Song H, Hu Z, Zhang S, Yang L, Liu Y, Wang T. Effectiveness and safety of tofacitinib combined with narrowband ultraviolet B phototherapy for patients with refractory vitiligo in real-world clinical practice. Dermatol Ther. 2022;35:e15821.
12. Mumford BP, Gibson A, Chong AH. Repigmentation of vitiligo with oral baricitinib. Australas J Dermatol. 2020;61(4):374–6.
13. Li X, Sun Y, Du J, Wang F, Ding X. Excellent repigmentation of generalized vitiligo with oral Baricitinib combined with NB-UVB phototherapy. Clin Cosmet Investig Dermatol. 2023;16:635–8.
14. Zhu Y, Shi Z, Xu Z, et al. Oral tofacitinib, baricitinib and upadacitinib monotherapy for steroid-resistant vitiligo: a prospective case series. J Eur Acad Dermatol Venereol. 2024; https://doi.org/10.1111/jdv.20109.
15. Ezzedine K, Peeva E, Yamaguchi Y, et al. Efficacy and safety of oral ritlecitinib for the treatment of active nonsegmental vitiligo: a randomized phase 2b clinical trial. J Am Acad Dermatol. 2023;88(2):395–403.
16. A phase 2b study to evaluate the efficacy and safety profile of PF-06651600 and PF-06700841 in active non-segmental vitiligo subjects; (2018). Available at: https://clinicaltrials.gov/ct2/show/NCT 03715829
17. Passeron T, Ezzedine K, Hamzavi I, et al. Efficacy and safety of Upadacitinib in a phase 2 randomized, double-blind, dose-ranging study of adults with extensive non-segmental vitiligo. Br J of Dermatol. 2024;190(2):65–6.
18. Efficacy and safety of povorcitinib for extensive vitiligo: 52-week results from a double-blinded, placebo-controlled, dose-ranging phase 2b study. Available from: https://eadvhighlights.com/medfyles/7-ezzedine-povorcitinib-in-vitiligo
19. Bordeaux UH. Evaluation of effect and tolerance of the association of baricitinib and phototherapy versus phototherapy in adults with progressive vitiligo (BARVIT). Available from:

Evaluation of Effect and Tolerance of the Association of Baricitinib and Phototherapy Versus Phototherapy in Adults With Progressive Vitiligo - Full Text View - ClinicalTrials.gov
20. Cohen S, Radominski SC, Gomez-Reino JJ, et al. Analysis of infections and all-cause mortality in phase II, phase III, and long-term extension studies of tofacitinib in patients with rheumatoid arthritis. Arthritis Rheumatol. 2014;66(11):2924–37.
21. Ytterberg SR, Bhatt DL, Mikuls TR, et al. Cardiovascular and cancer risk with Tofacitinib in rheumatoid arthritis. N Engl J Med. 2022;386(4):316–26.
22. Charles-Schoeman C, Buch MH, Dougados M, et al. Risk of major adverse cardiovascular events with tofacitinib versus tumour necrosis factor inhibitors in patients with rheumatoid arthritis with or without a history of atherosclerotic cardiovascular disease: a post hoc analysis from ORAL surveillance. Ann Rheum Dis. 2023;82(1):119–29.
23. Lin X, Meng X, Lin J. The possible role of Wnt/β-catenin signalling in vitiligo treatment. J Eur Acad Dermatol Venereol. 2023;37(11):2208–21.
24. Yamada T, Hasegawa S, Inoue Y, et al. Wnt/β-catenin and kit signaling sequentially regulate melanocyte stem cell differentiation in UVB-induced epidermal pigmentation. J Invest Dermatol. 2013;133(12):2753–62.
25. Han X, Chang L, Qiu Z, Lin M, Wang Y, Liu D, et al. Micro-injury induces hair regeneration and vitiligo repigmentation through wnt/b-catenin pathway. Stem Cells Dev. 2022;31(5–6):111–8.
26. Yang BJ, Fan SR, Zhang XF, et al. Design, synthesis and structure-activity relationship optimization of phenanthridine derivatives as new anti-vitiligo compounds. Bioorg Chem. 2022;119:105582.
27. Vanderweil SG, Amano S, Ko WC, et al. A double-blind, placebo-controlled, phase-II clinical trial to evaluate oral simvastatin as a treatment for vitiligo. J Am Acad Dermatol. 2017;76(1):150–151.e3.
28. Maschmeyer P, Petkau G, Siracusa F, et al. Selective targeting of pro-inflammatory Th1 cells by microRNA-148a-specific antagomirs in vivo. J Autoimmun. 2018;89:41–52.
29. Su M, Miao F, Jiang S, Shi Y, Luo L, He X, Wan J, Xu S, Lei TC. Role of the p53-TRPM1/miR-211-MMP9 axis in UVB-induced human melanocyte migration and its potential in repigmentation. Int J Mol Med. 2020;45(4):1017–26.
30. Alzhrani A, Bottomley M, Wood K, Hester J, Issa F. Identification, selection, and expansion of non-gene modified alloantigen-reactive Tregs for clinical therapeutic use. Cell Immunol. 2020;357:104214.
31. Zhang Q, Cui T, Chang Y, Zhang W, Li S, He Y, Li B, Liu L, Wang G, Gao T, Li C, Jian Z. HO-1 regulates the function of Treg: association with the immune intolerance in vitiligo. J Cell Mol Med. 2018;22(9):4335–43.
32. Zhang X, Liu D, He M, Lin M, Tu C, Zhang B. Polymeric nanoparticles containing rapamycin and autoantigen induce antigen-specific immunological tolerance for preventing vitiligo in mice. Hum Vaccin Immunother. 2021;17(7):1923–9.
33. Dellacecca ER, Cosgrove C, Mukhatayev Z, et al. Antibiotics drive microbial imbalance and vitiligo development in mice. J Invest Dermatol. 2020;140(3):676–687.e6.
34. Lim HW, Grimes PE, Agbai O, et al. Afamelanotide and narrowband UV-B phototherapy for the treatment of vitiligo: a randomized multicenter trial. JAMA Dermatol. 2015;151(1):42–50.
35. Toh JJH, Chuah SY, Jhingan A, Chong WS, Thng STG. Afamelanotide implants and narrowband ultraviolet B phototherapy for the treatment of nonsegmental vitiligo in Asians. J Am Acad Dermatol. 2020;82(6):1517–9.
36. Birol A, Kisa U, Kurtipek GS, Kara F, Kocak M, Erkek E, et al. Increased tumor necrosis factor alpha (TNF-alpha) and interleukin 1 alpha (IL1-alpha) levels in the lesional skin of patients with nonsegmental vitiligo. Int J Dermatol. 2006;45(8):992–3.
37. Simón JA, Burgos-Vargas R. Vitiligo improvement in a patient with ankylosing spondylitis treated with infliximab. Dermatology. 2008;216(3):234–5.
38. Alghamdi KM, Khurrum H, Taieb A, Ezzedine K. Treatment of generalized vitiligo with anti-TNF-α agents. J Drugs Dermatol. 2012;11(4):534–9.

39. Rigopoulos D, Gregoriou S, Larios G, Moustou E, Belayeva-Karatza E, Kalogeromitros D. Etanercept in the treatment of vitiligo. Dermatology. 2007;215(1):84–5.
40. Kim NH, Jeon S, Lee HJ, Lee AY. Impaired PI3K/Akt activation-mediated NF-kappaB inactivation under elevated TNF-alpha is more vulnerable to apoptosis in vitiliginous keratinocytes. J Invest Dermatol. 2007;127(11):2612–7.
41. Bae JM, Kim M, Lee HH, et al. Increased risk of vitiligo following anti-tumor necrosis factor therapy: a 10-year population-based cohort study. J Invest Dermatol. 2018;138(4):768–74.
42. Elkady A, Bonomo L, Amir Y, Vekaria AS, Guttman-Yassky E. Effective use of ustekinumab in a patient with concomitant psoriasis, vitiligo, and alopecia areata. JAAD Case Rep. 2017;3(6):477–9.
43. Katz K, Rupley K, Sink J, Shuley A, Gottlieb A. Interleukin-17 inhibition in a patient with psoriasis and concurrent vitiligo. J Psoriasis Psoriatic Arthritis. 2018;3(4):126–30.
44. Speeckaert R, Mylle S, van Geel N. IL-17A is not a treatment target in progressive vitiligo. Pigment Cell Melanoma Res. 2019;32(6):842–7.
45. Gilhar A, Zelickson B, Ulman Y, Etzioni A. In vivo destruction of melanocytes by the IgG fraction of serum from patients with vitiligo. J Invest Dermatol. 1995;105(5):683–6.
46. Ruiz-Argüelles A, Brito GJ, Reyes-Izquierdo P, Pérez-Romano B, Sánchez-Sosa S. Apoptosis of melanocytes in vitiligo results from antibody penetration. J Autoimmun. 2007;29(4):281–6.
47. Ruiz-Argüelles A, García-Carrasco M, Jimenez-Brito G, et al. Treatment of vitiligo with a chimeric monoclonal antibody to CD20: a pilot study. Clin Exp Immunol. 2013;174(2):229–36.
48. Ng CY, Chan YP, Chiu YC, et al. Targeting the elevated IFN-γ in vitiligo patients by human anti- IFN-γ monoclonal antibody hampers direct cytotoxicity in melanocyte. J Dermatol Sci. 2023;110(3):78–88.
49. Harris JE, Harris TH, Weninger W, Wherry EJ, Hunter CA, Turka LA. A mouse model of vitiligo with focused epidermal depigmentation requires IFN-γ for autoreactive $CD8^+$ T-cell accumulation in the skin. J Invest Dermatol. 2012;132(7):1869–76.
50. Maouia A, Sormani L, Youssef M, Helal AN, Kassab A, Passeron T. Differential expression of CXCL9, CXCL10, and IFN-γ in vitiligo and alopecia areata patients. Pigment Cell Melanoma Res. 2017;30(2):259–61.
51. Biswas KB, Takahashi A, Mizutani Y, et al. GPNMB is expressed in human epidermal keratinocytes but disappears in the vitiligo lesional skin. Sci Rep. 2020;10(1):4930.
52. Richmond JM, Masterjohn E, Chu R, Tedstone J, Youd ME, Harris JE. CXCR3 depleting antibodies prevent and reverse vitiligo in mice. J Invest Dermatol. 2017;137(4):982–5.
53. Tembhre MK, Parihar AS, Sharma VK, Sharma A, Chattopadhyay P, Gupta S. Alteration in regulatory T cells and programmed cell death 1-expressing regulatory T cells in active generalized vitiligo and their clinical correlation. Br J Dermatol. 2015;172(4):940–50.
54. Miao X, Xu R, Fan B, Chen J, Li X, Mao W, Hua S, Li B. PD-L1 reverses depigmentation in Pmel-1 vitiligo mice by increasing the abundance of Tregs in the skin. Sci Rep. 2018;8(1):1605.
55. Richmond JM, Strassner JP, Zapata L Jr, et al. Antibody blockade of IL-15 signaling has the potential to durably reverse vitiligo. Sci Transl Med. 2018;10(450):eaam7710.
56. Henning SW, Fernandez MF, Mahon JP, et al. $HSP70i_{Q435A}$-encoding DNA Repigments vitiligo lesions in Sinclair swine. J Invest Dermatol. 2019;139(4):977.
57. Mosenson JA, Zloza A, Nieland JD, et al. Mutant HSP70 reverses autoimmune depigmentation in vitiligo. Sci Transl Med. 2013;5(174):174ra28.

Chapter 14
Laser and Other Light-Based Therapies

Yng Sun, Ting-Ting Yang, and Cheng-Che Eric Lan

Abstract This chapter provides a comprehensive overview of the various phototherapy modalities used in treating vitiligo, including narrowband UVB (NB-UVB), excimer light, excimer laser, and psoralen plus UVA (PUVA). Phototherapy remains a cornerstone in vitiligo management, with each modality offering unique benefits and mechanisms to induce repigmentation. NB-UVB is highlighted for its efficacy and safety, serving as the first-line treatment for generalized vitiligo. Excimer laser and light, characterized by high irradiance, offer targeted treatments that show rapid and significant repigmentation, particularly in localized vitiligo. PUVA, while effective, is less favored due to its higher risk profile. The chapter also discusses factors influencing phototherapy protocols, the importance of combination therapies, and the need for personalized treatment plans. Emphasis is placed on the ongoing refinement of these therapies through relevant translational studies, aiming to enhance clinical outcomes and patient quality of life.

Keywords Vitiligo · Phototherapy · Narrowband ultraviolet B · Excimer

Y. Sun
Department of Dermatology, Kaohsiung Medical University Hospital, Kaohsiung Medical University, Kaohsiung, Taiwan

T.-T. Yang
Department of Dermatology, Kaohsiung Medical University Hospital, Kaohsiung Medical University, Kaohsiung, Taiwan

Department of Dermatology, Kaohsiung Medical University Gangshan Hospital, Kaohsiung, Taiwan

C.-C. Eric Lan (✉)
Department of Dermatology, Kaohsiung Medical University Hospital, Kaohsiung Medical University, Kaohsiung, Taiwan

Department of Dermatology, College of Medicine, Kaohsiung Medical University, Kaohsiung, Taiwan
e-mail: laneric@cc.kmu.edu.tw

R. Sarkar, V. Narayan R (eds.), *A Concise Guide to The Management of Vitiligo*,
https://doi.org/10.1007/978-981-95-3857-7_14

Key Points

- Different forms of phototherapy for vitiligo include narrowband UVB (NB-UVB), excimer light, excimer laser, and psoralen plus UVA.
- The main proposed mechanisms for inducing repigmentation in vitiligo by UV light involve the induction of T cell apoptosis and the stimulation of the proliferation/migration of functional melanocytes in perilesional skin and immature melanocytes in hair follicles.
- Optimizing NB-UVB requires the consideration of various factors that affect the phototherapy protocol.
- The Vitiligo Working Group consensus introduces possible answers to questions lacking evidence in the phototherapy of vitiligo.
- Phototherapy of vitiligo often encounters common obstacles, and there are strategies to overcome these challenges.
- Different forms of combination therapies are used with phototherapy in vitiligo, each showing various degrees of success.

14.1 Introduction

Vitiligo is an acquired autoimmune skin disorder marked by the disappearance of melanocytes from the skin, resulting in well-defined depigmented macules [1]. This condition, which affects 1–2% of the global population irrespective of sex, race, or age [2], can significantly impact an individual's physical appearance and lead to considerable psychosocial distress [3–6]. Consequently, vitiligo is not merely an aesthetic issue but also a disorder that necessitates active treatment for those seeking medical help. Phototherapy has emerged as a primary treatment modality for vitiligo, with various forms, including narrowband UVB (NB-UVB), excimer light and excimer laser, and psoralen plus UVA (PUVA). These therapies aim to halt disease progression and induce repigmentation through different pathogenic pathways, each with varying degrees of effectiveness [7].

14.2 Narrowband Ultraviolet B

NB-UVB phototherapy, characterized by polychromatic light with a peak emission wavelength usually around 311–313 nm, has been a cornerstone in the treatment of vitiligo since Westerhof and Nieuweboer-Krobotova first reported its efficacy in 1997 [8]. They found that after 4 months of treatment, 67% of patients receiving NB-UVB phototherapy twice a week developed significant repigmentation, compared to 46% of patients undergoing topical PUVA twice a week. Numerous studies have confirmed the superior efficacy of NB-UVB over PUVA [9–12], demonstrating its effectiveness in both adults and children [13–22].

A double-blind randomized study reported that 64% of patients receiving twice-weekly NB-UVB achieved more than 50% overall repigmentation, compared to 36% in the oral PUVA group [9]. A meta-analysis of 29 prospective studies further highlighted that after 6 months of NB-UVB therapy, 74.2% of patients achieved a mild response (≥25% repigmentation), 37.4% achieved a moderate response (≥50% repigmentation), and 19.2% achieved an excellent response (≥75% repigmentation) [23]. In a single-center cohort of Taiwanese vitiligo patients, 45.8% achieved ≥50% repigmentation, and 12.5% achieved ≥75% repigmentation after up to 1 year of treatment [19]. Lesions on the face and neck respond best to NB-UVB, followed by the trunk, arms, and legs, with the hands and feet being the least responsive [23].

NB-UVB phototherapy is now considered the first-line treatment for generalized vitiligo due to its superior efficacy and safety profile compared to other forms of phototherapy [2, 24, 25]. It has fewer adverse effects, primarily erythema, itching, and mild pain, which are generally well tolerated [23]. Current evidence does not show an increased risk of melanoma or nonmelanoma skin cancers in vitiligo patients treated with NB-UVB [26–28].

The mechanism by which NB-UVB induces repigmentation in vitiligo is multifaceted [29, 30]. In the active stage, NB-UVB's immunomodulatory actions stimulate the expression of interleukin-10 [31] and induce the apoptosis of T cells, which may inhibit melanocyte destruction [32]. In the stable stage, NB-UVB promotes the proliferation and migration of functional melanocytes from the perilesional skin and hair follicles, a process described as "biostimulation" [33]. This involves increased expression of endothelin-1, basic fibroblast growth factor, and matrix metalloproteinase-2 activity, enhancing melanocyte proliferation and migration [34–36].

Phototherapy with NB-UVB is recommended as the first-line treatment for pediatric and adult vitiligo patients with extensive (BSA ≥5–10%) or rapidly progressive disease and for those with insufficient response to topical treatments [37]. Traditionally, initiation typically involves a low dose (e.g., 200 mJ/cm^2) administered two to three times a week, with gradual increases until light pink erythema lasting less than 24 h is achieved. More recently, a low-dose protocol was shown to promote efficient repigmentation [38, 39].

Initiating NB-UVB therapy early is recommended to stop disease progression and promote repigmentation, especially for segmental and acral vitiligo, which becomes more resistant to treatment over time [37]. Research has shown that NB-UVB is effective in pediatric patients as young as 3 years old, provided that they can cooperate during treatment sessions [13, 40]. However, there is limited published evidence for treating children under 12 years old with vitiligo and should be administered with caution [41]. Treatment efficacy should be reassessed after 3–6 months of consistent therapy, as some patients may need prolonged treatment to see substantial results [42].

14.3 Adverse Effect

Patients treated with NB-UVB phototherapy may experience acute side effects, including skin pruritus, erythema, burn injury, and xerosis. [18, 24, 43] Eye protection is advised for those receiving treatment near the eyes though closing the eyes is sometimes deemed sufficient. The Vitiligo Working Group recommends closing the eyes and possibly using adhesive tape for eyelid lesions. Long-term effects include the darkening of normal skin and potential photoaging.

The potential risk of skin cancer from UV light phototherapy is a concern due to possible DNA damage and carcinogenic changes [44, 45]. However, studies have shown no increased risk of skin cancer in patients receiving BB-UVB or NB-UVB phototherapy for psoriasis. A study involving 3867 patients found no significant increase in squamous cell carcinoma or melanoma with NB-UVB phototherapy for various diseases [28]. The carcinogenic risk in vitiligo patients remains unclear though skin cancer development in vitiligo lesions is rare. NB-UVB is considered less carcinogenic than PUVA [46], and research suggests that it has a higher safety profile in higher skin phototypes [47].

14.4 Excimer Laser

The excimer laser, characterized by a wavelength of 308 nm generated using xenon and chlorine gases, emits monochromatic UVB radiation at high irradiance. With spot sizes varying between 15 and 30 mm, it allows the selective treatment of vitiligo lesional skin, minimizing hyperpigmentation of perilesional skin [43]. However, its small spot size makes it time-consuming and unsuitable for large body surface areas (>15%), and it is mainly used for localized vitiligo. The cost of excimer laser treatment is higher compared to other phototherapy devices [43].

The excimer laser was first reported as effective for treating vitiligo in 2001 [48, 49], and it has since shown promising results in inducing repigmentation [50–56]. Treatments are usually administered two to three times per week over 1–9 months. Although a higher frequency of treatments can speed up repigmentation, the total number of treatments determines the ultimate outcome [54]. The excimer laser may work similarly to NB-UVB due to its wavelength but is more effective in inducing T lymphocyte apoptosis [57, 58] and endothelin-1 secretion [59], which stimulates melanocytes.

The monochromatic excimer light (excimer lamp) also emits light at a 308-nm wavelength and has been shown to be effective in inducing repigmentation of vitiligo lesions [60]. The excimer lamp has a larger treatment field compared to the excimer laser, allowing irradiation of larger areas and shorter treatment times. Additionally, the cost of excimer lamp treatment is lower than that of laser devices.

The mechanism of action of both the excimer laser and excimer light in treating vitiligo is not well defined. Like NB-UVB, excimer light may have immunomodulatory effects by promoting T lymphocyte apoptosis [61] and stimulating the release of endothelin-1 from keratinocytes [59], thereby promoting melanocyte proliferation.

Excimer laser/light phototherapy is generally well tolerated, with common side effects, including erythema and occasional blistering. It is considered safer for pediatric patients due to its localized irradiation [43], which avoids total body exposure and reduces cumulative radiation doses. Studies suggest that the excimer laser is as effective as NB-UVB with a similar safety profile, although some report faster and greater repigmentation with the excimer laser [56]. A systematic review of seven RCTs including 390 vitiligo patients found no significant difference between excimer laser and NB-UVB or between excimer laser and excimer light in achieving ≥75% repigmentation, but more lesions achieved ≥50% repigmentation with excimer laser than with NB-UVB [62]. In a split-body RCT with 14 generalized vitiligo patients, 79.0% achieved ≥50% repigmentation with an excimer laser and 87.5% with excimer light after 20 treatments [63].

Excimer laser/light treatment is recommended for localized vitiligo [41, 42], with treatment typically starting at a low dose (e.g., 150 mJ/cm^2) two to three times per week, followed by incremental increases [64]. A low-dose protocol may be maintained once repigmentation is observed [39]. In a retrospective study, 50% of segmental vitiligo patients with lesions on the head and neck achieved ≥50% repigmentation with low-dose excimer light at a maximum dose of 300–400 mJ/cm^2 [39]. In a split-body RCT, the extent of repigmentation and the proportion of patients achieving ≥75% repigmentation were comparable between erythemal and suberythemal dose excimer laser regimens in patients with stable vitiligo on the face and neck [65]. Treatment should be re-evaluated after 3–6 months [38], as the number of sessions required varies individually. The long-term effects of excimer laser/light treatment have yet to be established. Relapses can occur, necessitating ongoing evaluation and possibly combining treatments for sustained results.

14.5 Excimer vs NB-UVB

Various studies have compared the therapeutic efficacy of excimer laser, excimer light, and NB-UVB in treating vitiligo [66–68]. Hong and colleagues [67] found that the excimer laser demonstrated greater efficacy than NB-UVB, inducing more rapid and significant repigmentation. A right-left comparison study at Cairo University Hospital over 24 weeks showed similar repigmentation scores between targeted NB-UVB and excimer light though the onset was 2 weeks earlier with excimer light. Recent meta-analyses indicate similar efficacy among excimer light, excimer laser, and NB-UVB for vitiligo treatment [62, 69, 70].

14.5.1 Irradiance of Phototherapy

Clinical studies have shown that excimer light has favorable efficacy compared to NB-UVB, likely due to its high irradiance. Experiments with cell models support this, showing that UVB radiation activates DNA and tryptophan, which in turn activates the aryl hydrocarbon receptor (AhR) cascade involved in melanoblast and melanocyte differentiation and homeostasis, contributing to pigmentation. Cultured melanoblasts treated with excimer light showed higher AhR-related activation and differentiation compared to NB-UVB. Reducing excimer light irradiance with a neutral density filter negated these effects, highlighting the importance of irradiance in repigmentation. Proper activation and differentiation of melanocyte stem cells near the hair follicle bulge are crucial for repigmenting vitiligo skin. The high irradiance UVB provided by excimer devices explains their superior efficacy in repigmenting vitiligo compared to NB-UVB [71]. See Fig. 14.1 for a schematic illustration.

14.6 Excimer for Segmental Vitiligo

Several studies have shown that patients with segmental vitiligo respond poorly to NB-UVB phototherapy compared to those with nonsegmental vitiligo. Anbar and colleagues [21] found that only 1 out of 13 patients (7.7%) with segmental vitiligo achieved greater than 25% repigmentation following 6 months of NB-UVB phototherapy. The efficacy of excimer laser and excimer light in treating segmental vitiligo is not well defined. In a study conducted in Korea involving 80 patients with segmental vitiligo treated with an excimer laser, Do and colleagues [72] found that 23.8% of patients achieved grade 4 (75–99%) and that 20% achieved grade 3 (50–74%) repigmentation. These findings suggest that excimer laser and excimer light may be effective phototherapy options for patients with segmental vitiligo.

14.7 PUVA

14.7.1 Oral PUVA

PUVA, or photochemotherapy, was the primary treatment for generalized vitiligo from the 1950s until it was replaced by NB-UVB [43, 73]. This treatment involves ingesting a photosensitizer, typically 8-methoxypsoralen (8-MOP), 2 h before UVA (320–400 nm) irradiation. Oral PUVA is usually administered to patients with generalized vitiligo twice weekly, with intervals of 24–48 h between sessions. The starting dose ranges from 0.5 to 1.0 J/cm^2, increasing until mild erythema develops [43, 74].

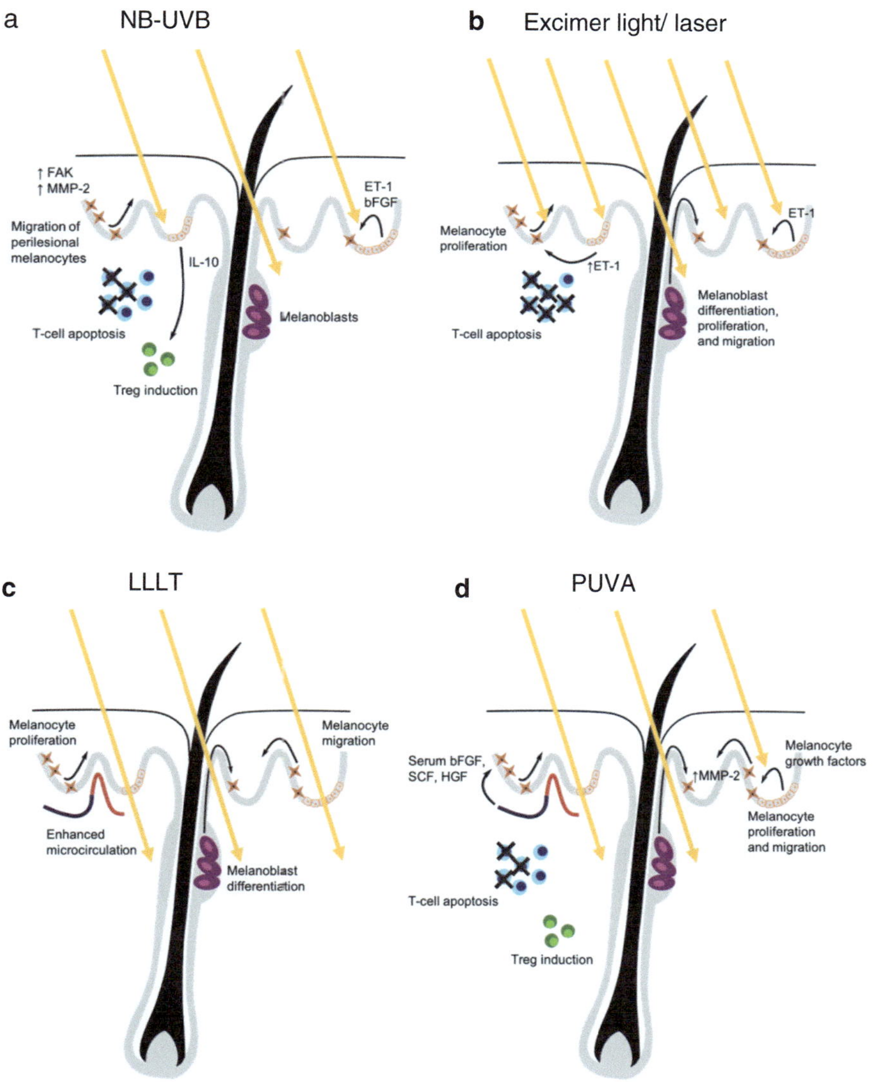

Fig. 14.1 Schematic illustration of the proposed mechanisms of different phototherapy devices in inducing vitiligo repigmentation. The proposed mechanisms include immunosuppression through T cell apoptosis and Treg induction, melanocyte proliferation through the release of melanocyte growth factors, enhanced melanocyte migration by increased MMP-2 and FAK expression, and induction of melanoblast maturation. Note that excimer laser/light offers targeted high-irradiance treatment, showing faster repigmentation than NB-UVB by increasing melanoblast activation capability

Methoxsalen, upon light activation, forms DNA adducts [74, 75], stimulates melanocyte growth factors, proliferation, migration, and melanogenesis, and reduces vitiligo-associated antigens [76–78]. It also induces lymphocyte apoptosis and T-regulatory lymphocyte differentiation [79, 80]. However, oral PUVA has been largely replaced by NB-UVB due to its superior efficacy and safety profile [81]. Oral PUVA poses risks of erythema, phototoxicity, xerosis, nausea, headache, photoaging, and an increased risk of skin cancers, making it less favorable compared to NB-UVB [42]. It is not recommended for children or pregnant women.

14.7.2 Topical PUVA

Topical PUVA is a suitable treatment for localized vitiligo, offering greater safety than oral PUVA due to the lower UVA dose and no systemic psoralen absorption. Treatment involves applying methoxsalen in solution or cream to vitiligo lesions 20–30 min before UVA exposure, typically administered one to three times a week [82, 83]. The starting UVA dose ranges from 0.25 to 0.5 J/cm^2 and is gradually increased until mild erythema appears. Posttreatment, the psoralen must be washed off with soap and water to prevent skin phototoxicity [82, 83].

In many patients, topical PUVA can cause perilesional tanning, which may be cosmetically unacceptable and hinder treatment continuation. The most common adverse effects are phototoxicity [84]. Despite the higher efficacy, color matching, and safety profile of NB-UVB, topical PUVA may still be considered for specific cases, such as acral vitiligo, resistant to other treatments, particularly in patients aged 12 years and older [81]. Further research is needed to determine the potential increased risk of skin cancer with topical PUVA [42].

A meta-analysis of nine prospective PUVA studies demonstrated that after 6 months of therapy, 23.5% of patients achieved a moderate response (≥50% repigmentation), and 8.5% achieved an excellent response (≥75% repigmentation) [23]. Topical psoralen followed by UVA exposure should be administered two to three times a week, and treatment should be re-evaluated after 6 months. Some patients may experience a delayed response and require over 12 months of continuous treatment to achieve maximum repigmentation [38].

14.8 Visible Light

Visible light, in the form of low-energy helium-neon laser (wavelength of 632.8 nm), is effective for segmental vitiligo, particularly in children with periorbital and perioral lesions [85–87]. In vitro studies demonstrate that the helium-neon (He-Ne) laser can induce repigmentation by stimulating melanocyte migration and promoting proliferation through keratinocytes [87, 88]. In a study of 30 segmental vitiligo patients, 60% achieved over 50% repigmentation with once- or twice-weekly He-Ne laser at 3.0 J/cm^2 [88]. Case reports also show significant repigmentation with a He-Ne laser and topical tacrolimus [89, 90]. This laser, particularly effective for periorbital and perioral lesions in children, works by enhancing melanocyte migration, proliferation, and microcirculation, with minimal adverse effects compared to NB-UVB, making it a favorable alternative [91].

14.9 Factors to Be Considered in Phototherapy

14.9.1 Activity of Vitiligo

NB-UVB can be initiated regardless of disease activity, as it has both stabilizing [12, 92] and repigmenting effects [15, 92–96]; however, its repigmenting effects are less advantageous in active cases [97]. Most vitiligo specialists prefer combining phototherapy with other stabilizing medications.

Practical Tip Disease activity should be monitored throughout the treatment course, and stabilizing treatments should be readministered if the disease becomes active.

14.9.2 Patient's Response to Light

A history or signs of photosensitivity should be considered before deciding on phototherapy. Caution is advised for patients showing signs of photo koebnerization [98], such as lesions concentrated on sun-exposed areas (e.g., dorsa of the hands, V-shaped area of the neck, forehead, nose), and those with a history of exacerbation after sunlight exposure.

Practical Tip In such cases, it is recommended to investigate and exclude systemic lupus erythematosus [99] and hepatitis C virus infection [100], as they may predispose to photosensitivity. Additionally, checking for a history of using photosensitizing medications is important [99].

14.9.3 Special Sites (Genitals)

It is recommended to cover male genitals during phototherapy sessions, a consensus also supported by the Vitiligo Working Group (VWG). However, there is no specific guideline for managing lesions in the genital area. While there is an old report of malignancy developing in exposed genitals, no further studies have confirmed or refuted the risk of phototherapy in these areas. Thus, excimer light may be suggested if topical treatments are ineffective.

14.10 Combination with Other Therapies

Combining NB-UVB with medical and/or surgical therapies can enhance treatment efficacy. [18] Combinations serve multiple purposes:

Induction of Stabilization Systemic steroids, particularly in oral-pulse and mini-pulse regimens, help achieve stabilization with minimal side effects [18, 101]. Other immunosuppressants like cyclosporine [102] and methotrexate [103] have been studied but show varying efficacies. Topical corticosteroids and calcineurin inhibitors are commonly used early in this disease because of their immunomodulatory effects [104]. The recent rise in the use of JAK inhibitors, such as tofacitinib and ruxolitinib, for vitiligo has shown promise in repigmentation, particularly in sun-exposed areas. A case series demonstrated that concomitant light exposure, either sunlight or low-dose NB-UVB, is essential for the efficacy of JAK inhibitors [105].

Overcoming Oxidative Stress Excessive oxidative stress is associated with vitiligo activity [106]. Systemic and topical antioxidants, such as pseudocatalase, vitamin E, vitamin C, ubiquinone, lipoic acid, Polypodium leucotomos, catalase/superoxide dismutase combinations, and *Ginkgo biloba*, are emerging therapies that help counteract this stress with high safety profiles [107–111].

Enhancement of Repigmentation Combining topical therapies like calcineurin inhibitors and vitamin D analogs with phototherapy can stimulate melanocyte proliferation and migration [18]. Afamelanotide, a synthetic analog of alpha-melanocyte-stimulating hormone (a-MSH), also stimulates melanogenesis [112]. Studies suggest that combining NB-UVB with an excimer laser can enhance treatment responses in resistant cases [113].

Improving the Melanocyte Environment Techniques such as dermabrasion, fractional lasers, 5-fluorouracil, and chemical peels can improve the environment for melanocytes, enhancing migration and proliferation [101–104, 112, 114–116]. These methods, alongside topical therapies, can reduce inflammatory cytokines and support better repigmentation.

14.11 Protocols for Phototherapy

Despite more than two decades of use, there is no universally accepted protocol for NB-UVB phototherapy. The Vitiligo Working Group reviewed existing recommendations and established a consensus through collaboration with six international institutions. The key points are summarized below.

14.11.1 Two vs Three Weekly Exposures

Both two- and three-weekly treatments are effective for vitiligo though no controlled trials have compared them directly. A one-year study at Cairo University Hospital found better compliance and lower equipment load with a twice-weekly regimen though repigmentation was slower. The VWG consensus recommends a thrice-weekly regimen for faster response.

Practical Tip Advise patients on the importance of adhering to a thrice-weekly regimen for quicker results.

14.11.2 Starting Dose

Measuring the minimal erythema dose (MED) is the most accurate way to determine the starting dose but is time-consuming. A fixed starting dose treating vitiligo as skin phototype I is often used [117]. However, darker skin types have additional photoprotective mechanisms, suggesting that a fixed starting dose for all skin types may not be optimal [118]. While using skin phototype to set starting doses increases the phototoxicity risk, it remains a practical method, especially for darker skin phototypes.

14.11.3 Erythema or Suberythema

Most studies [11, 21] use a 10–20% dose increase per session. The target erythema is debated; some protocols aim for rapid erythema [8, 9, 12, 21, 93], while others stop at suberythema (70% of MED) [119]. The VWG consensus recommends pink asymptomatic erythema ("carnation pink erythema") as the target. After reaching the target erythema, the dose can be maintained or increased until repigmentation begins. A more aggressive protocol may involve continuous dose increases as tolerated by the patient [22], with adjustments for darker skin phototypes [21]. Alternatively, a low-dose (suberythemic) NB-UVB protocol can be used, starting with a treatment dose of 200 mJ/cm^2 administered two to three times a week, with slow incremental increases. Once repigmentation is observed, the dose should be maintained at a constant level [39].

Practical Tip Patients with darker skin phototypes can usually tolerate a higher starting dose and larger incremental increases.

14.12 Summary

Phototherapy is a critical component in the management of vitiligo, encompassing a variety of modalities. Each treatment option has its unique benefits and mechanisms that aid in repigmentation. Excimer laser/light treatments are particularly effective due to their high irradiance. Ongoing research continues to refine and optimize these therapies, ensuring improved outcomes for vitiligo patients.

Conflicts of Interest None declared.

Funding Sources None.

References

1. Ezzedine K, Eleftheriadou V, Whitton M, van Geel N. Vitiligo. Lancet. 2015;386(9988):74–84.
2. Taieb A, Alomar A, Bohm M, Dell'anna ML, De Pase A, Eleftheriadou V, et al. Guidelines for the management of vitiligo: the European Dermatology Forum consensus. Br J Dermatol. 2013;168(1):5–19.
3. Ongenae K, Beelaert L, van Geel N, Naeyaert JM. Psychosocial effects of vitiligo. J Eur Acad Dermatol Venereol. 2006;20(1):1–8.
4. Ongenae K, Van Geel N, De Schepper S, Naeyaert JM. Effect of vitiligo on self-reported health-related quality of life. Br J Dermatol. 2005;152(6):1165–72.
5. Amer AA, Gao XH. Quality of life in patients with vitiligo: an analysis of the dermatology life quality index outcome over the past two decades. Int J Dermatol. 2016;55(6):608–14.
6. Krüger C, Schallreuter KU. Stigmatisation, avoidance behaviour and difficulties in coping are common among adult patients with vitiligo. Acta Derm Venereol. 2015;95(5):553–8.
7. Diotallevi F, Gioacchini H, De Simoni E, Marani A, Candelora M, Paolinelli M, et al. Vitiligo, from pathogenesis to therapeutic advances: state of the art. Int J Mol Sci. 2023;24(5):4910.
8. Westerhof W, Nieuweboer-Krobotova L. Treatment of vitiligo with UV-B radiation vs topical psoralen plus UV-A. Arch Dermatol. 1997;133(12):1525–8.
9. Yones SS, Palmer RA, Garibaldinos TM, Hawk JL. Randomized double-blind trial of treatment of vitiligo: efficacy of psoralen-UV-A therapy vs Narrowband-UV-B therapy. Arch Dermatol. 2007;143(5):578–84.
10. Parsad D, Kanwar AJ, Kumar B. Psoralen-ultraviolet A vs. narrow-band ultraviolet B phototherapy for the treatment of vitiligo. J Eur Acad Dermatol Venereol. 2006;20(2):175–7.
11. El Mofty M, Mostafa W, Esmat S, Youssef R, Azzam O, Hunter N, et al. Narrow band Ultraviolet B 311 nm in the treatment of vitiligo: two right-left comparison studies. Photodermatol Photoimmunol Photomed. 2006;22(1):6–11.

12. Bhatnagar A, Kanwar AJ, Parsad D, De D. Comparison of systemic PUVA and NB-UVB in the treatment of vitiligo: an open prospective study. J Eur Acad Dermatol Venereol. 2007;21(5):638–42.
13. Njoo MD, Bos JD, Westerhof W. Treatment of generalized vitiligo in children with narrow-band (TL-01) UVB radiation therapy. J Am Acad Dermatol. 2000;42(2 Pt 1):245–53.
14. Scherschun L, Kim JJ, Lim HW. Narrow-band ultraviolet B is a useful and well-tolerated treatment for vitiligo. J Am Acad Dermatol. 2001;44(6):999–1003.
15. Natta R, Somsak T, Wisuttida T, Laor L. Narrowband ultraviolet B radiation therapy for recalcitrant vitiligo in Asians. J Am Acad Dermatol. 2003;49(3):473–6.
16. Samson Yashar S, Gielczyk R, Scherschun L, Lim HW. Narrow-band ultraviolet B treatment for vitiligo, pruritus, and inflammatory dermatoses. Photodermatol Photoimmunol Photomed. 2003;19(4):164–8.
17. Kanwar AJ, Dogra S. Narrow-band UVB for the treatment of generalized vitiligo in children. Clin Exp Dermatol. 2005;30(4):332–6.
18. Yazdani Abyaneh M, Griffith RD, Falto-Aizpurua L, Nouri K. Narrowband ultraviolet B phototherapy in combination with other therapies for vitiligo: mechanisms and efficacies. J Eur Acad Dermatol Venereol. 2014;28(12):1610–22.
19. Chen GY, Hsu MM, Tai HK, Chou TC, Tseng CL, Chang HY, et al. Narrow-band UVB treatment of vitiligo in Chinese. J Dermatol. 2005;32(10):793–800.
20. Brazzelli V, Antoninetti M, Palazzini S, Barbagallo T, De Silvestri A, Borroni G. Critical evaluation of the variants influencing the clinical response of vitiligo: study of 60 cases treated with ultraviolet B narrow-band phototherapy. J Eur Acad Dermatol Venereol. 2007;21(10):1369–74.
21. Anbar TS, Westerhof W, Abdel-Rahman AT, El-Khayyat MA. Evaluation of the effects of NB-UVB in both segmental and non-segmental vitiligo affecting different body sites. Photodermatol Photoimmunol Photomed. 2006;22(3):157–63.
22. Nicolaidou E, Antoniou C, Stratigos AJ, Stefanaki C, Katsambas AD. Efficacy, predictors of response, and long-term follow-up in patients with vitiligo treated with narrowband UVB phototherapy. J Am Acad Dermatol. 2007;56(2):274–8.
23. Bae JM, Jung HM, Hong BY, Lee JH, Choi WJ, Lee JH, et al. Phototherapy for vitiligo: a systematic review and meta-analysis. JAMA Dermatol. 2017;153(7):666–74.
24. Nicolaidou E, Antoniou C, Stratigos A, Katsambas AD. Narrowband ultraviolet B phototherapy and 308-nm excimer laser in the treatment of vitiligo: a review. J Am Acad Dermatol. 2009;60(3):470–7.
25. Ling TC, Clayton TH, Crawley J, Exton LS, Goulden V, Ibbotson S, et al. British Association of Dermatologists and British Photodermatology Group guidelines for the safe and effective use of psoralen-ultraviolet A therapy 2015. Br J Dermatol. 2016;174(1):24–55.
26. Wu YH, Chou CL, Chang HC. Risk of skin cancer after ultraviolet phototherapy in patients with vitiligo: a systematic review and meta-analysis. Clin Exp Dermatol. 2022;47(4):692–9.
27. Weischer M, Blum A, Eberhard F, Röcken M, Berneburg M. No evidence for increased skin cancer risk in psoriasis patients treated with broadband or narrowband UVB phototherapy: a first retrospective study. Acta Derm Venereol. 2004;84(5):370–4.
28. Hearn RM, Kerr AC, Rahim KF, Ferguson J, Dawe RS. Incidence of skin cancers in 3867 patients treated with narrow-band ultraviolet B phototherapy. Br J Dermatol. 2008;159(4):931–5.
29. Alikhan A, Felsten LM, Daly M, Petronic-Rosic V. Vitiligo: a comprehensive overview Part I. Introduction, epidemiology, quality of life, diagnosis, differential diagnosis, associations, histopathology, etiology, and work-up. J Am Acad Dermatol. 2011;65(3):473–91.
30. Westerhof W, d'Ischia M. Vitiligo puzzle: the pieces fall in place. Pigment Cell Res. 2007;20(5):345–59.
31. Ponsonby AL, Lucas RM, van der Mei IA. UVR, vitamin D and three autoimmune diseases--multiple sclerosis, type 1 diabetes, rheumatoid arthritis. Photochem Photobiol. 2005;81(6):1267–75.

32. Ozawa M, Ferenczi K, Kikuchi T, Cardinale I, Austin LM, Coven TR, et al. 312-nanometer ultraviolet B light (narrow-band UVB) induces apoptosis of T cells within psoriatic lesions. J Exp Med. 1999;189(4):711–8.
33. Cui J, Shen LY, Wang GC. Role of hair follicles in the repigmentation of vitiligo. J Invest Dermatol. 1991;97(3):410–6.
34. Wu CS, Yu CL, Wu CS, Lan CC, Yu HS. Narrow-band ultraviolet-B stimulates proliferation and migration of cultured melanocytes. Exp Dermatol. 2004;13(12):755–63.
35. Hirobe T. Role of keratinocyte-derived factors involved in regulating the proliferation and differentiation of mammalian epidermal melanocytes. Pigment Cell Res. 2005;18(1):2–12.
36. Imokawa G. Autocrine and paracrine regulation of melanocytes in human skin and in pigmentary disorders. Pigment Cell Res. 2004;17(2):96–110.
37. van Geel N, Speeckaert R, Taieb A, Ezzedine K, Lim HW, Pandya AG, et al. Worldwide expert recommendations for the diagnosis and management of vitiligo: position statement from the International Vitiligo Task Force Part 1: towards a new management algorithm. J Eur Acad Dermatol Venereol. 2023;37(11):2173–84.
38. Taieb A, Alomar A, Böhm M, Dell'anna ML, De Pase A, Eleftheriadou V, et al. Guidelines for the management of vitiligo: the European Dermatology Forum consensus. Br J Dermatol. 2013;168(1):5–19.
39. Chiu SH, Liu IL, Chen YW, Lan CE. Low-dose UVB therapy is comparable with conventional UVB phototherapy for treatment of vitiligo: a pilot study. J Dermatol Sci. 2018;92(2):218–20.
40. Percivalle S, Piccinno R, Caccialanza M, Forti S. Narrowband ultraviolet B phototherapy in childhood vitiligo: evaluation of results in 28 patients. Pediatr Dermatol. 2012;29(2):160–5.
41. Eleftheriadou V, Atkar R, Batchelor J, McDonald B, Novakovic L, Patel JV, et al. British Association of Dermatologists guidelines for the management of people with vitiligo 2021. Br J Dermatol. 2022;186(1):18–29.
42. Seneschal J, Speeckaert R, Taieb A, Wolkerstorfer A, Passeron T, Pandya AG, et al. Worldwide expert recommendations for the diagnosis and management of vitiligo: position statement from the international Vitiligo Task Force-Part 2: specific treatment recommendations. J Eur Acad Dermatol Venereol. 2023;37(11):2185–95.
43. Pacifico A, Leone G. Photo(chemo)therapy for vitiligo. Photodermatol Photoimmunol Photomed. 2011;27(5):261–77.
44. Tzung TY, Rünger TM. Assessment of DNA damage induced by broadband and narrowband UVB in cultured lymphoblasts and keratinocytes using the comet assay. Photochem Photobiol. 1998;67(6):647–50.
45. Budiyanto A, Ueda M, Ueda T, Ichihashi M. Formation of cyclobutane pyrimidine dimers and 8-oxo-7,8-dihydro-2′-deoxyguanosine in mouse and organ-cultured human skin by irradiation with broadband or with narrowband UVB. Photochem Photobiol. 2002;76(4):397–400.
46. Ibbotson SH, Bilsland D, Cox NH, Dawe RS, Diffey B, Edwards C, et al. An update and guidance on narrowband ultraviolet B phototherapy: a British Photodermatology Group Workshop Report. Br J Dermatol. 2004;151(2):283–97.
47. Youssef R, Ossama S, Mashaly HM, Fathy M, Safwat M, Shaker O, et al. Phototherapeutic modalities pose no significantly increased risk of oxidative damage to DNA in dark skinned individuals. Indian J Dermatol Venereol Leprol. 2016;82(6):666–72.
48. Baltás E, Nagy P, Bónis B, Novák Z, Ignácz F, Szabó G, et al. Repigmentation of localized vitiligo with the xenon chloride laser. Br J Dermatol. 2001;144(6):1266–7.
49. Baltás E, Csoma Z, Ignácz F, Dobozy A, Kemény L. Treatment of vitiligo with the 308-nm xenon chloride excimer laser. Arch Dermatol. 2002;138(12):1619–20.
50. Spencer JM, Nossa R, Ajmeri J. Treatment of vitiligo with the 308-nm excimer laser: a pilot study. J Am Acad Dermatol. 2002;46(5):727–31.
51. Ostovari N, Passeron T, Zakaria W, Fontas E, Larouy JC, Blot JF, et al. Treatment of vitiligo by 308-nm excimer laser: an evaluation of variables affecting treatment response. Lasers Surg Med. 2004;35(2):152–6.

52. Hadi S, Tinio P, Al-Ghaithi K, Al-Qari H, Al-Helalat M, Lebwohl M, et al. Treatment of vitiligo using the 308-nm excimer laser. Photomed Laser Surg. 2006;24(3):354–7.
53. Zhang XY, He YL, Dong J, Xu JZ, Wang J. Clinical efficacy of a 308 nm excimer laser in the treatment of vitiligo. Photodermatol Photoimmunol Photomed. 2010;26(3):138–42.
54. Hofer A, Hassan AS, Legat FJ, Kerl H, Wolf P. Optimal weekly frequency of 308-nm excimer laser treatment in vitiligo patients. Br J Dermatol. 2005;152(5):981–5.
55. Hofer A, Hassan AS, Legat FJ, Kerl H, Wolf P. The efficacy of excimer laser (308 nm) for vitiligo at different body sites. J Eur Acad Dermatol Venereol. 2006;20(5):558–64.
56. Passeron T, Ortonne JP. Use of the 308-nm excimer laser for psoriasis and vitiligo. Clin Dermatol. 2006;24(1):33–42.
57. Novák Z, Bónis B, Baltás E, Ocsovszki I, Ignácz F, Dobozy A, et al. Xenon chloride ultraviolet B laser is more effective in treating psoriasis and in inducing T cell apoptosis than narrow-band ultraviolet B. J Photochem Photobiol B. 2002;67(1):32–8.
58. Novák Z, Bérces A, Rontó G, Pállinger E, Dobozy A, Kemény L. Efficacy of different UV-emitting light sources in the induction of T-cell apoptosis. Photochem Photobiol. 2004;79(5):434–9.
59. Noborio R, Morita A. Preferential induction of endothelin-1 in a human epidermal equivalent model by narrow-band ultraviolet B light sources. Photodermatol Photoimmunol Photomed. 2010;26(3):159–61.
60. Leone G, Iacovelli P, Paro Vidolin A, Picardo M. Monochromatic excimer light 308 nm in the treatment of vitiligo: a pilot study. J Eur Acad Dermatol Venereol. 2003;17(5):531–7.
61. Bianchi B, Campolmi P, Mavilia L, Danesi A, Rossi R, Cappugi P. Monochromatic excimer light (308 nm): an immunohistochemical study of cutaneous T cells and apoptosis-related molecules in psoriasis. J Eur Acad Dermatol Venereol. 2003;17(4):408–13.
62. Sun Y, Wu Y, Xiao B, Li L, Li L, Chen HD, et al. Treatment of 308-nm excimer laser on vitiligo: a systemic review of randomized controlled trials. J Dermatolog Treat. 2015;26(4):347–53.
63. Shi Q, Li K, Fu J, Wang Y, Ma C, Li Q, et al. Comparison of the 308-nm excimer laser with the 308-nm excimer lamp in the treatment of vitiligo--a randomized bilateral comparison study. Photodermatol Photoimmunol Photomed. 2013;29(1):27–33.
64. Choi KH, Park JH, Ro YS. Treatment of vitiligo with 308-nm xenon-chloride excimer laser: therapeutic efficacy of different initial doses according to treatment areas. J Dermatol. 2004;31(4):284–92.
65. Bae JM, Kwon SH, Ju HJ, Kang HY. Suberythemic and erythemic doses of a 308-nm excimer laser treatment of stable vitiligo in combination with topical tacrolimus: a randomized controlled trial. J Am Acad Dermatol. 2020;83(5):1463–4.
66. Casacci M, Thomas P, Pacifico A, Bonnevalle A, Paro Vidolin A, Leone G. Comparison between 308-nm monochromatic excimer light and narrowband UVB phototherapy (311–313 nm) in the treatment of vitiligo--a multicentre controlled study. J Eur Acad Dermatol Venereol. 2007;21(7):956–63.
67. Hong SB, Park HH, Lee MH. Short-term effects of 308-nm xenon-chloride excimer laser and narrow-band ultraviolet B in the treatment of vitiligo: a comparative study. J Korean Med Sci. 2005;20(2):273–8.
68. Le Duff F, Fontas E, Giacchero D, Sillard L, Lacour JP, Ortonne JP, et al. 308-nm excimer lamp vs. 308-nm excimer laser for treating vitiligo: a randomized study. Br J Dermatol. 2010;163(1):188–92.
69. Lopes C, Trevisani VF, Melnik T. Efficacy and safety of 308-nm monochromatic excimer lamp versus other phototherapy devices for vitiligo: a systematic review with meta-analysis. Am J Clin Dermatol. 2016;17(1):23–32.
70. Xiao BH, Wu Y, Sun Y, Chen HD, Gao XH. Treatment of vitiligo with NB-UVB: a systematic review. J Dermatolog Treat. 2015;26(4):340–6.
71. Yang TT, Chiu SH, Lan CE. The effects of UVB irradiance on vitiligo phototherapy and UVB-induced photocarcinogenesis. Photodermatol Photoimmunol Photomed. 2020;36(4):257–62.

72. Do JE, Shin JY, Kim DY, Hann SK, Oh SH. The effect of 308nm excimer laser on segmental vitiligo: a retrospective study of 80 patients with segmental vitiligo. Photodermatol Photoimmunol Photomed. 2011;27(3):147–51.
73. Kwok YK, Anstey AV, Hawk JL. Psoralen photochemotherapy (PUVA) is only moderately effective in widespread vitiligo: a 10-year retrospective study. Clin Exp Dermatol. 2002;27(2):104–10.
74. Gupta AK, Anderson TF. Psoralen photochemotherapy. J Am Acad Dermatol. 1987;17(5 Pt 1):703–34.
75. Averbeck D. Recent advances in psoralen phototoxicity mechanism. Photochem Photobiol. 1989;50(6):859–82.
76. Abdel-Naser MB, Hann SK, Bystryn JC. Oral psoralen with UV-A therapy releases circulating growth factor(s) that stimulates cell proliferation. Arch Dermatol. 1997;133(12):1530–3.
77. Lei TC, Vieira WD, Hearing VJ. In vitro migration of melanoblasts requires matrix metalloproteinase-2: implications to vitiligo therapy by photochemotherapy. Pigment Cell Res. 2002;15(6):426–32.
78. Kao CH, Yu HS. Comparison of the effect of 8-methoxypsoralen (8-MOP) plus UVA (PUVA) on human melanocytes in vitiligo vulgaris and in vitro. J Invest Dermatol. 1992;98(5):734–40.
79. Bulat V, Situm M, Dediol I, Ljubicić I, Bradić L. The mechanisms of action of phototherapy in the treatment of the most common dermatoses. Coll Antropol. 2011;35(Suppl 2):147–51.
80. El-Domyati M, Moftah NH, Nasif GA, Abdel-Wahab HM, Barakat MT, Abdel-Aziz RT. Evaluation of apoptosis regulatory proteins in response to PUVA therapy for psoriasis. Photodermatol Photoimmunol Photomed. 2013;29(1):18–26.
81. Wang E, Rodrigues M. An update and review of narrowband ultraviolet B phototherapy for vitiligo. Dermatolog Rev. 2022;3(5):257–350.
82. Grimes PE, Minus HR, Chakrabarti SG, Enterline J, Halder R, Gough JE, et al. Determination of optimal topical photochemotherapy for vitiligo. J Am Acad Dermatol. 1982;7(6):771–8.
83. Halpern SM, Anstey AV, Dawe RS, Diffey BL, Farr PM, Ferguson J, et al. Guidelines for topical PUVA: a report of a workshop of the British Photodermatology Group. Br J Dermatol. 2000;142(1):22–31.
84. Shenoi SD, Prabhu S, Indian Association of Dermatologists V, Leprologists. Photochemotherapy (PUVA) in psoriasis and vitiligo. Indian J Dermatol Venereol Leprol. 2014;80(6):497–504.
85. Lan CC, Wu CS, Chiou MH, Chiang TY, Yu HS. Low-energy helium-neon laser induces melanocyte proliferation via interaction with type IV collagen: visible light as a therapeutic option for vitiligo. Br J Dermatol. 2009;161(2):273–80.
86. Yu WT, Yu HS, Wu CS, Lee CH, Cheng YC, Lin WT, et al. Noninvasive cutaneous blood flow as a response predictor for visible light therapy on segmental vitiligo: a prospective pilot study. Br J Dermatol. 2011;164(4):759–64.
87. Lan CC, Wu CS, Chiou MH, Hsieh PC, Yu HS. Low-energy helium-neon laser induces locomotion of the immature melanoblasts and promotes melanogenesis of the more differentiated melanoblasts: recapitulation of vitiligo repigmentation in vitro. J Invest Dermatol. 2006;126(9):2119–26.
88. Yu HS, Wu CS, Yu CL, Kao YH, Chiou MH. Helium-neon laser irradiation stimulates migration and proliferation in melanocytes and induces repigmentation in segmental-type vitiligo. J Invest Dermatol. 2003;120(1):56–64.
89. Lan CC, Wu CS, Chen GS, Yu HS. Helium-neon laser and topical tacrolimus combination therapy: novel treatment option for vitiligo without additional photocarcinogenic risks. J Eur Acad Dermatol Venereol. 2009;23(3):344–5.
90. Byun JW, Babitha S, Kim EK, Shin J. A successful helium-neon laser and topical tacrolimus combination therapy in one child with vitiligo. Dermatol Ther. 2015;28(6):333–5.
91. Winkie MJ, Sakunchotpanit G, Salazar CE, Gunasekera NS, Buzney EA, Nambudiri VE. A focused review of visible light therapies for vitiligo. Photodermatol Photoimmunol Photomed. 2024;40(1):e12939.

92. Dawe RS, Cameron H, Yule S, Man I, Wainwright NJ, Ibbotson SH, et al. A randomized controlled trial of narrowband ultraviolet B vs bath-psoralen plus ultraviolet a photochemotherapy for psoriasis. Br J Dermatol. 2003;148(6):1194–204.
93. Kishan Kumar YH, Rao GR, Gopal KV, Shanti G, Rao KV. Evaluation of narrow-band UVB phototherapy in 150 patients with vitiligo. Indian J Dermatol Venereol Leprol. 2009;75(2):162–6.
94. Sapam R, Agrawal S, Dhali TK. Systemic PUVA vs. narrowband UVB in the treatment of vitiligo: a randomized controlled study. Int J Dermatol. 2012;51(9):1107–15.
95. Percivalle S, Piccino R, Caccialanza M, Forti S. Narrowband UVB phototherapy in vitiligo: evaluation of results in 53 patients. G Ital Dermatol Venereol. 2008;143(1):9–14.
96. Kanwar AJ, Dogra S, Parsad D, Kumar B. Narrow-band UVB for the treatment of vitiligo: an emerging effective and well-tolerated therapy. Int J Dermatol. 2005;44(1):57–60.
97. Bhatnagar A, Kanwar AJ, Parsad D, De D. Psoralen and ultraviolet A and narrow-band ultraviolet B in inducing stability in vitiligo, assessed by vitiligo disease activity score: an open prospective comparative study. J Eur Acad Dermatol Venereol. 2007;21(10):1381–5.
98. Ezzedine K, Lim HW, Suzuki T, Katayama I, Hamzavi I, Lan CC, et al. Revised classification/nomenclature of vitiligo and related issues: the Vitiligo Global Issues Consensus Conference. Pigment Cell Melanoma Res. 2012;25(3):E1–13.
99. Chen YT, Chen YJ, Hwang CY, Lin MW, Chen TJ, Chen CC, et al. Comorbidity profiles in association with vitiligo: a nationwide population-based study in Taiwan. J Eur Acad Dermatol Venereol. 2015;29(7):1362–9.
100. Esmat S, Elgendy D, Ali M, Esmat S, El-Nabarawy EA, Mahmoud SB, et al. Prevalence of photosensitivity in chronic hepatitis C virus patients and its relation to serum and urinary porphyrins. Liver Int. 2014;34(7):1033–9.
101. Radakovic-Fijan S, Furnsinn-Friedl AM, Honigsmann H, Tanew A. Oral dexamethasone pulse treatment for vitiligo. J Am Acad Dermatol. 2001;44(5):814–7.
102. Gupta AK, Ellis CN, Nickoloff BJ, Goldfarb MT, Ho VC, Rocher LL, et al. Oral cyclosporine in the treatment of inflammatory and noninflammatory dermatoses. A clinical and immunopathologic analysis. Arch Dermatol. 1990;126(3):339–50.
103. Singh H, Kumaran MS, Bains A, Parsad D. A randomized comparative study of oral corticosteroid minipulse and low-dose oral methotrexate in the treatment of unstable vitiligo. Dermatology. 2015;231(3):286–90.
104. Speeckaert R, Speeckaert MM, van Geel N. Why treatments do(n't) work in vitiligo: an autoinflammatory perspective. Autoimmun Rev. 2015;14(4):332–40.
105. Liu LY, Strassner JP, Refat MA, Harris JE, King BA. Repigmentation in vitiligo using the Janus kinase inhibitor tofacitinib may require concomitant light exposure. J Am Acad Dermatol. 2017;77(4):675–82.e1.
106. Karsli N, Akcali C, Ozgoztasi O, Kirtak N, Inaloz S. Role of oxidative stress in the pathogenesis of vitiligo with special emphasis on the antioxidant action of narrowband ultraviolet B phototherapy. J Int Med Res. 2014;42(3):799–805.
107. Elgoweini M, Nour El Din N. Response of vitiligo to narrowband ultraviolet B and oral antioxidants. J Clin Pharmacol. 2009;49(7):852–5.
108. Dell'Anna ML, Mastrofrancesco A, Sala R, Venturini M, Ottaviani M, Vidolin AP, et al. Antioxidants and narrow band-UVB in the treatment of vitiligo: a double-blind placebo controlled trial. Clin Exp Dermatol. 2007;32(6):631–6.
109. Yuksel EP, Aydin F, Senturk N, Canturk T, Turanli AY. Comparison of the efficacy of narrow band ultraviolet B and narrow band ultraviolet B plus topical catalase-superoxide dismutase treatment in vitiligo patients. Eur J Dermatol. 2009;19(4):341–4.
110. Bakis-Petsoglou S, Le Guay JL, Wittal R. A randomized, double-blinded, placebo-controlled trial of pseudocatalase cream and narrowband ultraviolet B in the treatment of vitiligo. Br J Dermatol. 2009;161(4):910–7.

111. Patel DC, Evans AV, Hawk JL. Topical pseudocatalase mousse and narrowband UVB phototherapy is not effective for vitiligo: an open, single-centre study. Clin Exp Dermatol. 2002;27(8):641–4.
112. Grimes PE, Hamzavi I, Lebwohl M, Ortonne JP, Lim HW. The efficacy of afamelanotide and narrowband UV-B phototherapy for repigmentation of vitiligo. JAMA Dermatol. 2013;149(1):68–73.
113. Shin S, Hann SK, Oh SH. Combination treatment with excimer laser and narrowband UVB light in vitiligo patients. Photodermatol Photoimmunol Photomed. 2016;32(1):28–33.
114. Shin J, Lee JS, Hann SK, Oh SH. Combination treatment by 10 600 nm ablative fractional carbon dioxide laser and narrowband ultraviolet B in refractory nonsegmental vitiligo: a prospective, randomized half-body comparative study. Br J Dermatol. 2012;166(3):658–61.
115. Dang YP, Li Q, Shi F, Yuan XY, Liu W. Effect of topical calcineurin inhibitors as monotherapy or combined with phototherapy for vitiligo treatment: a meta-analysis. Dermatol Ther. 2016;29(2):126–33.
116. Anbar TS, Westerhof W, Abdel-Rahman AT, Ewis AA, El-Khayyat MA. Effect of one session of ER:YAG laser ablation plus topical 5Fluorouracil on the outcome of short-term NB-UVB phototherapy in the treatment of non-segmental vitiligo: a left-right comparative study. Photodermatol Photoimmunol Photomed. 2008;24(6):322–9.
117. Jeon SY, Lee CY, Song KH, Kim KH. Spectrophotometric measurement of minimal erythema dose sites after narrowband ultraviolet B phototesting: clinical implication of spetrophotometric values in phototherapy. Ann Dermatol. 2014;26(1):17–25.
118. El-Khateeb EA, Ragab NF, Mohamed SA. Epidermal photoprotection: comparative study of narrowband ultraviolet B minimal erythema doses with and without stratum corneum stripping in normal and vitiligo skin. Clin Exp Dermatol. 2011;36(4):393–8.
119. Hamzavi I, Jain H, McLean D, Shapiro J, Zeng H, Lui H. Parametric modeling of narrowband UV-B phototherapy for vitiligo using a novel quantitative tool: the Vitiligo Area Scoring Index. Arch Dermatol. 2004;140(6):677–83.

Chapter 15
Complications of Medical Modalities of Vitiligo Therapy

Surabhi Sinha and Savitha Sharath

Abstract A plethora of drugs that target disease processes at various stages are used in the therapy of vitiligo with the aims of achieving arrest of disease progression and inducing repigmentation of existing lesions. The management of vitiligo requires long-term treatment with immunosuppressive and immunomodulatory agents, which could result in adverse effects. Routine monitoring is required to detect such adverse effects earlier and avoid any serious complications. We discuss frequent as well as uncommon side effects associated with various topical and oral agents and lasers, and light-based therapies employed in vitiligo treatment.

Keywords Vitiligo · Medical · Drugs · Topical · Immunosuppressive drugs
Complications · Phototherapy · Laser · Corticosteroids · JAK inhibitors
Tacrolimus

Vitiligo is a multifactorial disease characterized by limited or widespread depigmented macules, often associated with significant mental stress and social ostracizing of the patients. Several medical treatments are available and are used to arrest disease progression and induce repigmentation. These agents exhibit varying degrees of success, and the majority are safe and effective. Nevertheless, like all therapeutic modalities, these drugs are also associated with certain adverse effects, and a dermatologist should be mindful of these effects while charting the treatment plan for a patient.

We discuss the adverse effects of topical and systemic drugs and laser and light-based therapies in vitiligo.

S. Sinha (✉)
Department of Dermatology & STD, Lady Hardinge Medical College & associated hospitals, New Delhi, India

S. Sharath
Department of Dermatology & STD, Dr. Ram Manohar Lohia Hospital, New Delhi, India

R. Sarkar, V. Narayan R (eds.), *A Concise Guide to The Management of Vitiligo*,
https://doi.org/10.1007/978-981-95-3857-7_15

15.1 Topical Therapies

The complications associated with topical agents used in vitiligo are listed in Table 15.1.

15.1.1 Topical Corticosteroids

Topical corticosteroids (TCSs) remain the first-line therapy for focal vitiligo and give beneficial results in those with face and neck involvement and recent lesions. The use of high-potency TCS for longer durations is associated with side effects such as atrophy, hypopigmentation, telangiectasia, hypertrichosis, striae, acneiform eruptions, and perioral dermatitis. The incidence of such side effects is higher when applied on the face. The application of high-potency TCS on larger surface areas could lead to systemic absorption, resulting in adrenal suppression, particularly in children, and its use in intertriginous areas.

The use of class IV TCS, such as mometasone furoate cream, is recommended in patients with extrafacial vitiligo for a period of 3 months when prescribed daily or 6 months when given intermittently [1]. "Soft steroids" such as mometasone furoate and methylprednisolone aceponate have an advantage in minimizing systemic side effects while retaining anti-inflammatory effects. A cross-sectional study found no increased risk of ophthalmological complications (cataract, glaucoma, uveitis) in 19 vitiligo patients with periorbital use of TCS, including clobetasol propionate [2].

15.1.2 Topical Calcineurin Inhibitors

Tacrolimus 0.1% and pimecrolimus 1% ointment are extensively used as topical calcineurin inhibitors (TCIs) in the management of limited vitiligo, with optimal results in segmental vitiligo as well. TCIs have a good safety profile with only rare localized side effects, such as burning and itching sensations, and can lead to

Table 15.1 Adverse effects of topical therapies used in vitiligo

Corticosteroids	Atrophy, hypopigmentation, telangiectasia, hypertrichosis, striae, acneiform eruptions, and perioral dermatitis
Calcineurin inhibitors	Itching and burning sensation (FDA black box warning: carcinogenicity in children less than 2 years of age)
Vitamin D3 analogues	Local irritation
Basic fibroblast growth factor	Burning sensation and xerosis
JAK inhibitors	Erythema, pruritus, hyperpigmentation, and acneiform eruption

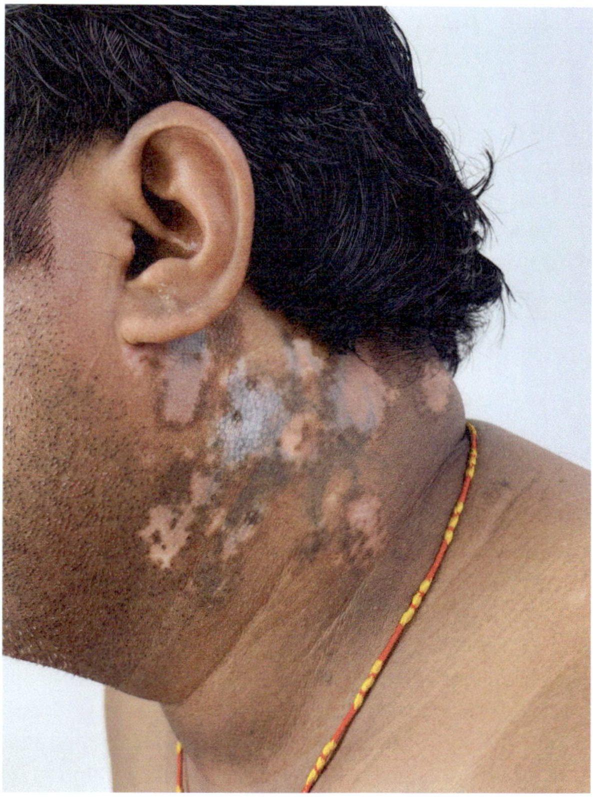

Fig. 15.1 A patient with segmental vitiligo treated with topical tacrolimus ointment 0.1% and micropigmentation (tattooing). Marginal hyperpigmentation following tacrolimus application and a bluish discoloration due to Tyndall effect (deeper migration of tattoo pigment) can be seen

erythema after alcohol consumption. Sometimes hyperpigmentation may be seen in some photoexposed vitiligo lesions after the application of tacrolimus ointment over a period of time [1] (Fig. 15.1). TCIs can increase susceptibility to infections such as herpes simplex and molluscum contagiosum. A study found topical tacrolimus to be well tolerated in vitiligo with irritation in a few cases (30%) [3]. However, the FDA black box warning of the potential carcinogenicity risk associated with TCI contraindicates its use in children less than 2 years of age, although recent long-term follow-up studies in children with atopic dermatitis refute the causal relationship between TCI use and the development of malignancies [4, 5].

15.1.3 Topical Vitamin D Analogues

Topical calcipotriene, calcipotriol, and tacalcitol have been used in combination with TCS or phototherapy in the management of vitiligo. While they can cause localized irritation, when used in combination with TCS, there is a reduction in the irritation potential of vitamin D analogues and the atrophogenic effects of TCS.

15.1.4 Basic Fibroblast Growth Factor (bFGF)-Derived Peptide

bFGF decapeptide 0.1% solution is used in the management of vitiligo, commonly as an adjunct modality, and it helps in repigmentation. It is generally well tolerated and can cause minor side effects, including xerosis, burning sensation, and irritation of the skin. Studies have demonstrated the excellent tolerability of this molecule, with infrequent and minor side effects that resolve without the discontinuation of the drug [6, 7].

15.1.5 Topical JAK Inhibitors

Tofacitinib 2% and ruxolitinib 1.5% creams have recently been used in vitiligo, and their side effects include erythema, pruritus, hyperpigmentation, and acneiform eruptions. Ruxolitinib 1.5% cream is FDA approved for nonsegmental vitiligo in adults and children >12 years of age. Two RCTs reported application site acne, application site pruritus, nasopharyngitis, headache, pyrexia and urinary tract infection as common adverse effects (>1%) with the use of topical rituximab in vitiligo, and infrequent adverse effects (0.5–1%) noted were application site dermatitis, folliculitis, hypertension, anxiety, diarrhea, ear infection, gastritis, hordeolum, influenza-like illness, insomnia, nasal congestion, and vomiting [8]. Recently, the novel JAKi delgocitinib (JAK1/2/3/TYK2 inhibitor) has been used in vitiligo with mixed results without any side effects [9].

15.1.6 Mycophenolate Mofetil (MMF)

A pilot study on the use of 15% MMF cream in active nonsegmental vitiligo found 25% repigmentation in 36% of patients, without any side effects [10].

15.2 Systemic Immunosuppressive and Immunomodulatory Agents

Immunosuppressive agents (ISAs), such as oral corticosteroids, methotrexate, azathioprine, mycophenolate mofetil, and cyclosporine, are used in the management of active and rapidly progressive vitiligo. ISAs are used mainly to limit the activity of the disease, and some agents might help in repigmentation as well. Side effects seen with the use of ISAs in vitiligo are enumerated in Table 15.2. These ISAs are associated with an increased risk of opportunistic infections and reactivation of latent

Table 15.2 Adverse effects of systemic agents used in the management of vitiligo

Immunosuppressive and immunomodulatory agents	
Oral corticosteroids	Acneiform eruptions, cushingoid habitus, atrophy, striae, hypertrichosis, impaired wound healing, hypertension, congestive heart failure, osteoporosis and spontaneous fracture, osteonecrosis, avascular necrosis of the femur, myopathy, hypothalamic-pituitary-adrenal axis suppression, secondary amenorrhea, hyperglycemia, hyperlipidemia, weight gain, headache, sleep disorders, and psychosis Ocular: glaucoma, cataract, peptic ulceration, and infections
Methotrexate	Constitutional: fatigue, anorexia Gastrointestinal: nausea, diarrhea, stomatitis, and hepatotoxicity Hematological: cytopenia Mucocutaneous: mucositis, radiation recall reactions, and alopecia Infections: reactivation of latent tuberculosis and hepatitis Reproductive: teratogenicity and oligospermia Pulmonary: pneumonitis and pulmonary fibrosis Oncogenicity: Epstein-related lymphoma and squamous cell carcinoma Neurological: headache, dizziness, and alterations in mood
Cyclosporine	Cutaneous: acneiform eruptions, gingival hyperplasia, and hypertrichosis CNS: paresthesias, tremors, headache, and rarely seizures CVS: hypertension Musculoskeletal: myalgia Dyselectrolytemia: hypomagnesemia and hyperkalemia Renal: hyperuricemia and nephrotoxicity
Azathioprine	Myelosuppression, hepatotoxicity, and gastrointestinal symptoms such as nausea, vomiting, and diarrhea
Mycophenolate mofetil	Gastrointestinal intolerance, myelosuppression, and hepatotoxicity
Minocycline	Cutaneous and nail hyperpigmentation, gastrointestinal discomfort, ototoxicity (dizziness and vertigo), pseudotumor cerebri, photosensitivity, serum sickness-like reaction, lupus-like syndrome, cutaneous polyarteritis nodosa, and hepatotoxicity
Small molecules	
Apremilast	Minor: headache, abdominal pain, nausea, and diarrhea Serious adverse effects: depression and suicidal attempt
JAK inhibitors	Common: nasopharyngitis, hyperlipidemia, acneiform eruptions, anemia, lymphocytopenia, and headache Less common: gastrointestinal perforations, thromboembolism, malignancies, myocardial infarction, stroke, and serious infections
Biologics (no side effects reported in vitiligo patients)	
TNF-α inhibitors	Serious infections, malignancies (lymphomas and nonmelanoma skin cancers), congestive heart failure, lupus-like syndrome, injection site reactions, and demyelinating disorders
Tildrakizumab	Infections, injection site reactions, and diarrhea

infections such as tuberculosis and hepatitis B and C. They are also carcinogenic and are linked with an increased risk of hematological malignancies and skin cancers.

15.2.1 Oral Corticosteroids

Oral corticosteroids (OCS) are administered in rapidly progressive vitiligo as daily therapy or oral mini-pulse (OMP) regimen and are usually given long term. They help in stabilizing the rapid progression of the disease and achieving repigmentation in some cases. However, OCS are associated with a higher adverse effect profile which includes:

(a) Dermatologic: Acneiform eruptions, cushingoid habitus, atrophy, striae, hypertrichosis, and impaired wound healing
(b) Cardiovascular: Hypertension and congestive heart failure
(c) Musculoskeletal: Osteoporosis and spontaneous fracture, osteonecrosis, avascular necrosis of the femur, and myopathy
(d) Endocrinologic and metabolic: Hypothalamic-pituitary-adrenal axis suppression, secondary amenorrhea, hyperglycemia, hyperlipidemia, and weight gain
(e) Neuropsychiatric: Pseudotumor cerebri, headache, sleep disorders, and psychosis
(f) ocular: Glaucoma and cataract
(g) Gastrointestinal: Fatty liver, peptic ulceration, and pancreatitis
(h) Infections

OMP with dexamethasone or betamethasone (5 mg two days a week) is used frequently in the management of unstable vitiligo; however, this regimen has only an adjunctive role. OMP is considered to have a good safety profile as compared to daily therapy. Studies on steroid pulse have reported side effects such as weight gain, headache, general weakness, and acneiform eruptions, of which weight gain is most commonly observed [11, 12]. In addition, sleeping problems, restlessness, irregular menstrual cycles, hypertrichosis, increased appetite, high blood pressure, elevated blood sugar levels, peptic ulcer disease, infections, palpitations, and striae were reported with the use of OMP [11].

15.3 Methotrexate

Methotrexate (MTX) is used in low doses (5–25 mg weekly) in vitiligo which acts by inhibition of T cells and reduction of TNF-α levels. It helps in halting the rapid progression of the disease. Common adverse effects with methotrexate include hepatotoxicity, pancytopenia, pulmonary toxicity, and gastrointestinal side effects. Severe nausea leading to discontinuation of MTX has been reported [13].

Nevertheless, few studies have shown good tolerability of MTX when used in vitiligo patients [14, 15]. MTX is a potential teratogen and abortifacient and FDA pregnancy category X drug. Rarely, malignancies (lymphomas and melanomas) are reported with the use of MTX, particularly in psoriasis patients.

15.3.1 Cyclosporine

Cyclosporine is used as an alternative therapy in rapidly progressive vitiligo cases where corticosteroids are ineffective, contraindicated, or not tolerated and is found to be effective in arresting disease progression in 60% of patients [16]. A randomized controlled trial comparing OMP and cyclosporine in active vitiligo found no statistically significant difference in adverse effects between the two groups [17]. The side effects observed in the cyclosporine group included paresthesia, gingival hyperplasia, myalgia, hypertension, headache, hyperuricemia, hyperbilirubinemia, and dyspepsia [17]. It can also cause tremors, diarrhea, hyperkalemia, hypomagnesemia, hypomagnesemia, and renal toxicity.

15.3.2 Azathioprine

Azathioprine not only arrests disease progression but also aids in the repigmentation of vitiligo. It is used in low doses (50 mg once daily) in vitiligo as compared to high-dose regimens in other inflammatory disorders and thus could be used long-term without any serious adverse effects [18]. The side effects of the use of azathioprine are minimal and include myelosuppression, hepatotoxicity, and gastrointestinal symptoms such as nausea, vomiting, and diarrhea. A randomized controlled trial comparing azathioprine and OMP found azathioprine to be safer (5.5% vs 50%), while both drugs demonstrated equal efficacy in the treatment of vitiligo, and the side effects reported with azathioprine included hair loss and leukopenia in one patient each [18]. Another study on vitiligo reported acute pancreatitis in one patient with the use of azathioprine [19].

15.3.3 Mycophenolate Mofetil

Mycophenolate mofetil (MMF) inhibits B and T cells and helps in stabilizing rapidly progressive vitiligo with no/minimal effect on repigmentation, the efficacy of which is comparable to OMP [20]. Gastrointestinal intolerance is the dose-limiting side effect of MMF. A randomized study reported nausea (24%) and diarrhea (16%) as common side effects associated with MMF use in vitiligo [20]. It can cause serious adverse effects such as pancytopenia and hepatotoxicity, which require discontinuation of the therapy and resolve after stopping the drug [20].

15.3.4 *Minocycline*

Minocycline is an anti-inflammatory and immunomodulatory antibiotic that helps in limiting disease progression and used at a dosage of 100 mg once daily. It can cause gastrointestinal discomfort, ototoxicity (dizziness and vertigo), pseudotumor cerebri, photosensitivity, serum sickness-like reaction, lupus-like syndrome, cutaneous polyarteritis nodosa, and hepatotoxicity. It can result in pigmentation of the nail, skin, and mucosa and staining of adult teeth. Hyperpigmentation (cutaneous, oral mucosal, and nail) was commonly reported with minocycline in previous studies; in some patients confined only to vitiligo lesions [21, 22]. It is contraindicated in children less than 9 years of age, as it affects bone growth and causes yellowish discoloration of teeth.

15.4 Small Molecules and Biologicals

15.4.1 *Apremilast*

Apremilast helps arrest the progression of vitiligo, and there is some evidence of its efficacy in the repigmentation of lesions. It has a good safety profile, with side effects occurring in some patients. Gastrointestinal intolerance limits the dosing of apremilast and could lead to discontinuation of the drug.

Other side effects include headache, weight loss, and depression. In a randomized study, diarrhea, nausea, weight loss, loss of appetite, fatigue, headache, insomnia, depression, and upper abdominal pain were higher among patients receiving apremilast as add-on therapy to standard therapy compared to those receiving standard therapy alone [23]. Another randomized trial comparing the efficacy of apremilast plus NB-UVB phototherapy versus placebo plus NB-UVB therapy found two serious adverse events in the former group, which included suicide attempts (attributable to treatment) and a benign tumor of the amygdala [24].

15.4.2 *JAK Inhibitors*

Oral tofacitinib has been tried with success in vitiligo. The most common reported side effects with the use of JAKi include upper respiratory tract infections and nasopharyngitis. The incidence of infections associated with JAKi is comparable with that of biologics, but the incidence of herpes zoster is much higher [25].

The black box warning for tofacitinib includes serious infections (active tuberculosis, invasive fungal infections, and viral infections), mortality, malignancy (including lymphomas and solid tumors), major adverse cardiovascular events (cardiovascular death, myocardial infarction, and stroke), and thrombosis [26]. Prothrombotic effects seem to be rare and dose dependent (20 mg). Other adverse effects include gastrointestinal perforations, hyperlipidemia, acneiform eruptions, anemia, lymphocytopenia, and headache. New-onset generalized vitiligo has been reported as a paradoxical reaction in a female patient with rheumatoid arthritis receiving tofacitinib therapy [27].

Other JAKis tried in vitiligo such as baricitinib (JAK1/2 inhibitor) and upadacitinib were well tolerated by the patients [28–31]. Acne was reported as a common side effect associated with the use of upadacitinib in vitiligo (xinhong su). More recently, a phase 2b trial demonstrated a good safety profile of ritlecitinib (JAK1/TEC inhibitor) in active nonsegmental vitiligo during a 48-week treatment period [32].

15.4.3 *Biologics*

Vitiligo shows increased levels of proinflammatory mediators including TNF-α and IL-12, IL-23, and IL-17, targeting which might be promising in the management [33]. Previous reports have shown no side effects with the use of TNF-α inhibitors in vitiligo [34, 35]. A single case report of tildrakizumab (IL-23 inhibitor) in rapidly progressive acrofacial vitiligo was also well tolerated by the patient [36].

15.5 Laser and Light-Based Therapies (Table 15.3)

Table 15.3 Adverse effects of lasers and light therapies used in the management of vitiligo

Light-based therapies	
NB-UVB phototherapy	Well tolerated Minor side effects: erythema, itching, and mild burning Long-term use: risk of skin malignancies
PUVA	Acute effects: phototoxicity, pruritus, blistering, nausea, and reactivation of herpes simplex; less commonly can lead to nail pigmentation, photo-onycholysis, and photoallergic reactions Chronic: photoaging, PUVA keratoses, PUVA lentigines, and skin cancers
Lasers	
Excimer	Erythema, blistering, and less commonly perilesional pigmentation
Ablative	Risk of scarring
Fractional	Safer
Q-switched	Purpura, oozing, crusting, and pain

15.5.1 Light-Based Therapies

15.5.1.1 Narrowband UVB

Narrowband ultraviolet B (NB-UVB) phototherapy is associated with minor side effects such as erythema, itching, and mild burning or pain, which are generally well tolerated and resolve spontaneously within a few hours of treatment in most instances. The risk of carcinogenicity is not well defined with NBUVB. Recent studies have shown conflicting results on the increased risk of skin cancer with the use of NBUVB in vitiligo. Retrospective review of NBUVB in vitiligo found an increased risk of skin malignancies (basal cell carcinoma and squamous cell carcinoma) with long-term use of NBUVB in Asian vitiligo patients, and the risk increased with greater cumulative and maximum doses of phototherapy and with the concomitant use of systemic therapy [37]. Another large retrospective study found NBUVB to be safe in vitiligo patients without any increased risk of skin malignancies, although there was an increased risk of the development of actinic keratosis [38].

15.5.1.2 Photochemotherapy

Topical or systemic photochemotherapy involves the administration of UVA combined with psoralen (PUVA). Vitiligo requires prolonged therapy with 100–200 sessions over months to achieve optimal melanogenesis. The acute effects of PUVA include phototoxicity, pruritus, blistering, nausea, and reactivation of herpes simplex, and less commonly can lead to nail pigmentation, photoonycholysis, and photoallergic reactions. The chronic effects of PUVA include photoaging, PUVA keratoses, PUVA lentigines, and skin cancers. The risk of squamous cell carcinoma (SCC) is dose dependent, and it is recommended to limit the number of lifetime exposures to less than 150 to 200 sessions with a cumulative dose less than 1000–1500 J/cm^2 [39].

15.5.1.3 Lasers

Excimer, ablative, fractional, and Q-switched (Qs) lasers have been used in the management of vitiligo. The side effect profile of the excimer laser is comparable to that of NB-UVB phototherapy, and no significant difference has been noted between the excimer laser and excimer lamp [40, 41]. Excimer lamp might be associated with a slightly higher frequency of side effects, as it induces more erythema at the same doses compared to excimer laser [42]. Side effects are rare, transient, and localized to the treatment site and include erythema, blistering, and less commonly perilesional pigmentation. However, the incidence of side effects increases with increasing frequency of treatment sessions (thrice per week) [43].

Ablative lasers such as CO_2 and Er:YAG lasers have been used in combination with NBUVB phototherapy to enhance repigmentation but are associated with significant downtime and a risk of scarring; thus, fractional ablative lasers are used as an adjunctive therapeutic modality in the management of stable nonsegmental vitiligo, which are considered much safer [44].

Qs lasers are used in extensive to nearly complete vitiligo patients to achieve depigmentation of the skin with residual pigmentation. Short-lasting side effects include purpura, oozing, crusting, and pain. However, no risk of scarring or long-term side effects has been reported.

15.6 Conclusion

Vitiligo is often associated with impaired quality of life and demands long-term treatment with immunosuppressive drugs, some of which have a higher side effect profile, particularly corticosteroids. Traditional ISA and newer therapeutic drugs such as JAK inhibitors and biologicals, although infrequent, are associated with grave side effects like serious infections and malignancies. The selection of appropriate candidates for ISAs and strict monitoring for adverse effects help mitigate foreseeable complications.

References

1. Sahni K, Gupta V, Khanna N. Hyperpigmentation in photo exposed patches of vitiligo following tacrolimus therapy. Ind Dermatol Online J. 2014;5(2):164–6.
2. Khurrum H, AlGhamdi KM, Osman E. Screening of glaucoma or cataract prevalence in vitiligo patients and its relationship with periorbital steroid use. J Cutan Med Surg. 2016;20(2):146–9.
3. Rokni GR, Golpour M, Gorji AH, Khalilian A, Ghasemi H. Effectiveness and safety of topical tacrolimus in treatment of vitiligo. J Adv Pharm Technol Res. 2017;8:29–33.
4. Margolis DJ, Abuabara K, Hoffstad OJ, Wan J, Raimondo D, Bilker WB. Association between malignancy and topical use of pimecrolimus. JAMA Dermatol. 2015;151:594–9.
5. Siegfried EC, Jaworski JC, Hebert AA. Topical calcineurin inhibitors and lymphoma risk: evidence update with implications for daily practice. Am J Clin Dermatol. 2013;14:163–78.
6. Sharma A, Majid I, Kumar HK, et al. The safety and effectiveness of decapeptide in patients with vitiligo: a real-world study. Cureus. 2023;15(7):e41418.
7. Ramaiah A, Kar HK, Garg VK, Bajaj N, Gupta L, Madhava AS. A double blind randomized phase IV clinical trial of basic fibroblast growth factor related Deca-peptide in vitiligo. Pigment Disord. 2015;3:S3–004.
8. Rosmarin D, Passeron T, Pandya AG, et al. TRuE-V Study Group. Two phase 3, randomized, controlled trials of ruxolitinib cream for vitiligo. N Engl J Med. 2022;387:1445–55.
9. Yagi K, Ishida Y, Otsuka A, Kabashima K. Two cases of vitiligo vulgaris treated with topical Janus kinase inhibitor delgocitinib. Australas J Dermatol. 2021;62(3):433–4.
10. Handjani F, Aghaei S, Moezzi I, Saki N. Topical mycophenolate mofetil in the treatment of vitiligo: a pilot study. Dermatol Pract Concept. 2017;7(2):31–3.

11. Jafarzadeh A, Pour Mohammad A, Khosravi M, et al. A systematic review of case series and clinical trials investigating systemic oral or injectable therapies for the treatment of vitiligo. Skin Res Technol. 2024;30(3):e13642.
12. Chavez-Alvarez S, Herz-Ruelas M, Raygoza-Cortez AK, et al. Oral mini-pulse therapy in vitiligo: a systematic review. Int J Dermatol. 2021;60(7):868–76.
13. Singh H, Kumaran MS, Bains A, Parsad D. A randomized comparative study of oral corticosteroid minipulse and low-dose oral methotrexate in the treatment of unstable vitiligo. Dermatology. 2015;231(3):286–90.
14. ElGhareeb MI, Metwalli M, AbdelMoneim N. Combination of oral methotrexate and oral mini-pulse dexamethasone vs either agent alone in vitiligo treatment with follow up by dermoscope. Dermatol Ther. 2020;33(4):e13586.
15. Tavitova A, Valle Y, Lomonosov K. Using methotrexate in the treatment of advanced vitiligo. J Cosmet Dermatol. 2023;22(3):1136–8.
16. Taneja A, Kumari A, Vyas K, Khare AK, Gupta LK, Mittal AK. Cyclosporine in treatment of progressive vitiligo: an open-label, single-arm interventional study. Indian J Dermatol Venereol Leprol. 2019;85(5):528–31.
17. Mehta H, Kumar S, Parsad D, Bishnoi A, Vinay K, Kumaran MS. Oral cyclosporine is effective in stabilizing active vitiligo: results of a randomized controlled trial. Dermatol Ther. 2021;34(5):e15033.
18. Jawade S, Saoji V, Madke B, Singh A. Comparison of oral azathioprine and oral mini pulse steroid in the treatment of vitiligo: an open-label randomized controlled trial. Indian J Dermatol. 2023;68:591–7.
19. Patra S, Khaitan BK, Sharma VK, Khanna N. A randomized comparative study of the effect of betamethasone oral mini-pulse therapy versus oral azathioprine in progressive nonsegmental vitiligo. J Am Acad Dermatol. 2021;85(3):728–9.
20. Bishnoi A, Vinay K, Kumaran MS, Parsad D. Oral mycophenolate mofetil as a stabilizing treatment for progressive non-segmental vitiligo: results from a prospective, randomized, investigator-blinded pilot study. Arch Dermatol Res. 2021;313(5):357–65.
21. Charoenpongpun N, Kamanamool N, Udompataikul M, Khunkhet S, Kanokrungsee S. A pilot study of combined oral minocycline and narrowband UVB phototherapy in vitiligo: a randomized, double-blind, placebo-controlled trial. Dermatol Ther. 2022;35(8):e15596.
22. Singh A, Kanwar AJ, Parsad D, Mahajan R. Randomized controlled study to evaluate the effectiveness of dexamethasone oral minipulse therapy versus oral minocycline in patients with active vitiligo vulgaris. Indian J Dermatol Venereol Leprol. 2014;80(1):29–35.
23. Sharma S, Bhardwaj A, Dwivedi P, et al. Apremilast add-on benefits over conventional drugs (ABCD) in unstable non-segmental vitiligo: a 12-week single-center randomized controlled trial. Cureus. 2023;15:e37180.
24. Khemis A, Fontas E, Moulin S, Montaudié H, Lacour JP, Passeron T. Apremilast in combination with narrowband UVB in the treatment of vitiligo: a 52-week monocentric prospective randomized placebo-controlled study. J Invest Dermatol. 2020;140(8):1533–1537.e2.
25. Shalabi MMK, Garcia B, Coleman K, Siller A Jr, Miller AC, Tyring SK. Janus kinase and tyrosine kinase inhibitors in dermatology: a review of their utilization, safety profile and future applications. Skin Therapy Lett. 2022;27:4–9.
26. XELJANJ (tofacitinib) [package insert]. Manhattan (NY): Pfizer Corporation; 2012. Available from https://www.accessdata.fda.gov/drugsatfda_docs/label/2021/203214s028,208246s013,213082s003lbl.pdf. Accessed 15 May 2024.
27. Nguyen JK, Schlichte MJ, Jogi R, Alikhan M, Patel AB. A case of new-onset vitiligo in a patient on tofacitinib and brief review of paradoxical presentations with other novel targeted therapies. Dermatol Online J. 2020;26:13030/qt1hk2x4j5.
28. Mumford BP, Gibson A, Chong AH. Repigmentation of vitiligo with oral baricitinib. Australas J Dermatol. 2020;61(4):374–6.
29. Dong J, Huang X, Ma LP, et al. Baricitinib is effective in treating progressing vitiligo in vivo and in vitro. Dose Response. 2022;20(2):15593258221105370.

30. Li X, Sun Y, Du J, Wang F, Ding X. Excellent repigmentation of generalized vitiligo with oral baricitinib combined with NB-UVB phototherapy. Clin Cosmet Investig Dermatol. 2023;16:635–8.
31. Su X, Luo R, Ruan S, et al. Efficacy and tolerability of oral upadacitinib monotherapy in patients with recalcitrant vitiligo. J Am Acad Dermatol. 2023 Dec;89(6):1257–9.
32. Ezzedine K, Peeva E, Yamaguchi Y, et al. Efficacy and safety of oral ritlecitinib for the treatment of active nonsegmental vitiligo: a randomized phase 2b clinical trial. J Am Acad Dermatol. 2023;88(2):395–403.
33. Custurone P, Di Bartolomeo L, Irrera N, et al. Role of cytokines in vitiligo: pathogenesis and possible targets for old and new treatments. Int J Mol Sci. 2021;22:11429.
34. Alghamdi KM, Khurrum H, Taieb A, Ezzedine K. Treatment of generalized vitiligo with anti-TNF-α agents. J Drugs Dermatol. 2012;11:534–9.
35. Rigopoulos D, Gregoriou S, Larios G, Moustou E, Belayeva-Karatza E, Kalogeromitros D. Etanercept in the treatment of vitiligo. Dermatology. 2007;215:84–5.
36. Jerjen R, Moodley A, Sinclair R. Repigmentation of acrofacial vitiligo with subcutaneous tildrakizumab. Australas J Dermatol. 2020;61(4):e446–8.
37. Chia BKY, Yew YW, Zhao X, Chong WS, Thng TGS. Incidence of skin malignancies in patients with vitiligo or psoriasis who received narrowband ultraviolet B phototherapy (308 nm/311 nm): a retrospective review of 3730 patients. Photodermatol Photoimmunol Photomed. 2023;39(4):343–50.
38. Bae JM, Ju HJ, Lee RW, et al. Evaluation for skin cancer and precancer in patients with vitiligo treated with long-term narrowband UV-B phototherapy. JAMA Dermatol. 2020;156(5):529–37.
39. McKenna K, Ibbotson S. Principles of phototherapy. In: Griffiths C, Barker J, Bleiker T, Hussain W, Simpson R, editors. Rook's textbook dermatology. 10th ed. Hoboken: Wiley; 2024. p. 21.13–4.
40. Lopes C, Trevisani VF, Melnik T. Efficacy and safety of 308-nm monochromatic excimer lamp versus other phototherapy devices for vitiligo: a systematic review with meta-analysis. Am J Clin Dermatol. 2016;17(1):23–32.
41. Sun Y, Wu Y, Xiao B, et al. Treatment of 308-nm excimer laser on vitiligo: a systemic review of randomized controlled trials. J Dermatolog Treat. 2015;26:347–53.
42. Le Duff F, Fontas E, Giacchero D, et al. 308-nm excimer lamp vs. 308-nm excimer laser for treating vitiligo: a randomized study. Br J Dermatol. 2010;163(1):188–92.
43. Alhowaish AK, Dietrich N, Onder M, Fritz K. Effectiveness of a 308-nm excimer laser in treatment of vitiligo: a review. Lasers Med Sci. 2013;28(3):1035–41.
44. Chiu YJ, Perng CK, Ma H. Fractional CO_2 laser contributes to the treatment of non-segmental vitiligo as an adjunct therapy: a systemic review and meta-analysis. Lasers Med Sci. 2018;33(7):1549–56.

Part IV
Surgical Therapy

Chapter 16
Patient Selection and Counseling

Vignesh Narayan R and Rashmi Sarkar

Abstract Effective vitiligo therapy hinges on meticulous patient selection, emphasizing stable disease for surgical interventions. Surgical treatment shows optimal results in localized or segmental vitiligo due to underlying neurochemical mediators, whereas generalized vitiligo typically responds poorly. Stability assessment, defined by no new or expanding lesions for a year, is critical. Methods like digital photography, mini graft testing, and evaluation of the Koebner phenomenon are used to confirm stability. Small to medium depigmented areas are best treated with tissue grafts, while extensive lesions require cellular grafts. Anatomical location significantly influences outcomes, with favorable results in the neck and presternal regions and poor outcomes in the joints and acral areas.

Preoperative psychological assessment ensures realistic patient expectations, crucial for satisfaction. Counseling addresses preoperative anxiety, postoperative care, and relapse management, fostering patient-surgeon rapport and compliance. Techniques like cognitive behavioral therapy and relaxation therapy mitigate surgical anxiety. Effective communication and informed consent are pivotal, ensuring that patients comprehend the procedure and potential outcomes. In high-volume settings, counsellors aid by providing detailed information, addressing patient concerns, and ensuring follow-up adherence. This holistic approach, encompassing medical, psychological, and logistical factors, enhances the success of vitiligo surgery, leading to better patient outcomes and satisfaction.

Keywords Vitiligo surgery · Counseling · Patient selection

V. Narayan R
Department of Dermatology, Venereology and Leprology, New Varalakshmi Hospital, Bangalore, Karnataka, India

R. Sarkar (✉)
Department of Dermatology, Venereology and Leprology, Lady Hardinge Medical College and Hospitals, New Delhi, Delhi, India

R. Sarkar, V. Narayan R (eds.), *A Concise Guide to The Management of Vitiligo*,
https://doi.org/10.1007/978-981-95-3857-7_16

16.1 Patient Selection

Strict patient selection is crucial for achieving a favorable response to vitiligo therapy. Surgical treatment should be initiated only in patients with stable disease [1]. Various surgical options are available, and the type of therapy must be tailored to each patient's specific needs. The choice of intervention depends on the type of vitiligo, the location of the lesion, the extent of the disease, and the patient's motivation to adhere to postoperative instructions.

16.1.1 Type of Vitiligo

The best response to surgical treatment is observed in patients with localized or segmental vitiligo. In contrast, the response is usually poor in generalized vitiligo. This difference is likely due to the neurochemical mediators underlying segmental vitiligo, whereas nonsegmental vitiligo is characterized by periods of clinical quiescence.

16.1.2 Stability of Disease

Active vitiligo requires medical management to halt disease activity. According to the IADVL task force, vitiligo is considered stable when there is no growth of old lesions and no new lesions for a period of 1 year. Various modalities can be used to assess disease stability:

1. **Photography**: Digital photography provides an objective measurement of surface area and monitors changes over time.
2. **Mini Graft Testing**: This involves transplanting 1–1.5 mm tissue punches from a donor site into the vitiliginous patch. A positive test is indicated by pigment spread of more than 1 mm from the transplanted graft (Fig. 16.1).
3. **Koebner Phenomenon**: The spread of depigmented patches at trauma sites, ascertainable via history or experimentally induced, indicates disease instability (Fig. 16.2).

16.1.3 Area of Depigmentation

Small to medium-sized areas of depigmentation can be effectively covered with tissue grafting methods, whereas extensive lesions are better treated with cellular grafts. [2]

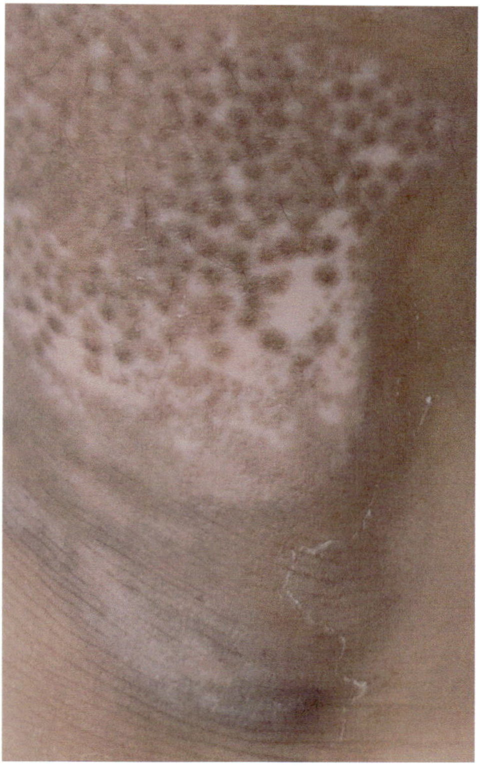

Fig. 16.1 Positive mini punch test with perigraft pigmentation

16.1.4 Location of Lesions

Excellent results are seen with transplantation on the neck and presternal region. Joints, however, show poor results due to difficulty in immobilization and graft attachment. Acral areas also support transplanted melanocyte survival and growth less effectively. Success is higher with mini punch grafting compared to split-thickness skin grafts and epidermal blister roofs. When multiple areas are involved, therapy is prioritized for exposed and more visible areas. Difficult-to-treat areas include the genital folds, joints, and acral areas like the palms and soles [3].

16.1.5 Age of Patients

There is no minimum age for vitiligo surgery. Techniques like seed grafting may be preferable in children [4]. Emphasis must be placed on the importance of aftercare to achieve optimal pigmentation.

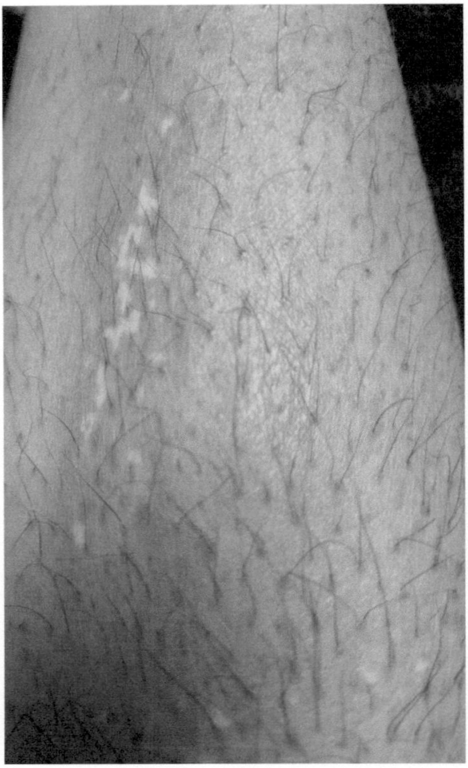

Fig. 16.2 Linear patches of depigmentation at sites of trauma indicating active disease

16.1.6 Newer Markers of Disease Stability

Immunohistochemical analysis of perilesional punch biopsy specimens can measure the number of CD8+ and CD45 RO cells per high-power field. Better survival and successful repigmentation are associated with fewer than 7 CD8+ cells and 11 CD45 RO cells [5]. An alternative method involves creating suction blisters; higher CXCL-9 levels in blister fluid correlate with active disease and a poor response to therapy [6].

16.1.7 Role of Phototherapy

Pretransplantation phototherapy serves as a form of priming and increases the chances of pigmentation postsurgery. Hence, an assessment is required to determine if the patient can meet the requirement of frequent visits to the phototherapy center. [7]

16.1.8 Preoperative Psychological Assessment

The quality of surgery is not the only factor determining patient satisfaction; the level of doctor-patient communication plays a crucial role. A comprehensive preoperative psychological assessment is essential to ensure that patients have realistic expectations and are well prepared for the procedure. This process includes several key steps [8]:

1. Assess the Patient's Request: Engage in a detailed discussion to understand the patient's specific concerns and the problems they wish to address with surgery.
2. Physical Examination and Surgical Planning: Conduct a thorough physical examination and develop a tailored surgical plan.
3. Evaluate Medical Conditions: Identify any medical contraindications for surgery.
4. Evaluate Psychological State: Continuously assess the patient's psychological readiness from the initial visit through to the follow-up period.

16.1.8.1 Understanding Patient Expectations [9]

Patients must have a reasonable understanding of what can be achieved with the planned procedure. It is crucial to gauge their comprehension of the wound healing process and the potential need for additional procedures. During the preoperative assessment, explore the patients' expectations and motivations. Patients with internal motivations, such as a desire to improve their self-image to meet personal standards, typically respond more positively to surgery than those with external motivations, who may attribute their physical appearance to their life problems (e.g., relationship or occupational issues).

Patients should not expect surgery to achieve physical perfection or solve unrelated personal issues. They should be given sufficient time to consider the implications of surgery, allowing them to make an informed decision and address any new questions or doubts that arise.

16.1.8.2 Identifying Poor Surgical Candidates

Indicators of a poor surgical candidate include:

- Multiple Previous Surgeries: A history of numerous unsatisfactory surgeries
- Surgeon Shopping: Indecisive patients who cannot commit to a surgeon or procedure, often leading to postsurgical regret
- Sudden Whim for Surgery: Impulsive decisions to undergo surgery without thorough consideration

If underlying psychopathology is suspected, a psychiatrist consultation and evaluation are advisable.

16.1.9 Contraindications

Contraindications include the presence of unrealistic expectations, hypertrophic scarring or a keloidal tendency, and positive viral serology for HIV, HBsAg, and HCV, since viral particles may become aerosolized during procedures such as dermabrasion or laser ablation [10].

Patient selection and disease stability assessment are critical for successful vitiligo surgery. Personalized approaches considering the type and location of vitiligo, as well as patient motivation and compliance, significantly enhance treatment outcomes.

16.2 Counseling in Vitiligo Surgery

Surgery, regardless of its complexity, often involves multiple stressful components. The stress begins before the surgical procedure and includes anxiety about the condition, the anticipated surgery, the potential pain, and the recovery period. What might be considered a minor procedure by the surgeon can provoke a strong emotional response and fear in the patient. Presurgical distress and anxiety can be associated with greater postoperative complications and prolonged recovery time. Therefore, psychosocial assessment and intervention play a crucial role in managing surgical patients.

Patients may fear that surgery could adversely alter their physical appearance or functionality. Insufficient communication can heighten patient anxiety, potentially leading to insomnia, which further exacerbates anxiety. It is essential to provide patients with a clear roadmap of the procedures they can expect and the possible outcomes.

Patients look for someone with whom they can objectively discuss their issues. This is especially important for patients with prior negative surgical experience. Effective counseling can alleviate scepticism toward treatment, helping patients feel more relaxed and confident in their surgeon. Counseling is particularly crucial in cases of disease relapse. Patients should be informed about the possibility of relapse and ways to minimize its chances. Good communication establishes a rapport with patients, reducing the likelihood of malpractice suits.

Counseling should emphasize the need for adherence to postoperative treatments, medications, and follow-ups. The treatment provider should also assess the patient's motivation for surgery. Presurgical counseling typically focuses on the surgical process, the chance of success, and the speed of recovery, while postoperative counseling centers on the further course of action and support. Fear of possible role changes postsurgery should also be addressed. An individualized care plan for both the patient and their family is beneficial.

16.2.1 Presurgical Anxiety and Preparation

During the surgical waiting period, patients often experience anticipatory fears, including feelings of helplessness and depression. A moderate amount of worry is optimal, as it ensures that patients process preoperative instructions and information adequately. Those with a moderate level of fear are more likely to be attentive to information and instructions, preparing them for postoperative recovery [11, 12].

16.2.2 Preparatory Information

Patients who are well prepared for what to expect during and after surgery tend to show better postoperative adjustment and recovery. Providing video recordings of the procedure can help patients prepare for what is to come [13].

16.2.3 Social Support

Social support significantly alleviates anxiety. This support can come from other patients who are about to undergo surgery or from those who have already undergone the procedure. This peer interaction provides firsthand accounts of the surgery and the postoperative period, offering a role model for recovery and alleviating fears [14].

16.2.4 Methods to Manage Surgical Anxiety

Managing surgical anxiety and fear can include cognitive behavioral therapy (CBT) and relaxation therapy. CBT involves mental exercises to change the patient's perspective on a situation to reduce anxiety. Techniques include distraction, identifying negative automatic thoughts, and replacing them with positive coping mechanisms. Relaxation techniques aim to produce a physiological state opposite to the stress response [15].

16.2.5 Counseling Children

Children should be informed about their illness and proposed treatment in a manner they can understand. Encouraging them to ask questions and express their emotions is important. Showing videos of other children undergoing the same procedure can be effective [16].

16.2.6 Challenges in Developing Countries

In developing countries, the high patient load often makes it challenging to provide adequate counseling and address anxiety and apprehension. However, addressing patient misconceptions and anxiety is critical. Easy access to the internet and social media has led to numerous patient doubts, which, if not adequately addressed, can lead to feelings of being let down. Patients may require repeated information and may ask the same questions during follow-up visits, posing a challenge for busy doctors.

16.2.7 Role of Counselors

In settings with high patient loads, counselors can reduce the time constraints on surgeons by providing adequate information to patients. They can address common queries, pacify patients during the recovery period, and ensure proper follow-up and posttreatment adherence. A good counselor should be a good listener, able to explain procedures in simple yet effective language, and adept at using audiovisual tools. However, certain information should be confirmed with the treating surgeon before being advised by the counselor [17, 18].

16.2.8 Effective Counseling Practices

Effective counseling involves several key practices [18]:

- Break the ice and show courtesy.
- Listen and understand the patient's problems before providing information and explanations.
- Consider the patient as a whole, including their social role and economic situation.
- Ensure confidentiality and privacy.

- Provide undivided attention.
- Acknowledge risks and respond promptly to doubts.

By following these guidelines, healthcare providers can enhance the surgical experience for patients, leading to better outcomes and greater patient satisfaction.

16.2.8.1 Counseling During Surgery

As many procedures are performed under local anesthesia, patients are conscious and aware of conversations during surgery. Intraoperative issues should be managed efficiently and discreetly. The surgeon should maintain a positive attitude toward the outcome and view the surgery as a positive experience.

16.2.8.2 Postoperative Counseling

If complications arise postsurgery and the patient is dissatisfied, it is important to listen empathetically rather than argue. Many patients seek reassurance and follow-up care even if they are disappointed. Providing frequent visits and dedicating more time to these patients can help restore their confidence. This support is crucial for patients to be receptive to any necessary secondary corrective procedures. Patients may need time to adjust to their new appearance and body image. Pre- and postoperative photographs can help patients appreciate the benefits of surgery.

16.2.8.3 Informed Consent

A proper informed consent process offers several advantages:

- Adequate Information: Ensures that the patient understands the disease and the procedure
- Greater Autonomy: Helps manage patient expectations
- Legal defense: Provides legal protection for the healthcare provider

An informed consent discussion should last between 15 and 30 min and cover all necessary details. The mnemonic DORIS can be used to summarize the requirements (Table 16.1). [19]

the disease, which may become active again. While photographs of previous results can be shown, it must be emphasized that individual variation exists. The technical procedure should be explained in simple terms, including the concept of taking tissue from another healthy site, such as the thigh. Potential adverse effects, such as scarring, incomplete pigmentation, and lack of graft survival, should also be discussed.

Table 16.1 The mnemonic DORIS, summarizing the various requirements of presurgical counseling

Acronym	Expansion	Meaning
D	Diagnosis	Explanation of the diagnosis and the likely natural history of the condition if left untreated
O	Options	Includes surgical, nonsurgical, and observation For surgical procedures, the description, sequalae, recovery, and follow-up must be discussed
R	Risks	Cover the general medical and surgical complications, with specific risk of the surgery chosen
I	Individual factors	Give consideration to the patients social and economic obligations and role
S	Shared decision	Share the outcome of the discussion with the patient

By following these guidelines, dermatologists can ensure that patients are well prepared, reducing anxiety and enhancing overall satisfaction with the surgical experience.

Acknowledgments None.

Conflicts of Interest None.

Source of Funding None.

Ethics Statement Written informed consent obtained from patient.

References

1. Sahni K, Parsad D. Stability in vitiligo: is there a perfect way to predict it? J Cutan Aesthet Surg. 2013;6(2):75–82.
2. Thakur V, Narayan RV, Parsad D. Transplantation procedures in vitiligo: what's new. Dermatol Rev. 2022;3(5):276–83.
3. Thakur V, Vinay K, Dogra S. Surgical modalities of treatment in vitiligo. Cosmoderma. 2021;1:13.
4. Sharma CK, Sharma M, Aggarwal B, Sharma V. Different advanced therapeutic approaches to treat vitiligo. J Environ Pathol Toxicol Oncol. 2015;34(4):321–34.
5. Bassiouny DA, El Tahlawy S, El Tawdy A, Abdellatif M, Amin DIE. Prediction of response to surgical therapy in nonsegmental vitiligo based on an immunohistochemical cutoff value. J Egypt Women's Dermatol Soc. 2020;17(1):19–24.
6. Lin F, Hu W, Xu W, Zhou M, Xu AE. CXCL9 as a key biomarker of vitiligo activity and prediction of the success of cultured melanocyte transplantation. Sci Rep. 2021;11(1):18298.
7. Bae JM, Jung HM, Hong BY, Lee JH, Choi WJ, Lee JH, et al. Phototherapy for vitiligo: a systematic review and meta-analysis. JAMA Dermatol. 2017;153(7):666–74.

8. Grochocka M, Wełniak A, Białczyk A, Marek-Jozefowicz L, Tadrowski T, Czajkowski R. Management of stable vitiligo-a review of the surgical approach. J Clin Med. 2023;12(5):1984.
9. Roenigk RK, Ratz JL, Roenigk HH. Preoperative psychological evaluation. In: Gloster Jr HM, Roenigk RK, editors. Roenigk's dermatologic surgery. Boca Raton: CRC Press; 2016. p. 53–8.
10. Dellatorre G, Antelo DAP, Bedrikow RB, Cestari TF, Follador I, Ramos DG, et al. Consensus on the treatment of vitiligo—Brazilian Society of Dermatology. An Bras Dermatol. 2020;95(Suppl 1(Suppl 1)):70–82.
11. Johnson JE. Psychological interventions and coping with surgery. In: Handbook of psychology and health, volume IV. London: Routledge; 2020. p. 167–87.
12. Johnston M, Carpenter L. Relationship between pre-operative anxiety and post-operative state. Psychol Med. 1980;10(2):361–7.
13. Krouse HJ. Video modelling to educate patients. J Adv Nurs. 2001;33(6):748–57.
14. Krohne HW, Slangen KE. Influence of social support on adaptation to surgery. Health Psychol. 2005;24(1):101–5.
15. Wang R, Huang X, Wang Y, Akbari M. Non-pharmacologic approaches in preoperative anxiety, a comprehensive review. Front Public Health. 2022;10:854673.
16. Ioannis K. Perioperative counseling in children. Rostrum Asclepius/Vima tou Asklipiou. 2012;11(4):523–30.
17. Watts SJ, Zijlker HVTD. Patient counselling and selection. Facial plastic and reconstructive surgery. 2012:1.
18. Desebbe O, Lanz T, Kain Z, Cannesson M. The perioperative surgical home: an innovative, patient-centred and cost-effective perioperative care model. Anaesth Crit Care Pain Med. 2016;35(1):59–66.
19. Ricketts D, Roper T, Rogers B, Phadnis J, Elsayed S, Sokol D. Informed consent: the view from the trenches. Ann R Coll Surg Engl. 2019;101(1):44–9.

Chapter 17
Tissue Grafting Techniques in Vitiligo Surgery

Madhulika Mhatre and Amit Jain

Abstract Vitiligo surgeries are evolving treatment modalities aimed at the repigmentation of stable vitiligo lesions. The surgeries have been classified into tissue and cellular grafts on the basis of the nature of the autologous graft transplanted. Tissue grafting techniques are more cost-effective and less labor and instrumentation-intensive. This chapter discusses various autologous tissue grafting techniques with basic principles and recent innovations to make these surgeries easier, more practical, and cost-effective for treating physicians and patients, leading to better cosmetic outcomes, satisfaction, and ease of doing the procedure for both the doctor and the patient.

Keywords Tissue grafting in vitiligo · Mini-punch grafting · Suction blister grafting · Split thickness grafting · Vitiligo surgery

17.1 Introduction

Vitiligo is a chronic, common dermatological disorder characterized by depigmented macules on the skin and the absence of functional melanocytes in the lesions involved histologically. It can be a source of great psychological and emotional distress among affected individuals; the presence of white spots in a person of color can give rise to significant social stigmas [1]. Various treatment options in the form of medical and surgical modalities exist for controlling and reversing the disease process. Medical modalities aimed at controlling the spread and repigmentation of these patches may not always be able to achieve complete repigmentation in certain

M. Mhatre (✉)
Skin Saga Centre for Dermatology, Mumbai, India

A. Jain
Department of Dermatology, Venereology and Leprosy, Bharati Vidyapeeth (Deemed to be university) Medical College, Pune, Maharashtra, India

R. Sarkar, V. Narayan R (eds.), *A Concise Guide to The Management of Vitiligo*, https://doi.org/10.1007/978-981-95-3857-7_17

patches, as the rate of repigmentation and resolution of lesions may vary according to the size, duration, and location of the aforementioned patches [2].

Surgical interventions, particularly skin grafting techniques, offer effective solutions for patients with stable vitiligo in cases where medical treatment offers only a limited response.

17.2 Concept of Stability in Vitiligo

"Stability" in vitiliginous disease has emerged as one of the most important prerequisites in case selection for vitiligo surgeries. Stable vitiligo refers to the absence of new lesion incidence along with no spread of old lesions for a selected period of time; however, a consensus regarding the actual duration of this period does not exist and may vary from 4 months to 2 years according to various schools of thought [3–6]. In a recent publication regarding standard care in vitiligo, a time period of 1 year with the absence of new lesions, koebnerization, and no increase in the size of old lesions was considered acceptable [7]. Alternatively, a 6-point Vitiligo Disease Activity (VIDA) Score can be used to assess the activity of the disease, with surgeries being performed only with a VIDA score of -1 or 0 [7]. Another method for establishing stability could be "test grafting" [2].

17.3 Basic Principles of Tissue Grafting Surgeries

Surgical interventions in vitiligo are aimed toward achieving repigmentation, which is appropriate for aesthetic standards, by transplanting autologous melanocytes from normal, unaffected pigmented skin into the vitiliginous lesion itself. It will not control unabetted disease activity but can give excellent results in the cases of stable vitiligo recalcitrant to treatment with medical modalities. Various surgical options are available for this, the choice of which will depend not only on the site, extent, and type of vitiligo but also on the availability of equipment, skill of the surgeon, and financial affordability of the patients.

Different surgical methods used for skin grafting techniques in vitiligo are mentioned in Table 17.1.

This chapter provides an in-depth overview of the tissue grafting techniques used in vitiligo surgery, highlighting their principles, methods, innovations, and outcomes.

Indications

- Stable vitiligo recalcitrant to medical therapies alone
- Segmental vitiligo
- Other depigmenting diseases including chemical leukoderma, burns, and piebaldism

Table 17.1 Classification of Vitiligo Surgery Techniques: techniques in vitiligo

Tissue grafts	Cellular grafts
Mini-punch grafting	Noncultured epidermal cell suspensions
Suction blister grafting	Cultured melanocytes/keratinocyte grafts
Thin split thickness grafting	
Hair follicle grafts	
Mesh grafts	
Flip-top pigment transplantation	

Contraindication (Relative)

- Active disease
- Childhood vitiligo
- Keloidal tendency

17.4 Types of Tissue Grafting Techniques

17.4.1 Mini-punch Grafting

17.4.1.1 Summary of Procedure

Principles and Technique

Mini-punch grafting involves the transplantation of small, circular punch grafts from pigmented donor skin to depigmented recipient sites (Figs. 17.1 and 17.2). This technique is minimally invasive and relatively simple. Mini-punch grafting is the transplantation of pigmented, autologous, normal skin in a vitiliginous patch in the form of multiple miniature punches. Flabella, in 1983, used mini-punch grafting successfully to treat segmental vitiligo. However, initially, it was believed that true vitiligo is not treatable by transplantation of normally pigmented autologous skin. A lot has changed since then: not only has the high effectiveness of this therapy been established but also different parameters of mini-punch grafting have evolved over the years. It has emerged as one of the fastest, easiest, cheapest, and least aggressive therapies. It works well with patients' advantages [8].

Procedure

1. Donor Site Preparation: A site with normal pigmentation is selected.
2. Graft Harvesting: Using a punch biopsy tool (1–2 mm), small grafts are harvested.
3. Recipient Site Preparation: Corresponding holes are created in the vitiliginous area using the same punch tool.

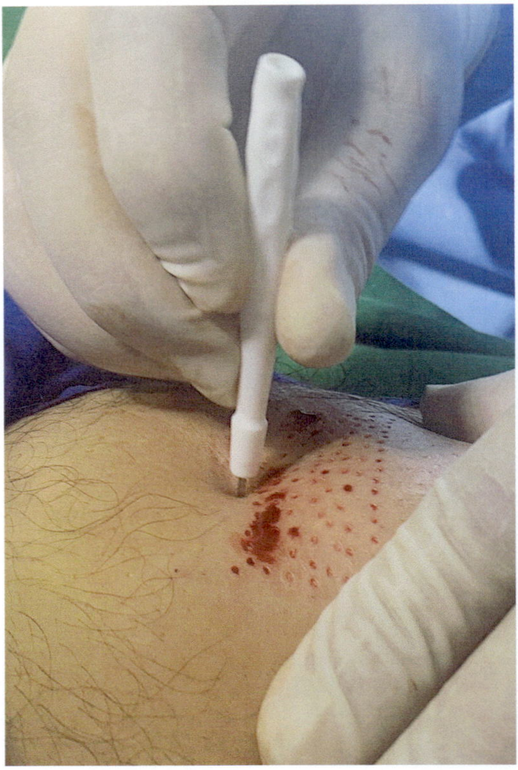

Fig. 17.1 Procedure of graft harvesting from a pigmentated donor site

4. Graft Placement: The harvested grafts are inserted into the recipient holes and secured with adhesive dressings.

Outcomes and Complications

- Efficacy: High repigmentation rates particularly effective in stable, localized vitiligo
- Complications: Cobblestoning, hyperpigmentation, and occasional graft rejection

The Method of Mini-grafting

1. The instruments required are 1.5 or 1.2 mm punches, small jeweler or graft holding forceps, and small curved tip scissors.
2. The recipient area is prepared first. Two percent lignocaine with or without adrenaline is infiltrated as a local anesthetic.

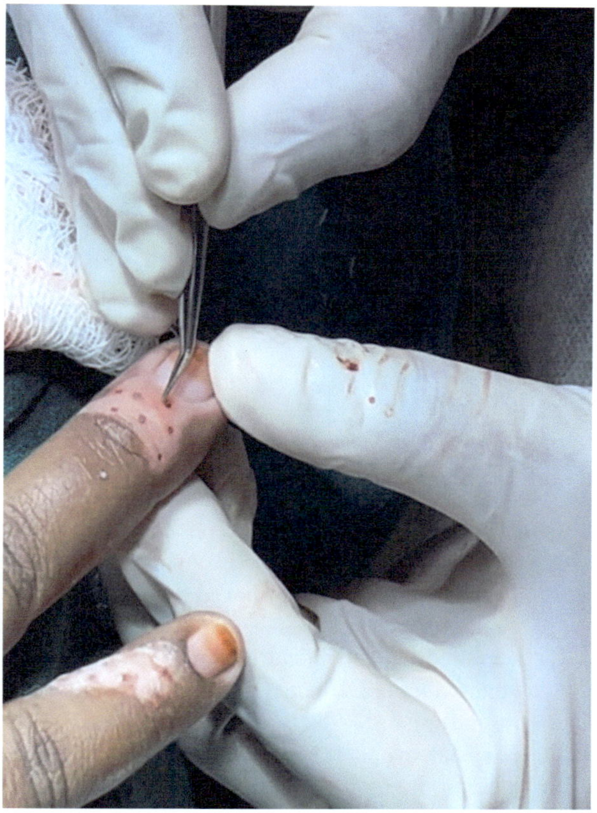

Fig. 17.2 Transplantation of the autologous graft to the depigmented areas

3. To minimize the chance of developing any perigraft halo, the initial recipient chambers are made on or very close to the border of the lesion. The punched out chambers are spaced according to the result of test grafting or at a gap of 5–10 mm from each other.
4. The donor area is either the upper lateral portion of the thigh or the gluteal area. Punch impressions are made very close to each other so that a maximum number of grafts can be taken from a small area.
5. Same-sized punches are used for both the donor and recipient areas.
6. The grafts are placed directly from the donor (buttock/upper thigh) to the recipient areas. This speeds up the procedure and lessens the chance of infection. Care is taken to ensure that the graft edges are not folded and that the tissue is not crushed or placed upside down. The needle of the syringe or the tip of the scissors is used for the proper placement of grafts in the recipient chambers.
7. Hemostasis is achieved by pressing a saline-soaked gauze piece over the area.
8. For the recipient area, the three layers of dressing from inside to out are paraffin-embedded, nonadherent sterile gauze (Jelonet®), sterile Surgipad®, and bio-occlusive Micropore®.
9. For the donor area, only Surgipad® and Micropore® are used.

10. The recipient area may be immobilized if necessary. Proper instructions for special areas like the lips are necessary. To secure the recipient area, these patients are advised to be on a liquid diet for the first 24 h, preferably with a straw. Patients are allowed a normal diet after this period.
11. Sometimes dressings are opened after 24 h to look for any dislodgement of grafts; if any are found, they are replaced.
12. Finally, after 4–7 days, the dressings are removed.

Innovations

1. Wedge insertion

   Although punch grafting can be performed universally over the body, certain areas can be more challenging to perform the procedure because of the risk of scarring or loss of cutaneous structures or skin thickness as well. To prevent scarring and loss of hair over the eyebrows, one such modification can be used here: rather than taking micro-punches, small wedges of pigmented skin are placed in an incision over the lesion over the eyebrow; the depth of the incision is 2 mm; the eyebrows are shaved beforehand and skin wedges are put in a way so the dermal portion goes deep in while epithelial sided remain up. The area can be anchored with stay sutures; this prevents patchy loss of hair following scarring caused by micro-punch grafting over the area [9].
2. Micrografting

   Thin skin over certain areas like eyelids can give rise to difficulties in the case of being grafted with thicker skin from the rest of the body; in these scenarios, the donor punches taken from the thicker parts of the body can be further divided into smaller pieces.

   These smaller grafts are later placed in the recipient's thinner area by creating pockets at the dermoepidermal junctions with a wide-bore syringe [9].
3. Follicular unit transplant [10]

   The following clinical features regarding the treatment of vitiligo have been observed:

   - Leucotrichia on a patch is a poor prognostic sign.
   - Pigmentation in a vitiligo patch often starts at the follicular opening.
   - Areas devoid of hair, e.g., palms and soles, are difficult to repigment.

   - The aforementioned clinical observations form a principle for using follicular units in the treatment of vitiligo. It is believed that the melanocyte reservoir present in the external root sheath can become activated and help in repigmenting the lesions of vitiligo. The donor hair can be taken from the selected areas by using a 1 mm punch and can be transplanted into the recipient areas using an 18 G needle with a 33 mm gap between the follicles [10].

4. Motorized punch (Fig. 17.3)

   Harvesting each graft manually can be a time taking process more so for larger vitiliginous lesions; for such cases, a motorized power punch can be used to increase the speed of surgery, reducing the number of sessions required to cover the lesion itself and greatly benefitting the patients in the process [11]. As an innovation, micro-punch grafting can be done with motorized punch with 0.5–0.9 mm grafts, further enhancing the quality of repigmentation.
5. Graft fixation

   During mini-punch grating to reduce the chances of graft dislodgment, Fevikwik cyanoacrylate gel can be used at the corners of the mini-graft; this can be achieved by attaching a wide-bore needle to the orifice of the cyanoacrylate gel, which can also achieve a controlled output from the tube itself [12] (Fig. 17.4).

Fig. 17.3 Motorized punch, which is being used to fasten the process of preparing the recipient site for graft transplantation

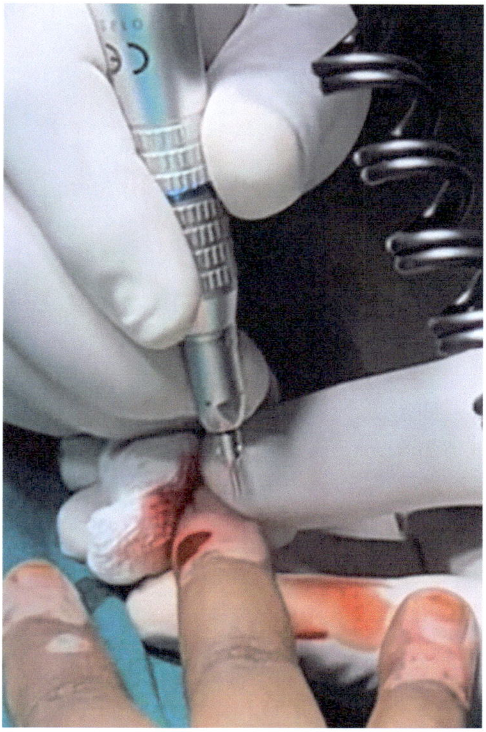

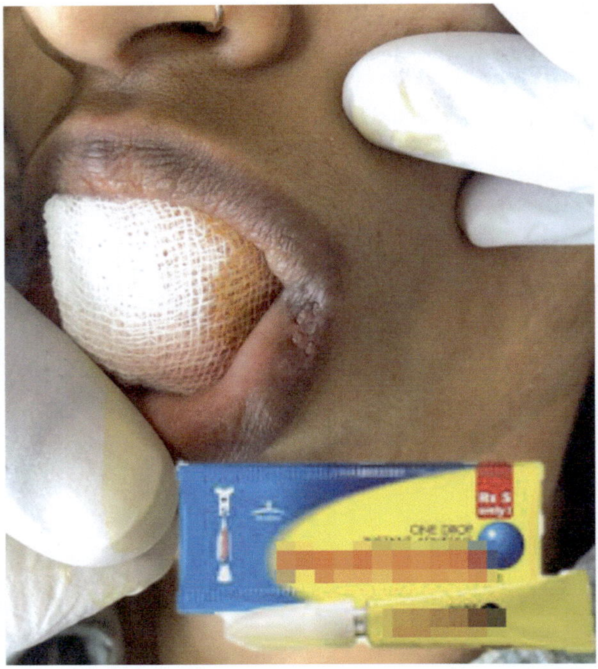

Fig. 17.4 Use of cyanoacrylate gel over a very mobile site to prevent the graft dislodgement

17.4.2 Suction Blister Epidermal Grafting

17.4.2.1 Summary of Procedure

Principles and Technique

Suction blister epidermal grafting involves creating blisters on the donor site using a suction device and transplanting the blister roofs, which contain melanocytes, to the depigmented areas.

Procedure

1. Donor Site Preparation: A suction device or syringes are applied to pigmented skin to form blisters.
2. Blister Harvesting: The epidermal roof of the blister is carefully separated.
3. Recipient Site Preparation: The depigmented area is prepared by superficial dermabrasion or laser ablation.
4. Graft Placement: The epidermal grafts are transplanted onto the prepared recipient site and covered with dressings.

Innovations

- Automated Suction Devices: Development of automated suction devices to create uniform blisters quickly and efficiently
- Advanced Dressing Materials: Use of silicon gel sheets and other advanced materials to secure grafts and enhance healing
- Use of hair dryer/UV to speed blister formation
- -Hijama cups

Outcomes and Complications

- Efficacy: Excellent repigmentation rates with minimal complications
- Complications: Postinflammatory hyperpigmentation, secondary infection, and occasional donor site scarring

17.4.2.2 Suction Blister Grafting (SBG)

Principle and Technique

In this procedure, the graft for autologous transplantation on the vitiliginous skin is harvested from the donor site by raising a blister. The blister is raised by using various modalities in an attempt to separate the donor epidermis from the dermis at the donor site, which is later transplanted as an epithelial graft; this is done to maximize the cosmetic result, as the harvested epidermis, devoid of the donor site dermis, will take the characteristics of the dermis of the recipient site and will result in a better color match at the recipient site and hence a better aesthetic result [2].

Procedure

Harvesting sites

Usually, covered parts like gluteal region or thighs are the area of choice to minimize the risks associated with donor site changes.

Preparation of the donor sites

- Surgical cleansing
- Topical anesthesia/infiltration of local anesthetic agent [lidocaine (2%) with epinephrine (1:200000) and xylocaine (1%)] and creating a regional block; the infiltrated local aesthetic may have an added advantage of a reduced blister induction time (BIT) [2]

Preparation of recipient sites

- The donor area is sterilized; local anesthesia (topical/intralesional) is given and dermabraded using a manual dermabrader.

Graft harvesting and transplantation

- For the creation of blisters, various devices can be used, which function on the principle of creation of negative pressure: suction cups/pumps, cutaneous negative pressure suction chambers, and syringes (10, 20, 50 ml) can be used (Fig. 17.5). The ideal pressure required is 300 mm of Hg [13].
- BIT for larger syringes (>20 ml) is usually longer, while blisters created by smaller syringes (<10 ml) require more skill to handle. A unilocular, nonhemorrhagic blister is considered ideal. Intradermal saline injections (~5 ml) can be used to increase the size of smaller blisters [2].
- The roofs are blisters, formed by aforementioned techniques, and then gently separated using iris scissors. Care is taken to avoid contact with the floor of the blister, which may give rise to the sensation of pain. Roofs obtained as a consequence are then spread on a slide with the dermal side up to obtain their maximum extent. Normal saline can be used for this purpose, which will also keep the grafts moist, increasing the vitality of the tissue for a limited time. The graft is now ready to be transplanted [2].
- Considering that the lateral pigment spreads from the grafts, a gap of 0.5 cm can be kept between the two grafts, which are secured by a nonadherent dressing and bandaged.
- The dressing over the recipient sites is removed after a week; meanwhile, the patient is asked to maintain immobility of the transplanted side. The grafts usually fall off in 10–14 days, essentially making this procedure a method for the transfer of autologous melanocyte.
- Dressing on the donor sites is done as well and could be changed every day.

Follow-ups

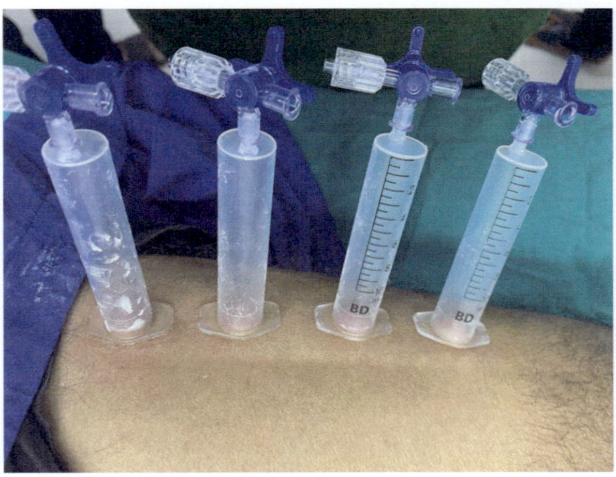

Fig. 17.5 Blister development in its various stages with 10 ml BD syringes and a three-way valve to maintain pressure and vacuum

- Excimer laser, topical/oral PUVASOL, or psoralene-UVA is recommended.
- Excellent repigmentation seen in 3–6 months.

Outcomes and Complications

- Efficacy: Excellent repigmentation rates with minimal complications
- Complications: Postinflammatory hyperpigmentation, secondary infection, and occasional donor site scarring

Innovations

Microdermabrasion (MDA) machine as a suction device

An MDA machine with a vacuum pump can also be used as a suction device. After removing the handpiece and powder-delivering tube, the vacuum tube of the machine can be connected to the three-way connector, which is already connected to a 20 cc syringe. The syringe placement for the blister is as usual. The MDA machine is only turned on for 30 s or so at a pressure of 200–400 mm of mercury, after which the connector is locked, and the pressure is maintained till the desired time. The machine gives a smooth, calibrated, and controlled suction, which is easily adjustable within the range of 0–760 mm of Hg, which is easily measurable. The tubing of the machine can also fit well to the connector, and the adverse effects on the machine's life are negligible because it is turned on only for 30 s or so [14].

Reduction of blister induction time

Long BIT can be a limitation in SBG surgeries; to overcome this obstacle, various physical modalities can be used. It has been previously demonstrated that the BIT is supposed to be directly related to the diameter of the suction device used. The other factors that may affect BIT are the site of the blister, age of the patient, amount of vacuum created, temperature, corticosteroid-induced atrophy, and pretreatment of the site with psoralene with ultraviolet A [13]. This information can further be the basis of the use of novel modalities to decrease BIT. On the basis of such findings, nowadays, light in the form of UV radiation (340–400 nm), Wood's lamp, and infrared devices, and other modalities such as cryotherapy and infiltration with local anesthesia are also used to decrease the BIT; local anesthesia has the added advantage of dulling the sensation of pain [13]. Similarly, in a recently conducted study, a household hairdryer was used to increase the temperature of the donor skin to 44'c to decrease the BIT. The ideal temperature described for the blister formation is 40–45'c in various studies [15].

Graft transfer

- This accounts for a very important part of the SBG process. The ideal transfer surface is of utmost importance for successful transfer, which should be a firm and flexible instrument permitting easy manipulation of the smallest size of the grafts; for this purpose, various modalities like spatula, gauge, microscopic slides, and acetate sheets have also been used (Fig. 17.6). In a conducted study, a gloved sterile finger was used as a transport platform, resulting in easy manipulation and excellent placement of the grafts [16].

Resizing the blister roof graft

Inspite of a good technique, blister formation at the end can be unpredictable to ameliorate these situations, we can resize the graft by putting the graft on the surface of the paper that sandwiches the sterile petroleum-soaked gauze. The graft is harvested by putting the sticky surface on the donor area; hence, the graft is obtained on the paper with the dermal side up, and the paper, along with the obtained blister roof, can now be easily cut and used in any desirable shape and placed over the recipient area [17].

Innovations in recipient area preparation

For the transplantation of the graft in suction blister grafting/split thickness grafting, a mechanical or manual dermabrader is usually used to dermabrade the area; the former requires a certain level of experience in handling, considering the cosmetic importance of certain areas while the latter can pose some concerns regarding its maneuverability at times because the dermatologist's comfort regarding an instrument may vary (Fig. 17.7). However, these are no longer the only available modalities anymore; these modalities mentioned below can be equally effective, manageable, and comfortable, in preparing the area and giving good aesthetic results:

- -Medium-grade sandpaper [18]

This has been documented previously as well; it can be used after sterilizing with ethylene oxide in the following ways:

1. Tied to the index finger of the treating physician with surgical suture material
2. On a disposable tongue depressor after cutting the paper to match the size of the depressor

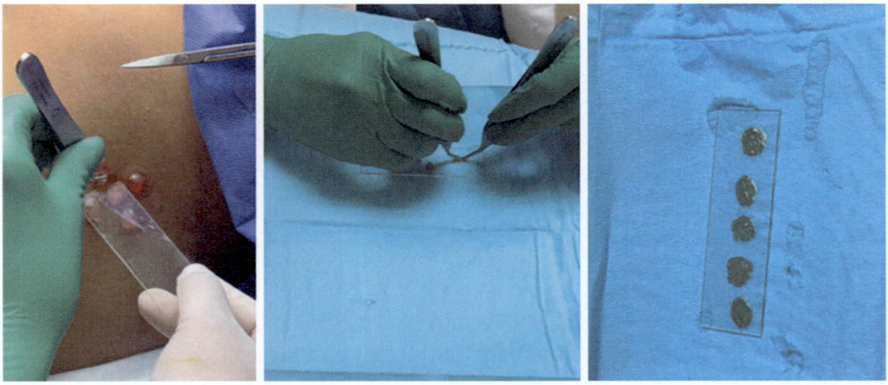

Fig. 17.6 Use of glass slides for better transfer of blister roof grafts

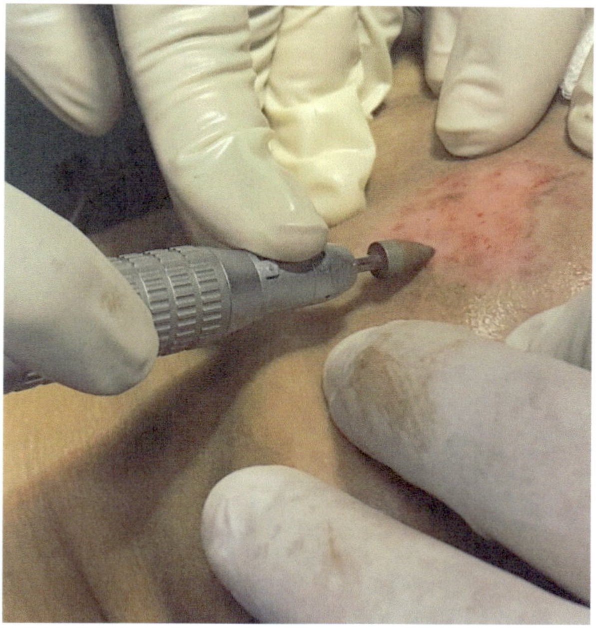

Fig. 17.7 Use of mechanical dermabrader to prepare the recipient areas. Note the pin point bleeding at places, which is required to access the depth of the dermabrasion

3. Held between the index finger and the tongue

This has the advantage of being very easily effective and very cost-effective.

Since the paper can be cut into the shapes and sizes desired, it can make dermabrading the difficult areas like the lid margin more manageable.

Hypodermic needle for dermabrasion

Dermabrasion using a hypodermic needle can be particularly beneficial in cases where the depigmented area is small, and protection of the surrounding skin is crucial. This technique is especially useful in vitiligo surgeries where complete repigmentation has not been achieved, leaving some depigmented patches. To preserve the already repigmented areas and prevent them from undergoing further dermabrasion, this method allows for precise, targeted treatment. It helps limit the dermabrasion area and reduces the size of the graft needed [19].

- Trichloroacetic acid (25%) application can also be used to dermabrade the recipient area [20].

Dressing for blister grafts on mobile areas

Vitiligo graft transplantation on mobile areas like the lips can give rise to a varying degree of success owing to graft displacement due to the mobility of the area and due to the absence of natural adhesive forces in the area. To overcome this, an aerosol spray consisting of polyvinyl polymer, cetrimide, and benzocaine can be used, and the spray will provide adhesive strength as well [21].

CELLUTOME epidermal harvesting system:

A novel method of harvesting suction blister grafts in which epidermal grafts are obtained by use of an automated system. This system uses temperatures of 37–41’C and a suction pressure of 400–500 mm Hg of pressure to create blisters that are called microdomes. It takes 45–50 min for the formation of these blisters. A simple dressing such as tegaderm™ can be used to harvest these grafts, which can be directly transferred to the recipient areas. The recipient area needs to be prepared with dermabrasion for graft transplantation. The system is completely automated, and no local anesthesia is needed to be given before harvesting the epidermal grafts [22].

17.4.2.3 Split Thickness Skin Grafting

Split thickness skin grafting involves the transplantation of a thin layer of skin from a pigmented donor area to a depigmented recipient site. This technique is suitable for larger vitiliginous patches.

Procedure

Graft harvesting is done from a pigmented stable site. The gluteal area is considered the best for graft harvesting despite being a difficult area to take a graft from. Other areas like the thighs and arms can be used as well. The area is anesthetized first either by using topical or infiltration anesthesia, and the skin is surgically cleaned and prepared for harvesting. At the time of harvesting, the skin is stretched to make sure the taken graft is as thin as possible (Fig. 17.8). Graft can be harvested by a sterile razor blade mounted on a Kocher’s forceps, a blade-holding instrument, a hand dermatome, a Humby knife, a silver knife, or an air-driven power dermatome (Zimmer Inc., Warsaw, IN, USA), which can be used according to the skill of the dermatologist, availability of instruments, and financial constraints [2].

The recipient area can be prepared by cleaning and dermabrading using the various methods discussed before.

The graft is carefully placed over the denuded recipient site, with the dermal surface facing down (Fig. 17.9). Immobilization of the graft is most important and is achieved by using surgical adhesive, octyl-2-cyanoacrylate, and pressure dressing.

After the transfer of graft, the three important biological processes take place, which are as follows:

Graft adherence

- In the first 3 days, the adherence is by fibrin.
- Graft appears pink.
- The first 3 days are the most crucial days and hence are important to avoid mobility, bleeding and superinfection of these sites; failure to do so will result in graft failure.

Revascularization

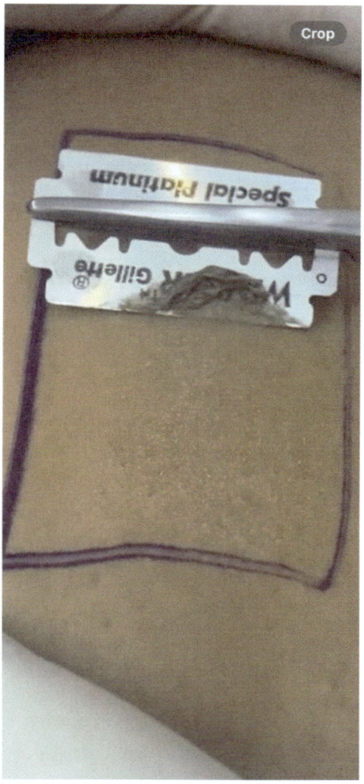

Fig. 17.8 Recent innovation where a razor blade mounted on a forceps is being used to harvest a thin skin graft. This provides the treating physician with a great deal of control over depth of the graft

- Interconnection between the graft and recipient vessels and the development of new vessels occur in this stage. It is important to have a proper compression dressing to avoid the development of a hematoma, seroma, or very dense fibrin layer.

Contraction

- After proper harvesting and even after placement of the graft, some degree of contraction is expected. Keeping the graft edges close to each other in these cases is important to avoid a perigraft halo and achromic fissures.

Follow-up

- First followup is at 24 h to look for serous collection/hematoma, to be drained if found.
- After that, the dressing changes at 7th day after healing.
- Prophylactic oral antibiotics.
- NB UVB in cases of depigmentation or achromic fissures if needed.

Advantages

- Larger areas can be treated in a short amount of time.

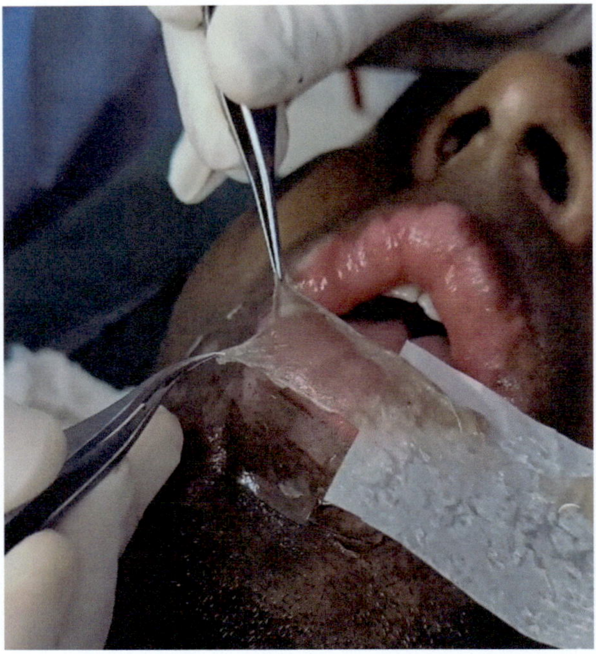

Fig. 17.9 A thin split thickness graft being placed on the recipient site; note how the use of an acetate sheet makes it more convenient to do so

- Relative ease of treatment for difficult areas such as eyelids, inner canthus of the eyes, areola, nipples, and genitals.
- Pigmentation achieved is uniform.
- Faster repigmentation.

Disadvantages

- Prolonged hyperpigmentation can occur.
- Postsurgery stuck-on appearance or milia formation (Fig. 17.10).
- Large areas require multiple sittings due to the limitation of the donor site.
- Surgical skill is required to take thin even grafts freehand.
- 1:1 Donor:recipient ratio needed.

Innovations

- Resizing the graft [17]
- Meek's original concept states that the sum of the perimeters of smaller grafts is larger than that of the harvested graft and that the smaller the graft size is, the greater the potential for regeneration.
- Hence, micrografting or cutting a larger graft into smaller pieces and then transplanting them give a better degree and quality of repigmentation.
- Smash grafting

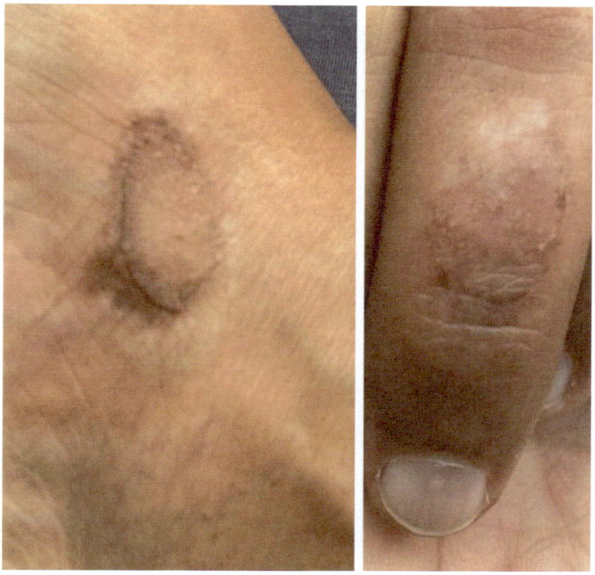

Fig. 17.10 Stuck on appearance. This is not a cosmetically ideal outcome; however, it can be managed further. Note the complete repigmentation

- In this method, the split skin graft obtained is "smashed" manually using sterile curved suture cutting scissors to obtain the smashed graft. No part of the graft taken is wasted. This smashed graft can cover ten times the recipient area. After applying it on recipient area, it is left undisturbed for 30 min so that it can naturally adhere to the dermabraded recipient area, after which it is covered with nonadherent gauze, and a dressing is done. This process has been known to produce good results [23].

17.5 Jodhpur Technique

Named after the city where it was conceptualized, it is similar to the epidermal curettage technique. The Jodhpur technique involves using noncultured, nontrypsinized melanocyte, keratinocyte epidermal cell transfer, applied to dermabraded vitiliginous areas. This is prepared by collecting shavings from the dermabrasion of a suitable donor area without taking a graft. Mupirocin ointment was added to the donor site to prevent spraying of the particles and to increase the yield. It is particularly noted for its simplicity, cost-effectiveness, and minimal donor site morbidity, making it accessible and practical for widespread use in clinical settings [24].

17.6 Flip-Top Grafting

Devised by McGovern et al., this technique has the advantage of minimal scarring and is economical. The inner aspect of the thigh or retroauricular region is chosen as the donor area.

A 10–15 mm graft containing the epidermis and minimal dermis was obtained using a razor. This graft is placed on gauze soaked in isotonic sodium chloride and divided into small pieces of 3–5 mm each. A flap of 6–8 m is raised within the epidermis and papillary dermis at the recipient site, and the grafts are placed juxtapositioning the dermis of the recipient area [25].

17.7 Conclusion

Tissue grafting techniques offer promising surgical options for patients with stable vitiligo. The choice of technique depends on various factors, including the size and location of the vitiliginous patches, available facilities, and patient preferences. Innovations in these techniques continue to improve outcomes, making them more accessible and effective. Future advancements in tissue engineering and regenerative medicine may further enhance the efficacy and scope of these treatments, providing hope for better management of vitiligo.

References

1. Parsad D, Dogra S, Kanwar AJ. Quality of life in patients with vitiligo. Health Qual Life Outcomes. 2003;1:58. https://doi.org/10.1186/1477-7525-1-58. Published 2003 Oct 23.
2. Khunger N, Kathuria SD, Ramesh V. Tissue grafts in vitiligo surgery—past, present, and future. Indian J Dermatol. 2009;54(2):150–8. https://doi.org/10.4103/0019-5154.53196.
3. Das SS, Pasricha JS. Punch grafting as a treatment for residual lesions in vitiligo. Indian J Dermatol Venereol Leprol. 1992;58:315–9.
4. Boersma BR, Westerhof W, Bos JD. Repigmentation in vitiligo vulgaris by autologous minigrafting: results in nineteen patients. J Am Acad Dermatol. 1995;33:990–5.
5. Olsson M, Juhlin L. long-term follow-up of leukoderma patients treated with transplants of autologous cultured melanocytes, ultrathin epidermal sheets and basal cell layer suspension. Br J Dermatol. 2002;47:893–904.
6. Falabella R. Surgical treatment of vitiligo: why, when and how. J Eur Acad Dermatol Venereol. 2003;17:518–20.
7. Parsad D, Gupta S. Standard guidelines of care for vitiligo surgery. Indian J Dermatol Venereol Leprol. 2008;74:37–45.
8. Lahiri K. Evolution and evaluation of autologous mini punch grafting in vitiligo. Indian J Dermatol. 2009;54(2):159–67. https://doi.org/10.4103/0019-5154.53195.
9. Ahmad TJ, Rashid T, Rani Z. Modifications in punch grafting. J Pak Assoc Dermatol. 2003;13(3):146–7.

10. Sacchidanand S, Thakur P, Purohit V, Sujaya SN. Follicular unit extraction as a therapeutic option for vitiligo. J Cutan Aesthet Surg. 2013;6(4):229–31. https://doi.org/10.4103/0974-2077.123413.
11. Chandrashekar B, Madura C, Varsha D. Autologous mini punch grafting: an experience of using motorized power punch in 10 patients. J Cutan Aesthet Surg. 2014;7(1):42–5. https://doi.org/10.4103/0974-2077.129977. PMID: 24761099; PMCID: PMC3996790.
12. Mutalik S, Pai GS, Talwar S. Dermatosurgery made easy—tips for beginners. In: ACS (I) textbook on cutaneous and aesthetic surgery. New Delhi: Jaypee; 2012. p. 912–26.
13. Kaliyadan F, Venkitakrishnan S, Manoj J. Use of a wood's lamp as a Ultra-Violet light source to improve the speed and quality of suction blister harvesting. Indian J Dermatol Venereol Leprol. 2010;76:429.
14. Kaliyadan F, Manoj J, Venkitakrishnan S. Using a microdermabrasion machine as a suction blister device. Indian J Dermatol Venereol Leprol. 2008;74:392.
15. Arora S, Kar BR. Reduction of blister formation time in suction blister epidermal grafting in vitiligo patients using a household hair dryer. J Cutan Aesthet Surg. 2016;9(4):232–5.
16. Laxmisha C, Thappa DM. Surgical pearl: gloved finger as a transport platform for epidermal graft of suction blister. J Am Acad Dermatol. 2007;57(5):S118–9.
17. Ashique KT, Srinivas CR. Resizing blister roof grafts for vitiligo surgery. J Am Acad Dermatol. 2014;71(2):e39–40.
18. Ashique KT, Kaliyadan F, George RR. Dermabrasion of the recipient skin in vitiligo surgery: an easier way out. Indian J Dermatol Venereol Leprol. 2018;84:498–9.
19. Gupta S, Gupta S, Kumar A. The hypodermic needle as a dermabrading device for recipient area preparation for skin grafting in vitiligo. J Am Acad Dermatol. 2015;72(4):e105–6.
20. Razmi M, Kumaran SM, Parsad D. Trichloroacetic acid 25% peel to facilitate dermabrasion at difficult sites in vitiligo surgery. Dermatologic Surg. 2019;45(5):750–2.
21. Subramaniyan R, Donaparthi N, Kumar R. An innovative use of an aerosol spray in surgical management of lip vitiligo: our experience. J Am Acad Dermatol. 2020;83(3):e183–4.
22. Veliu S, Kröpfl J, Vrbnjak D. CELLUTOME™ epidermal harvesting system. Albanian J Trauma Emerg Surg. 2018;2(2):163–73.
23. Krishnan A, Kar S. Smashed skin grafting or smash grafting–a novel method of vitiligo surgery. Int J Dermatol. 2012;51(10):1242–7.
24. Kachhawa D, et al. The Jodhpur Technique: non-cultured epidermal cell suspension transplantation in vitiligo. J Cutan Aesthet Surg. 2014;7(1):23–8.
25. McGovern TW, Bolognia J, Leffell DL. Flip-top pigment transplantation. Arch Dermatol. 1999;135:1305–7.

Chapter 18
Cellular Grafting Methods

Anubha Dev

Abstract Medical therapies often have limited effectiveness in stable vitiligo patches. This has prompted the exploration of advanced modalities like cellular transplantation surgery. In this chapter, we discuss the current methodologies and outcomes of cellular transplantation techniques in the treatment of vitiligo. Various approaches can be taken such as noncultured epidermal cell suspension (NCES), cultured melanocyte transplantation, and hair follicle cell transplantation, among which NCES is the most widely used technique. Apart from the technical aspects of graft preparation and transplantation per se, it is crucial to emphasize the careful selection of patients and lesions, as well as proper preparation of both donor and recipient sites.

Keywords Vitiligo · Surgery · NCES · Stable · Melanocyte · Repigmentation

18.1 Introduction

Stable vitiligo patches often do not respond to topical or oral therapies, as they usually do not have residual melanocytes or their precursors [1]. Surgical management is required to achieve repigmentation in such lesions. This entails supplying the lesional skin with tissues that contain melanocytes, melanocytes per se or melanocyte precursors like stem cells, which produce melanin [1]. Various mechanisms of repigmentation have been postulated in the context of vitiligo surgeries like:

(a) Melanocytes reposition in the basal layer and proliferate after injury by recipient site preparation. This migration is facilitated by matrix metalloproteinases, heparanases, and the downregulation of E-cadherin.

A. Dev (✉)
Department of Dermatology, Venereology, Leprology, PGIMER, Chandigarh, India

R. Sarkar, V. Narayan R (eds.), *A Concise Guide to The Management of Vitiligo*,
https://doi.org/10.1007/978-981-95-3857-7_18

(b) The injury caused stimulates growth factors such as hepatocyte growth factor, basal fibroblast growth factor (bFGF), and keratinocyte growth factor, which promote melanogenesis [2].

Vitiligo surgery was first attempted by Haxthausen in 1947 in the form of split-thickness skin grafting [3]. The initial procedures that followed were predominantly tissue grafting techniques, which included mini-punch grafting, suction blister grafting, flip-top grafting, and smash grafting [2]. Cellular techniques were pioneered by Gauthier in 1992 in the form of epidermal cell suspension transplantation [4].

18.2 Patient Selection

The most important parameter to establish eligibility for vitiligo surgery is disease stability. Though there is no consensus regarding the definition of stability, the IADVL task force has suggested a duration of 1 year to establish stability [5]. This is defined as no new lesions, no increase in the size of preexisting lesions, no Koebner phenomenon for at least 1 year or a vitiligo disease activity score of −1 or 0. The mini-punch grafting test, initially proposed by Falabella, is also a useful technique for assessing disease stability in those who will have a good response [6]. Four to six minigrafts of 1.0–1.2 mm size are transplanted within the lesions, and the test is labeled positive if repigmentation occurs >1 mm from the margin of the graft in 3 months. However, the utility of this test is challenged as it can be positive even in unstable disease. There are reports of the assessment of stability by reflectance confocal microscopy; detection of cellular markers, like IL-17, CXCL-9, and 10; and perilesional CD8 T cell count [2]. However, these methods are more appropriate for research settings and are not feasible in clinical practice. Though controversial, it is generally believed that lesional stability is more important than overall disease stability in the context of vitiligo surgery. This can also be assessed clinically, as stable lesions have well-defined concave borders with or without areas of repigmentation.

Both segmental vitiligo and stable nonsegmental vitiligo that is refractory to medical management are indications for surgery. It can also be used for difficult-to-treat areas, like acral areas; however, the response of such lesions is to a lesser extent. Lesions which respond well are facial lesions, focal vitiligo, segmental vitiligo, and lesions in younger patients. A very important aspect is to manage patients' expectations and counsel regarding the prognosis.

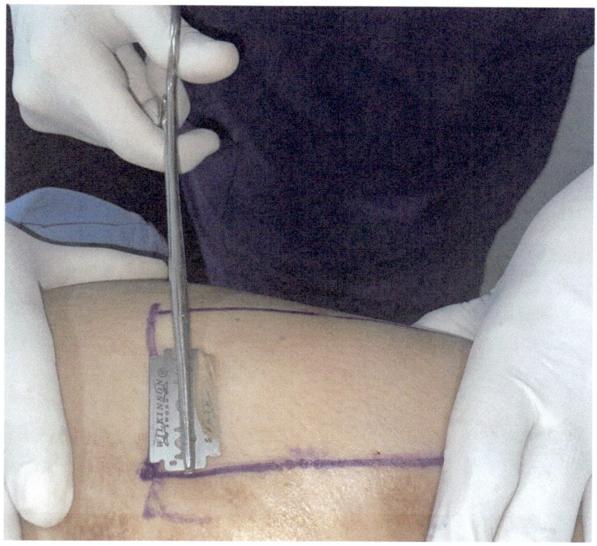

Fig. 18.1 A split-thickness skin graft is harvested with the help of a razor blade and artery forceps from the upper lateral thigh of the patient

18.3 Donor Site

The ideal donor site is the upper lateral aspect of the thigh [2]. Other sites that may be used are the medial aspect of the forearm, arm, abdomen, and gluteal area. The postauricular area can be used for facial lesions as it gives a good color match. With respect to cellular techniques, a split-thickness skin graft is harvested with the help of a razor blade and artery forceps (Fig. 18.1).

18.4 Recipient Site Preparation

Preparation of the recipient site is essential prior to cellular grafting procedures so that the underlying structures can be accessed for the adherence and nutrition of melanocytes [7]. The epidermis should be separated from the dermis at the dermo-epidermal junction up to the point when pinpoint bleeding is seen. This helps in plasmatic imbibition during the first 1–2 days post grafting, when vascularity also increases and provides nutrition to cells. This is a critical step in achieving successful repigmentation because dermabrasion and suction blisters alone without grafting can also cause repigmentation:

(a) Dermabrasion: This is the most widely used method for recipient site preparation, with the most common device being Manekshaw's manual dermabrader. It is effective, rapid, has minimal scarring risks, and is more economical. However, it is difficult to perform on concave surfaces like periorbital areas and softer tissues like genitalia. Motor dermabrasion can also be used in which a diamond fraise, a wire brush, or a serrated wheel is used. Figure 18.2a shows Manekshaw's manual dermabrader of different sizes, and Fig. 18.2b shows the manual dermabrasion being performed on the lesion. Pinpoint bleeding points can be visualized.

(b) Electrofulguration (EF): It is a type of radiofrequency ablation that uses a markedly dampened current. The electrode is held such that it maintains a slight distance from the skin surface. Though it has not been used traditionally, there have been multiple reports of good response of EF recently [8–10]. A hyfrecator with a ball-tip electrode in low output and monopolar mode provides good results [11]. This technique has multiple benefits: it is less labor intensive; requires less time; margins can be delineated better; control over uniformity and depth; easy preparation of sites like neck, eyelids and axillae; bleeding is minimal; and chances of inflammation and scarring are lower.

(c) Suction blisters: It is more useful for small recipient sites and is done using generating a suction pressure of up to 150 mm of mercury through a 20 ml syringe. The cell suspension can be injected into the blister cavity after aspirating the blister fluid and keeping the roof intact.

(d) Liquid nitrogen: It is used to create a blister which is then deroofed [12]. Complications include peripheral hyperpigmentation or hypopigmentation and hypertrophic scarring.

(e) Lasers: CO_2 and Er:YAG are traditionally used. The advantages are similar to electrofulguration. The endpoint is a "chamois" yellow appearance that is observed on reaching the reticular dermis. The Er:YAG has lesser penetration than the CO_2 laser, which allows more precise tissue ablation without any thermal necrosis.

(f) Dermasanding: This method uses sterile sandpaper.

(g) Dermarolling [12].

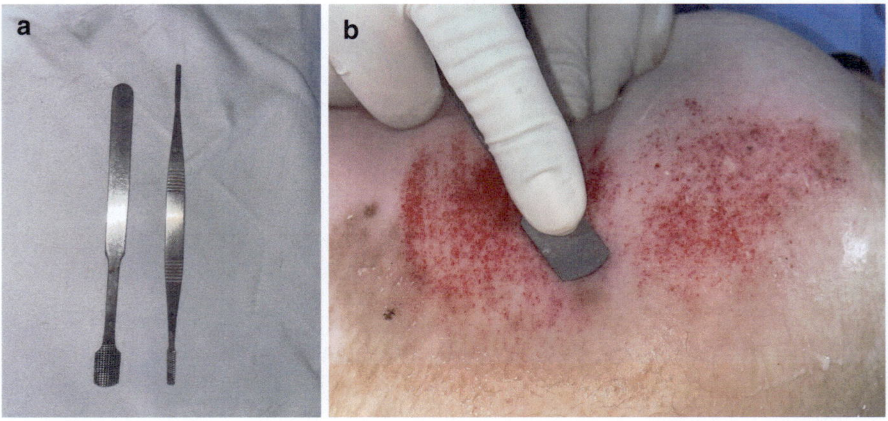

Fig. 18.2 (**a**) Manekshaw's manual dermabrader of different sizes. (**b**) Manual dermabrasion being performed on the lesion. The epidermis is gently abraded in circular motion until pinpoint bleeding points can be visualized uniformly over the field

(h) Chemical preparation using trichloroacetic acid [13] or PUVA.

18.5 Cultured Melanocyte Transplantation

It was not possible to cultivate melanocytes initially, as keratinocytes had a preferential growth over melanocytes in culture. The introduction of melanocyte mitogens in 1982 was a breakthrough. Subsequently, in 1989, Brysk et al. and Falabella et al. successfully treated stable vitiligo using a cocultured solution of melanocytes and keratinocytes [14, 15]. They used bFGF, which is an important factor that promotes the survival and proliferation of melanocytes. Earlier, 12-O-tetradecanoylphorbol-13-acetate, which was tumorigenic, was used.

A donor-recipient area ratio of 1:60 to 1:100 is maintained, and melanocytes are cultured for 3 weeks in the laboratory in Eagle's minimal essential medium. Melanocytes are detached from the culture plates, and the suspension is transplanted onto the denuded recipient area at a density of 1000–2000 melanocytes/mm^2.

Cultured epidermal grafts, which organize themselves into a sheet-like basal layer, can also be used [16]. A major advantage of cultured cell techniques is that large areas can be treated, and the cells can be cryopreserved for use in the future. However, the scope of application is limited by strict laws on the culture of stem cells for use in patients. Other limitations are that it is time consuming, labor intensive, and costly.

18.6 Noncultured Epidermal Cell Suspension (NCES)

NCES is the current standard of care for vitiligo surgery. In this method, melanocytes and keratinocytes are transplanted to the recipient area without being cultured. The donor-to-recipient area ratio for the NCES is 1:5 to 1:10. Gauthier et al. pioneered this procedure in vitiligo using scalp skin as a donor site using a process called cold trypsinization [4]. In this, the epidermal graft was transferred to a 0.25% trypsin-0.02% EDTA solution in a Petri dish and incubated for 18 h at 4 °C. Subsequently over the years, many modifications have been reported to optimize the procedure. Hot trypsinization reduces the time taken to prepare the suspension by incubating the graft for 1 h at 37 °C in 5% CO_2 [17]. However, cold trypsinization has a better outcome in terms of repigmentation, as it provides a higher number of viable cells [18]. A melanocyte count of 210–250 cells per mm^2 is ideal and can be measured prior to transplantation. After the cells were separated and washed, the suspension was centrifuged at 1000 rpm for 5 min to form a pellet containing melanocytes and keratinocytes. The pellet was then resuspended in phosphate-buffered saline (PBS) or Dulbecco's modified Eagle's medium and transferred to a 1 ml tuberculin syringe. The suspension is then transferred onto the prepared recipient site as a thin and uniform layer using a wide-bore 16-gauge needle. Figure 18.3 shows the cell pellet in a PBS solution in a centrifuge tube, ready to be grafted.

The substitution of melanocyte culture media with PBS brings down the cost of the procedure, improves melanocyte survival by preventing osmosis-induced cell death, and removes excess trypsin [19]. Hyaluronic acid has also been used as a suspension medium to increase the viscosity of the cell suspension and improve its adherence to the recipient site [20]. The use of platelet-rich plasma or the patient's own serum has also been reported.

Recently, the ReCell-kit was described with good repigmentation [21]. It is a single-use battery-operated device that automates cell harvesting. Other techniques that have been described include the "6-well plate" technique [22] and the four-compartment or 4C method. In this, ultrathin skin grafts were taken in a Petri dish with four compartments [23]. In the first compartment, hot trypsinization was done. In compartments 2 and 3, the trypsinized skin graft was washed in PBS twice to remove extra trypsin. In the fourth compartment, the melanocytes were dislodged into PBS. The Jodhpur technique involves harvesting donor cells using dermabrasion till pinpoint bleeding occurs [24]. This creates a paste-like material of the epidermis, which is removed with a spatula and spread directly over the recipient site without trypsinization.

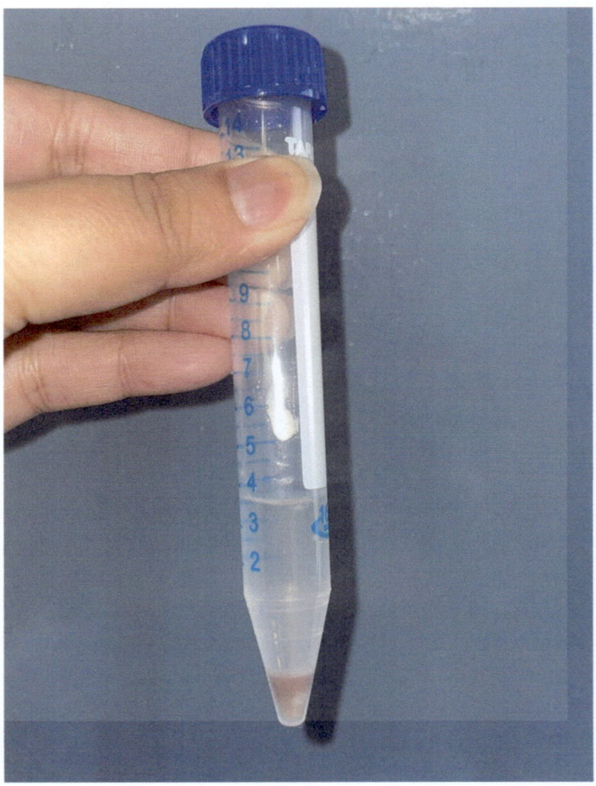

Fig. 18.3 Cell pellet containing melanocytes and keratinocytes in PBS solution in a centrifuge tube ready to be grafted

The adverse effects that one must be wary of include color mismatch, halo phenomenon, scarring, and secondary infection [10].

18.7 Noncultured Outer Root Sheath Hair Follicle Cell Suspension (NCORSHFS) Transplantation

Hair follicles are a very good source of melanocytes and their precursors. These stem cells are concentrated in the outer layer of the outer root sheath of the infundibulum, the midfollicle region, and the matrix of the hair bulb [25]. The follicular-melanin unit ratio is 1:5, which is significantly higher than the epidermal-melanin unit that is 1:36. Follicular melanocytes are also less affected by autoimmune destruction, but they are more affected by aging. This reservoir of cells is otherwise important in the therapy of vitiligo, as proven by the fact that repigmentation pattern in the initial stages is mostly perifollicular and patches present in areas that lack hair follicles, e.g., palms, often do not respond to medical therapies. Both follicular unit extraction and follicular cell suspension (FCS) can be done. Hair follicles are extracted from the occipital area of the scalp using small punches ($\leq$1 mm) and then subjected to the same process as NCES, except that the follicles are washed in PBS three times and transferred to a new tube of trypsin every 30 min [25].

18.8 Transplantation of Combined Epidermal and Hair Follicle Cell Suspensions

Studies have shown that combined NCES and FCS showed superior repigmentation, as compared to either NCES or FCS alone in acral vitiligo and difficult-to-treat vitiligo [26]. This was attributed to higher levels of growth factors and OCT4+ stem cells in the combined suspensions.

18.9 Transplantation of Combined Epidermal and Dermal Cell Suspensions

Dermal mesenchymal stem cells (DMCs) inhibit T cell proliferation and induce apoptosis. Hence, it has been postulated that the immunoregulatory properties of DMCs from noncultured dermal cell suspension (NDCS) can be used to improve the outcome of NCES. It is prepared by separating the epidermis from the dermis from a punch biopsy of the skin and then incubating the dermis overnight in collagenase at room temperature. A suspension containing both components (NCES and NDCS) is transplanted in a 1:1 ratio. In a pilot study by Thakur et al., it was observed

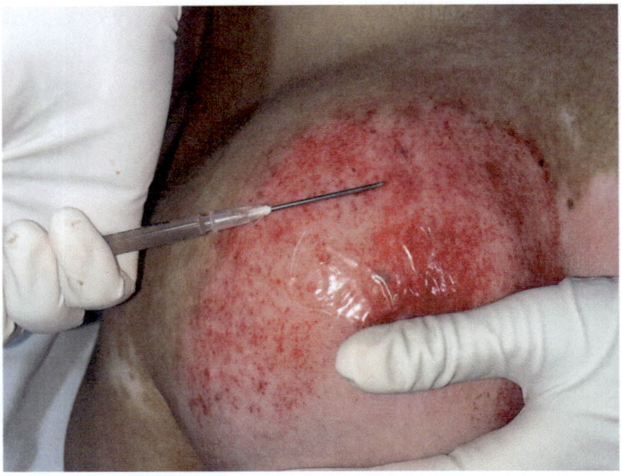

Fig. 18.4 Application of the suspension with a tuberculin syringe and a 16 G needle, followed by the application of a collagen sheet dressing

that in patients with shorter disease stability (3–6 months), combined NCES and NDCS had better repigmentation rates as compared to NCES alone [27].

18.10 Postoperative Care and Dressings

After transplantation of the suspension, proper dressings are required to keep the cells in position and to allow adequate time and milieu for the transplanted cells to be integrated into the recipient bed [28]. It also prevents infection, promotes wound healing, and soaks excess fluid. The first layer of dressings is a collagen sheet that promotes reepithelialization, followed by an antiseptic impregnated mesh dressing, cotton pad, polyurethane film and finally an elastic adhesive bandage. Figure 18.4 demonstrates application of the suspension, followed by a collagen sheet dressing on the prepared recipient site.

On uneven and curved surfaces, there is a risk of run-off of the suspension due to its fluidity, which results in poor repigmentation over such areas. A putty material in the shape of a body part has been successfully used to prepare a cast to hold the suspension in its place [29].

18.11 Follow-Up and Prognosis

Posttransplantation and healing of lesions, NBUVB, or PUVA can be used to augment the onset of repigmentation [30]. Initial hyperpigmentation is expected, which gradually resolves to an even color match after a few months. Figure 18.5a shows a pretreatment image of a stable vitiligo patch on the forehead, and Fig. 18.5b shows significant repigmentation at 6 months postsurgery.

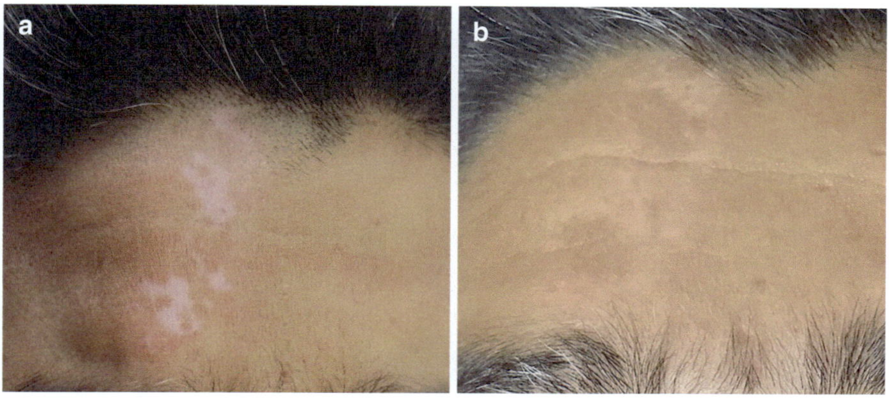

Fig. 18.5 (**a**) Pretreatment image of a stable vitiligo patch on the forehead. (**b**) Significant repigmentation (>90%) can be observed at 6 months postsurgery

A six-year follow-up study by Altalhab et al. in patients with vitiligo treated with NCES showed that 84.3% achieved good to excellent repigmentation at 6 months and 18.6% of patients had relapse [31]. Factors associated with relapse included male gender, age at surgery ≥23 years, nonsegmental vitiligo, age at onset of vitiligo >13 years and fingertip involvement, whereas an affected body surface area <1% and mechanical dermabrasion were associated with lower rates of relapse. Overall, cultured cell transplantation has better repigmentation rates as compared to noncultured techniques [32].

18.12 Conclusion

Cellular grafting techniques are the mainstay of management of stable vitiligo. Though good to excellent repigmentation is seen in the majority of patients, careful patient selection, adequate recipient site preparation, adherence to techniques to maintain the melanocyte count in the transplanted suspension, and facilitating uptake and proper postop care are important to improve outcomes.

References

1. Razmi TM, Afra TP, Parsad D. Vitiligo surgery: a journey from tissues via cells to the stems! Exp Dermatol. 2018;28(6):690–4.
2. Gamal AM, El-Barbary RA, Moftah NH. Updates in surgical treatment of vitiligo. J Recent Adv Med. 2021;2(1):118–27.
3. Haxthausen H. Studies on the pathogenesis of morphea, vitiligo, and acrodermatitis atrophicans by means of transplantation experiments. Acta Derm Venereol. 1947;27(5):352–67.

4. Gauthier Y, Surleve-Bazeille JE. Autologous grafting with noncultured melanocytes: a simplified method for treatment of depigmented lesions. J Am Acad Dermatol. 1992;26(2 Pt 1):191–4.
5. Parsad D, Gupta S. Standard guidelines of care for vitiligo surgery. Indian J Dermatol Venereol Leprol. 2008;74(Suppl(7)):S37–45.
6. Falabella R, Arrunategui A, Barona MI, Alzate A. The minigrafting test for vitiligo: detection of stable lesions for melanocyte transplantation. J Am Acad Dermatol. 1995;32(2 Pt 1):228–32.
7. Hamzavi I, Al-Hadidi N, Griffith J, Al-Jamal M. Role of recipient-site preparation techniques and post-operative wound dressing in the surgical management of vitiligo. J Cutan Aesthetic Surg. 2015;8(2):79–87.
8. Bishnoi A, Gupta M, Parsad D, Vinay K. Electrofulguration-assisted dermabrasion for recipient-site preparation in noncultured epidermal cell suspension type vitiligo surgery. J Am Acad Dermatol. 2019;80(6):e149–50.
9. Kumar S, Vinay K, Parsad D, et al. Comparison of recipient-site preparation by electrofulguration-assisted manual dermabrasion versus conventional manual dermabrasion in non-cultured epidermal cell suspension procedure for stable vitiligo: an open-label comparison study. J Eur Acad Dermatol Venereol. 2020;34(7):e337–9.
10. Dev A, Vinay K, Kumaran MS, et al. Electrofulguration-assisted dermabrasion is comparable to manual dermabrasion in patients undergoing autologous non-cultured epidermal cell suspension for treatment of stable vitiligo: a randomized controlled trial. J Cosmet Dermatol. 2022;21(4):1574–81.
11. Kaliyadan F. Using the ball-shaped attachment of a radiofrequency ablation device for preparation of recipient site in vitiligo surgery. Indian J Dermatol. 2011;56(4):459–60.
12. Subburaj K, Thakur V, Kumaran MS, Vinay K, Srivastava N, Parsad D. A prospective, randomized clinical study to compare the efficacy of recipient site preparation using dermabrasion, cryoblister, and dermaroller in autologous noncultured epidermal cell suspension in stable vitiligo. Dermatol Ther. 2021;34(1):e14683.
13. Razmi TM, Kumaran SM, Parsad D. Trichloroacetic acid 25% peel to facilitate dermabrasion at difficult sites in vitiligo surgery. Dermatologic Surg. 2019;45(5):750–2.
14. Brysk MM, Newton RC, Rajaraman S, et al. Repigmentation of vitiliginous skin by cultured cells. Pigment Cell Res. 1989;2(3):202–7.
15. Falabella R, Escobar C, Borrero I. Treatment of refractory and stable vitiligo by transplantation of in vitro cultured epidermal autografts bearing melanocytes. J Am Acad Dermatol. 1992;26(2):230–6.
16. Guerra L, Capurro S, Melchi F, et al. Treatment of "stable" vitiligo by timedsurgery and transplantation of cultured epidermal autografts. Arch Dermatol. 2000;136(11):1380–9.
17. Olsson MJ, Juhlin L. Leucoderma treated by transplantation of a basal cell layer enriched suspension. Br J Dermatol. 1998;138(4):644–8.
18. Awasti S, Vinay K, Thakur V, et al. Comparison of efficacy of cold trypsinization versus warm trypsinization in preparation of autologous non-cultured epidermal cell suspension for treatment of stable vitiligo. J Eur Acad Dermatol Venereol. 2019;33(6):e237–9.
19. Holla AP, Kumar R, Parsad D, Kanwar A. Modified procedure of noncultured epidermal suspension transplantation: changes are the core of vitiligo surgery. J Cutan Aesthetic Surg. 2011;4(1):44–5.
20. van Geel N, Ongenae K, De Mil M, Naeyaert JM. Modified technique of autologous noncultured epidermal cell transplantation for repigmenting vitiligo: a pilot study. Dermatol Surg Off Publ Am Soc Dermatol Surg Al. 2001;27(10):873–6.
21. Mulekar SV, Ghwish B, Al Issa A, Al Eisa A. Treatment of vitiligo lesions by ReCell vs. conventional melanocyte-keratinocyte transplantation: a pilot study. Br J Dermatol. 2008;158(1):45–9.
22. Goh BK, Chua XM, Chong KL, de Mil M, van Geel NAC. Simplified cellular grafting for treatment of vitiligo and piebaldism: the "6-well plate" technique. Dermatol Surg Off Publ Am Soc Dermatol Surg Al. 2010;36(2):203–7.

23. Mrigpuri S, Razmi TM, Sendhil Kumaran M, Vinay K, Srivastava N, Parsad D. Four compartment method as an efficacious and simplified technique for autologous non-cultured epidermal cell suspension preparation in vitiligo surgery: a randomized, active-controlled study. J Eur Acad Dermatol Venereol. 2019;33(1):185–90.
24. Lamoria A, Agrawal A, Rao P, Kachhawa D. A comparative study between follicular unit transplantation and autologous non-cultured non-trypsinized epidermal cells grafting (Jodhpur technique) in stable vitiligo. J Cutan Aesthetic Surg. 2020;13(3):204.
25. Vinay K, Dogra S, Parsad D, et al. Clinical and treatment characteristics determining therapeutic outcome in patients undergoing autologous non-cultured outer root sheath hair follicle cell suspension for treatment of stable vitiligo. J Eur Acad Dermatol Venereol. 2015;29(1):31–7.
26. Razmi TM, Parsad D, Kumaran SM. Combined epidermal and follicular cell suspension as a novel surgical approach for acral vitiligo. J Am Acad Dermatol. 2017;76(3):564–7.
27. Thakur V, Kumar S, Kumaran MS, Kaushik H, Srivastava N, Parsad D. Efficacy of transplantation of combination of noncultured dermal and epidermal cell suspension vs epidermal cell suspension alone in vitiligo: a randomized clinical trial. JAMA Dermatol. 2019;155(2):204–10.
28. Thakur V, Narayan R V, Vinay K, et al. Surgical modalities of treatment in vitiligo. Cosmoderma. 2021;1:13.
29. Akshi B, Shilpa K, Harish P. A novel point of care technique to improve graft uptake in melanocyte-keratinocyte transplantation procedure for vitiligo of contoured areas like external ear. J Am Acad Dermatol. Published online June 2020.
30. Lommerts JE, Uitentuis SE, Bekkenk MW, de Rie MA, Wolkerstorfer A. The role of phototherapy in the surgical treatment of vitiligo: a systematic review. J Eur Acad Dermatol Venereol. 2018;32(9):1427–35.
31. Altalhab S, AlJasser MI, Mulekar SV, et al. Six-year follow-up of vitiligo patients successfully treated with autologous non-cultured melanocyte–keratinocyte transplantation. J Eur Acad Dermatol Venereol. 2019;33(6):1172–6.
32. Ju HJ, Bae JM, Lee RW, et al. Surgical interventions for patients with vitiligo: a systematic review and meta-analysis. JAMA Dermatol. 2021;157(3):307–16.

Chapter 19
Nongrafting Methods (Dermabrasion, Excision, Therapeutic Wounding, and Cryotherapy)

Vignesh Narayan R, Shyamanta Barua, and Rashmi Sarkar

Abstract Vitiligo is a chronic skin condition characterized by depigmented patches resulting from the loss of melanocytes. Nongrafting surgical techniques offer alternative treatment options for patients with localized vitiligo. This review explores several key nongrafting approaches, including microneedling, dermabrasion, excision, and cryotherapy. Microneedling involves the use of fine needles to create microchannels in the skin, stimulating melanocyte migration and enhancing repigmentation. Dermabrasion, which removes the outer layers of skin, is effective for resurfacing depigmented areas and promoting pigment restoration when combined with medical therapies. Excision entails the surgical removal of vitiligo-affected skin, often followed by grafting or adjunctive treatments to facilitate pigment integration. Cryotherapy, utilizing liquid nitrogen, induces controlled freezing of lesions to destroy abnormal cells and encourage repigmentation through inflammatory responses. Each technique has distinct mechanisms, procedural protocols, and outcomes, making patient selection and personalized treatment planning crucial. This review also discusses the benefits, risks, and success rates associated with these techniques and highlights future directions for research and technological advancements. Nongrafting approaches remain valuable for managing localized vitiligo and offer various options for achieving cosmetic improvement in affected individuals.

Keywords Nongrafting methods · Dermabrasion · Cryotherapy

V. Narayan R
Department of Dermatology, Venereology and Leprology, Bangalore Medical College and Research Institute, Bangalore, Karnataka, India

S. Barua
Department of Dermatology, Assam Medical College & Hospital, Dibrugarh, India

R. Sarkar (✉)
Department of Dermatology, Venereology and Leprology, Lady Hardinge Medical College and Hospitals, New Delhi, Delhi, India

R. Sarkar, V. Narayan R (eds.), *A Concise Guide to The Management of Vitiligo*,
https://doi.org/10.1007/978-981-95-3857-7_19

19.1 Introduction

Nongrafting approaches in vitiligo surgery are primarily based on the goal of achieving repigmentation without the need for tissue transplantation or grafting, which can be more invasive and technically demanding. These methods leverage the body's natural healing processes and regenerative capacity to stimulate melanocyte migration or proliferation. Techniques such as needling, microneedling, dermabrasion, and laser-assisted repigmentation create controlled injury to the skin, promoting the release of growth factors and cytokines that can enhance melanocyte activation or migration from adjacent pigmented areas. These nongrafting approaches are particularly useful for patients with stable vitiligo, where the disease is not actively progressing and where the depigmented areas are not extensive enough to require large-scale skin grafting. Moreover, nongrafting methods offer a less invasive option, with fewer risks of complications such as scarring or graft rejection, which are sometimes seen in grafting procedures [1].

The rationale behind these techniques is also supported by their ability to be combined with other therapeutic modalities, such as topical immunomodulators or phototherapy, to enhance repigmentation. For instance, procedures like needling or laser treatments can create microchannels in the skin that improve the penetration of topical treatments, such as tacrolimus, which may further stimulate melanocyte activity. Additionally, these methods are generally less resource intensive, requiring minimal equipment and shorter recovery times compared to grafting surgeries. For many patients, nongrafting techniques provide a more accessible and convenient option for managing stable vitiligo, particularly in areas like the face or joints where cosmetic outcomes and functional preservation are important considerations.

19.2 Patient Selection

The selection of nongrafting techniques for vitiligo treatment depends on several key criteria, the most important being the stability of the disease. Nongrafting methods are typically indicated for patients with stable vitiligo, defined as the absence of new lesions or the progression of existing lesions for at least 12 months. Stability ensures that the treated areas will not experience depigmentation postprocedure, which undermines the effectiveness of these techniques. Additionally, the type and location of vitiligo play a crucial role. Nongrafting approaches are often chosen for focal, segmental, or limited nonsegmental vitiligo where small, localized areas of depigmentation are present. In such cases, these techniques can effectively trigger repigmentation without the need for larger interventions like grafting.

Another important criterion is the overall health and skin condition of the patient. Nongrafting techniques are less invasive and are therefore suitable for patients who may not be ideal candidates for more aggressive surgical procedures due to underlying health conditions or concerns about potential scarring. Patients with vitiligo in cosmetically sensitive areas, such as the face or hands, where scarring must be minimized, are often good candidates for nongrafting options. Additionally, patient preference and tolerance for postprocedure recovery are important considerations, as nongrafting methods generally have shorter recovery times and fewer complications compared to grafting. Factors like the patient's ability to undergo combination treatments, such as phototherapy or topical immunomodulators, also influence the decision to use nongrafting techniques, as these adjunctive therapies can significantly enhance the success of nongrafting interventions.

19.3 Nongrafting Surgical Techniques: An Overview

Nongrafting techniques for vitiligo can be broadly classified into the following categories based on their mechanism of action and procedural approach:

(a) **Needling-Based Techniques**

- **Needling/Microneedling**: Involves creating microinjuries in the depigmented areas using fine needles. This triggers the release of growth factors, promotes melanocyte migration from surrounding pigmented skin, and enhances repigmentation.
- **Dermaroller**: A variation of microneedling, using a rolling device with multiple fine needles to cover larger areas in a shorter time.

(b) **Ablative Techniques**

- **Dermabrasion**: A mechanical method that involves controlled removal of the epidermis and papillary dermis to stimulate repigmentation. It is often used in combination with phototherapy or topical agents.
- **Chemical Peeling**: The application of caustic agents like phenol or trichloroacetic acid (TCA) to induce controlled exfoliation of the skin. This process stimulates melanocyte migration and is sometimes combined with phototherapy or topical treatments.

(c) **Laser-Based Techniques**

- **Ablative Lasers (e.g., CO_2 or Erbium)**: These lasers create controlled thermal damage to the skin, triggering a wound-healing response that can stimulate melanocyte activity.
- **Nonablative Lasers (e.g., Fractional Lasers)**: Use of fractional laser technology to stimulate skin regeneration and melanocyte migration without removing the epidermis.

(d) **Phototherapy-Augmented Techniques**

- **Excimer Laser or Narrowband UVB (NB-UVB)**: Although not traditionally surgical, these light-based therapies are often used postprocedure to enhance the effects of nongrafting techniques like needling or dermabrasion by stimulating melanocyte activity.

19.4 Needling/Microneedling

19.4.1 Mechanism of Action in Repigmentation

Needling or microneedling involves creating microinjuries to the skin using fine needles, which penetrate the epidermis and superficial dermis. This mechanical disruption stimulates a wound-healing response that triggers the release of growth factors and cytokines, promoting melanocyte migration from surrounding pigmented areas into the depigmented patches. The microinjuries also enhance the penetration of topical agents applied to the skin, such as immunomodulators or growth factor-stimulating agents, further promoting repigmentation. Additionally, the procedure stimulates the release of melanocyte-stimulating factors and increases the vascular supply, which can help in restoring pigment to vitiligo-affected areas [2].

19.4.2 Procedure Protocol and Variations

The microneedling procedure typically begins with cleansing and numbing the affected area using topical anesthetics. A dermaroller or dermapen equipped with fine needles is then rolled or stamped across the depigmented skin, creating controlled microwounds (Fig. 19.1). The depth of the needles can vary depending on the skin's thickness and the targeted area, usually ranging from 0.5 to 2.0 mm. Multiple passes are made to ensure uniform coverage. Variations in the technique may include using different needle lengths or applying additional pressure in difficult-to-treat areas. The procedure may need to be repeated every 4–6 weeks for several sessions, depending on the size and response of the treated area.

19.4.3 Combination Therapies (e.g., with Topical Agents or Light Therapy)

Microneedling is often combined with other therapies to improve outcomes. Topical immunomodulators like tacrolimus or pimecrolimus are commonly applied immediately after microneedling to take advantage of increased skin permeability. It may also be combined with modalities like 5-fluorouracil [3] (Fig. 19.2). These agents help suppress the autoimmune component of vitiligo while promoting melanocyte migration. Phototherapy, particularly narrowband UVB (NB-UVB) or excimer laser

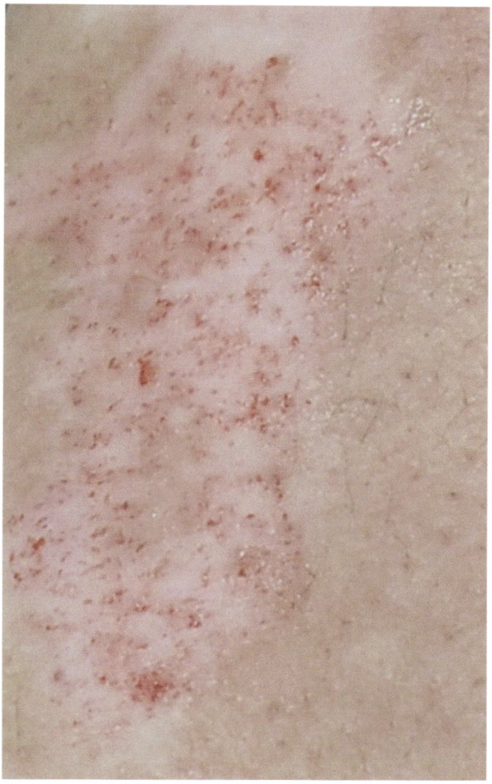

Fig. 19.1 Microchannel injuries created with microneedling using a dermapen

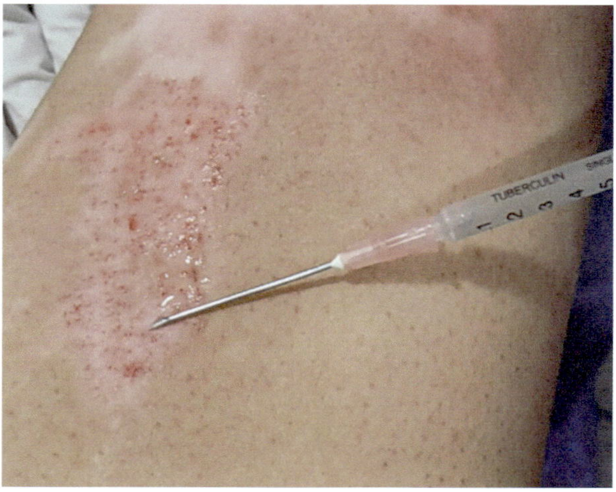

Fig. 19.2 Application of topical 5-FU solution over microchannels

therapy, is frequently used in conjunction with microneedling. Phototherapy is typically initiated after the skin has healed, usually 2–3 days postprocedure, to further stimulate melanocytes and enhance repigmentation. The combination of these treatments is often more effective than using microneedling or topical therapy alone, as microneedling enhances the efficacy of both topical agents and phototherapy by allowing deeper penetration and stimulating melanocyte activity.

19.4.4 Case Examples and Success Rates

Several studies have shown promising results with microneedling for vitiligo, particularly in stable cases. For example, a study involving patients with stable vitiligo who underwent microneedling combined with topical tacrolimus showed significant repigmentation in over 50% of cases after 6 months [4]. Another study demonstrated that patients who combined microneedling with NB-UVB achieved faster and more pronounced repigmentation compared to those who used NB-UVB alone [5]. Success rates are generally higher in areas with thinner skin, such as the face and neck, and lower in thicker, more resistant areas like the hands and feet. Outcomes are also more favorable in segmental vitiligo and focal vitiligo, where the disease is more localized. The results are patient dependent, but overall, microneedling has been shown to be a safe and effective option, particularly when combined with other therapies.

19.5 Dermabrasion

19.5.1 Concept of Epidermal Removal in Vitiligo

Dermabrasion involves controlled mechanical ablation of the epidermis and superficial dermis to initiate a reparative wound-healing response conducive to melanocyte migration and repigmentation in vitiligo (Fig. 19.3). The procedure disrupts the depigmented skin, removing the nonfunctional epidermis and creating an environment that facilitates melanocyte migration from the surrounding pigmented margins into the depigmented zones. This method relies on the regenerative potential of the epidermis to reestablish pigment through melanocyte reactivation. The success of dermabrasion is predicated on the stability of the vitiligo, where active disease processes are not undermining repigmentation [6].

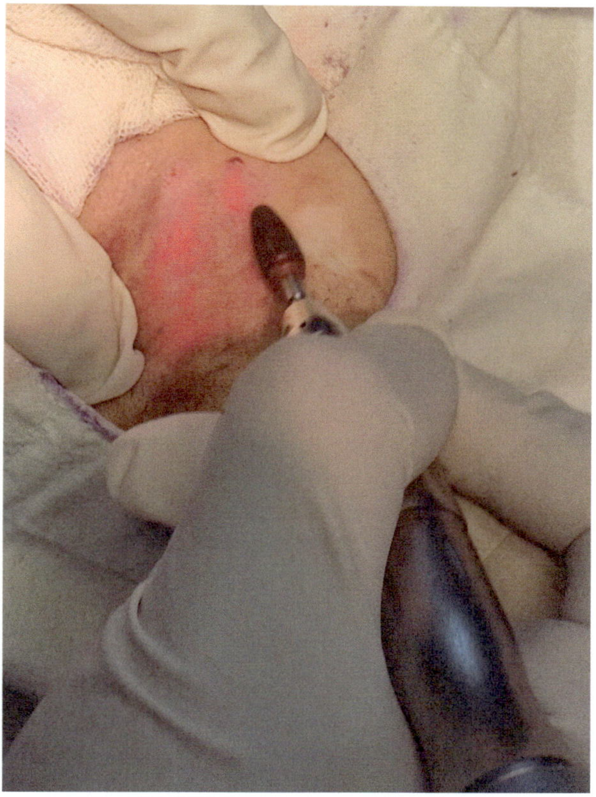

Fig. 19.3 Dermabrasion of a vitiligo patch using a Marathon™ motor carbide burr

19.5.2 Use in Combination with Medical Therapy

Dermabrasion is frequently employed as an adjunct to medical treatments, capitalizing on the enhanced transdermal delivery of topical agents' postprocedure. The disruption of the epidermal barrier allows for improved penetration of topical immunomodulators such as tacrolimus, pimecrolimus, and corticosteroids, which can suppress the underlying autoimmune response implicated in vitiligo [7]. Additionally, ablated skin responds more robustly to **narrowband UVB (NB-UVB)** or **excimer laser** therapy, which are integral to promoting melanocyte proliferation and migration [8]. In the immediate postoperative phase, phototherapy can be initiated once the re-epithelialization process begins, enhancing the overall efficacy of the repigmentation process. The combination of dermabrasion and adjunctive therapies is particularly effective in stable vitiligo, facilitating more uniform and sustained repigmentation.

19.5.3 Risks and Benefits

The key advantage of dermabrasion is its ability to induce repigmentation by mechanically creating an environment favorable for melanocyte proliferation without the need for autologous grafting. It offers a viable option for patients with stable, localized vitiligo, especially in areas where cosmetic outcomes are a priority. In combination with topical immunomodulators and phototherapy, it provides a multifaceted approach for repigmentation, with superior results reported in patients with segmental or focal vitiligo.

However, dermabrasion carries inherent risks, particularly with deeper procedures. The potential for hypertrophic scarring, keloid formation, and postinflammatory hyper- or hypopigmentation is elevated in cases where the dermis is breached. Other risks include infection, prolonged healing, and the exacerbation of disease activity if performed in patients with unstable vitiligo [9]. Proper patient selection, procedural expertise, and postoperative care are essential for mitigating these risks and optimizing therapeutic outcomes. Despite these potential complications, dermabrasion remains an effective, minimally invasive option in the armamentarium for managing stable vitiligo when combined with appropriate adjunct therapies.

19.5.4 Excision as a Treatment for Vitiligo

Excision is a surgical technique used in vitiligo treatment, primarily for localized and stable vitiligo lesions. The procedure involves the complete removal of the affected skin using a scalpel or surgical laser, followed by primary closure or skin grafting. The rationale behind excision is that it targets the depigmented areas directly, eliminating the pathologically altered skin and allowing for the repigmentation of the surrounding or transplanted healthy skin (Fig. 19.4). This approach is particularly effective in cases where vitiligo is confined to small, well-defined areas, as it can provide rapid and significant cosmetic improvement by reintroducing normal pigment to the affected region [10].

19.5.5 Cryotherapy

Cryotherapy involves the application of extreme cold to target vitiligo lesions, typically using liquid nitrogen. This technique induces controlled freezing of the skin, which leads to localized destruction of the affected epidermal cells. The freezing process causes the formation of ice crystals within the cells, resulting in cell necrosis and a subsequent inflammatory response. This can be used as a modality to depigment residual normal pigmented skin in universal vitiligo, and it has equal efficacy as a 755 nm laser in this regard [11].

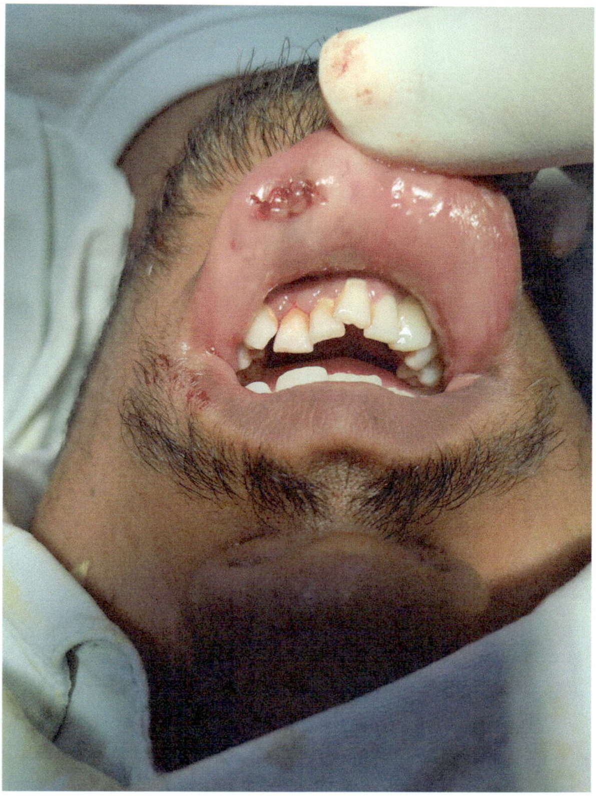

Fig. 19.4 Excision and suturing of the vitiligo from the lip

19.6 Laser-Assisted Nongrafting Techniques

19.6.1 Use of Ablative and Nonablative Lasers in Vitiligo

Laser-assisted nongrafting techniques in vitiligo aim to stimulate repigmentation by inducing controlled skin injury and promoting melanocyte migration and proliferation. Ablative lasers, such as **fractional CO_2** and **erbium** lasers, create microscopic thermal injuries by vaporizing tissue, promoting re-epithelialization, and stimulating wound healing processes that encourage melanocyte migration from adjacent healthy skin. Nonablative lasers, on the other hand, deliver energy that induces dermal remodeling without removing the epidermis, stimulating collagen production and melanocyte activity indirectly.

Ablative lasers are typically preferred when more aggressive treatment is needed to break down fibrotic barriers in chronic, stable vitiligo lesions, while nonablative lasers are employed in areas where minimal damage to the epidermis is desired or for combination therapy with topical agents or phototherapy. These techniques are particularly useful for patients who may not be candidates for surgical grafting procedures but have stable, localized lesions that have not responded well to other therapies [12].

19.6.2 Fractional CO_2 Laser, Erbium, and Others

Fractional CO_2 Laser This laser creates microscopic columns of thermal injury through the epidermis and dermis, promoting a wound-healing response that facilitates melanocyte migration and the production of growth factors like TGF-β and PDGF. It is often used for resistant lesions, particularly on acral surfaces, and is combined with phototherapy or topical immunomodulators to enhance melanocyte activity [13].

Erbium Laser Similar to the fractional CO_2 laser but with more superficial ablation, the erbium laser creates precise epidermal injury with minimal thermal damage to surrounding tissues. This makes it more suitable for thinner or more sensitive skin, such as on the face. Erbium laser is also used in conjunction with other repigmentation therapies to accelerate outcomes [14].

Excimer Laser (308 nm) Although primarily nonablative, the excimer laser uses UVB light to directly stimulate melanocytes and induce localized repigmentation. It is particularly effective for segmental and focal vitiligo, and it has a well-documented safety profile when combined with other treatments like microneedling or superficial ablative lasers [15].

19.6.3 Mechanisms and Protocols

The mechanism of laser-assisted therapies in vitiligo involves creating controlled damage to the skin, thereby activating the wound-healing cascade. Ablative lasers (e.g., fractional CO_2) create microthermal zones (MTZs) in the epidermis and dermis, prompting keratinocyte and melanocyte migration from surrounding healthy skin. These MTZs enhance the delivery of topical agents by increasing skin permeability, which is particularly useful when combined with immunomodulators (e.g., tacrolimus or pimecrolimus).

The typical protocol for ablative lasers involves pretreatment with topical anesthetics to minimize discomfort. Fractional CO_2 or erbium lasers are applied in multiple passes to cover the affected area. Posttreatment, topical agents are applied immediately to optimize their absorption, followed by phototherapy (e.g., narrowband UVB or excimer laser) initiated 1–2 weeks after healing. Sessions are generally spaced 3–4 weeks apart, with three to six treatments recommended depending on patient response.

Nonablative lasers like the excimer laser target specific wavelengths of UV light to stimulate melanocytes directly, with no epidermal disruption. Protocols typically include two to three sessions per week for 3–4 months, often combined with topical corticosteroids or calcineurin inhibitors to enhance repigmentation [16].

19.6.4 Patient Outcomes and Considerations

Laser-assisted nongrafting techniques have demonstrated significant efficacy in inducing repigmentation, particularly in patients with stable vitiligo. Ablative lasers have shown success in repigmenting difficult-to-treat areas, such as the hands, feet, and elbows, where other therapies often fail. Studies have reported up to 60–70% repigmentation in patients treated with fractional CO_2 or erbium lasers, especially when combined with topical agents and phototherapy. Nonablative excimer lasers have shown high success rates in segmental vitiligo, with repigmentation observed in over 50% of treated cases within 3–4 months.

However, patient selection is crucial. Laser therapy is most effective in stable, localized vitiligo and may not be appropriate for patients with widespread or actively spreading disease. The risk of side effects, such as postinflammatory hyperpigmentation, scarring, and prolonged erythema, is higher with ablative lasers, particularly in patients with darker skin types. Nonablative lasers have a more favorable safety profile but may require more sessions for visible results. Patient expectations must be managed, as complete repigmentation may not always be achievable, and maintenance sessions may be necessary to sustain results. Overall, laser-assisted techniques, when carefully selected and combined with adjunctive therapies, offer a promising option for stable vitiligo management.

19.7 Patient Counseling and Follow-Up

19.7.1 Managing Expectations

Effective patient counseling is critical in managing expectations before initiating nongrafting surgical techniques for vitiligo. Patients must be informed that these procedures aim to stimulate repigmentation, but outcomes can vary significantly based on individual factors such as disease stability, lesion location, and skin type. It is essential to explain that full repigmentation may not always be achievable, particularly in areas with poor melanocyte reservoirs (e.g., hands and feet) or long-standing lesions. Patients should understand that nongrafting techniques, such as needling, dermabrasion, or laser therapies, often require multiple treatment sessions and that repigmentation may be gradual over weeks to months. Additionally, the need for adjunctive treatments like topical immunomodulators or phototherapy should be emphasized to optimize outcomes.

Counseling must also address the possibility of partial or incomplete repigmentation and the risk of color mismatch between treated areas and the surrounding skin. It is important to set realistic expectations about the cosmetic outcome, particularly for lesions on visible areas like the face or neck. Recurrence of depigmentation, though less likely in stable vitiligo, can still occur, and long-term maintenance treatments may be necessary. By clearly discussing these points, patients can approach treatment with a realistic understanding of what to expect, leading to better satisfaction with the results.

19.7.2 Postprocedure Care and Long-Term Follow-Up

Post-procedure care plays a vital role in the success of nongrafting vitiligo treatments. After procedures like microneedling, dermabrasion, or laser therapy, patients should be advised to avoid direct sun exposure and use broad-spectrum sunscreen to protect the treated areas from UV damage, which can exacerbate depigmentation or cause postinflammatory hyperpigmentation. Topical medications, such as tacrolimus or corticosteroids, may be prescribed to promote melanocyte migration and suppress local immune responses. It is important to instruct patients on the proper application of these agents to enhance repigmentation.

Wound care is essential following ablative techniques, particularly dermabrasion and fractional laser treatments. Patients should be counseled on keeping the treated areas clean and moist with ointments like petroleum jelly to promote healing and minimize the risk of infection or scarring. Monitoring for signs of complications, such as prolonged erythema, infection, or excessive scarring, is crucial during the initial posttreatment phase.

Long-term follow-up is necessary to assess the success of repigmentation and to monitor for any recurrence of vitiligo. Follow-up visits should be scheduled at regular intervals (e.g., every 4–6 weeks) to evaluate the response to treatment and make adjustments as needed. Patients undergoing combination therapy with phototherapy will require more frequent visits for UVB or excimer sessions. Even after successful repigmentation, continued follow-up may be required to manage potential recurrences and to provide maintenance treatments to preserve the pigment.

19.7.3 Addressing Complications and Recurrence

Despite the minimally invasive nature of nongrafting techniques, complications can arise, especially in ablative methods like dermabrasion and laser treatments. Patients should be counseled about potential risks, including postinflammatory hyperpigmentation (PIH), hypopigmentation, scarring, and infection. Darker skin types are particularly prone to PIH, and preventive measures such as strict sun protection and the use of depigmenting agents (e.g., hydroquinone) may be necessary.

In cases of complications such as scarring or infection, patients should be advised to seek prompt medical evaluation. Superficial infections can often be managed with topical or systemic antibiotics, but deeper infections may require more intensive intervention. If scarring occurs, treatments such as silicone gel or fractional laser resurfacing may be considered.

Recurrence of depigmentation is a concern, especially in patients with a history of unstable vitiligo. Patients should be informed that while nongrafting procedures can stimulate repigmentation, they do not cure the underlying autoimmune process that drives vitiligo. Recurrence can occur months or years after treatment, and maintenance therapies such as periodic phototherapy or topical immunomodulators may be required to preserve the repigmentation achieved. Counseling on long-term maintenance and the possibility of recurrence ensures that patients remain engaged in their care and are prepared for future management strategies if needed.

19.8 Future Directions in Nongrafting Surgical Techniques

19.8.1 Emerging Techniques and Technologies

The field of nongrafting surgical techniques for vitiligo is rapidly evolving, with emerging technologies aiming to enhance repigmentation outcomes and reduce treatment time. One promising area is the development of **robotic and automated microneedling devices**, which allow for precise control of needle depth and speed, optimizing the procedure's efficacy while minimizing trauma to the surrounding skin [17]. Additionally, **laser-assisted drug delivery (LADD)** is gaining attention as a technique to enhance the penetration of topical agents following laser treatment [18]. By using fractional ablative lasers to create microchannels in the skin, LADD increases the absorption of topical therapies like calcineurin inhibitors or corticosteroids, significantly improving their effectiveness.

The combination of **nanotechnology-based delivery systems** with nongrafting techniques is also being explored. Nanocarriers can encapsulate active compounds (e.g., immunomodulators or melanocyte-stimulating agents) and release them in a controlled manner when combined with microneedling or laser treatments, enhancing therapeutic outcomes [19].

19.8.2 Potential Improvements in Current Procedures

While current nongrafting techniques like microneedling, dermabrasion, and laser therapy are effective in stable vitiligo, there are opportunities for refinement. One area for improvement is the **standardization of protocols** to reduce variability in outcomes. Studies are focusing on optimizing the depth and intensity of microneedling or laser treatment based on skin type, lesion location, and disease duration to ensure more predictable results.

Combination therapies are also being revisited, particularly the timing and sequence of topical agents and phototherapy after nongrafting procedures. Refining the delivery of **growth factors**, **stem cell-stimulating compounds**, or **exosome therapies** as adjuncts to microneedling and laser treatments could significantly improve repigmentation rates. These biologically active substances can be delivered through the microchannels created during the procedure, enhancing the natural wound healing and repigmentation process. Additionally, **gene therapy** and the targeting of specific molecular pathways involved in melanocyte destruction or dysfunction (e.g., JAK inhibitors) hold promise in improving repigmentation results.

19.8.3 Future Research Areas

Several key research areas could shape the future of nongrafting surgical techniques in vitiligo. One major area is the exploration of **biomarkers** to predict which patients will respond best to nongrafting interventions. Identifying genetic or molecular markers associated with melanocyte resilience or autoimmune activity could guide personalized treatment plans, improving success rates and reducing the trial-and-error approach currently used [20].

Another area of interest is the **long-term durability of repigmentation** achieved through nongrafting methods. While the initial results may be promising, recurrence remains a significant concern. Research into the use of **immunomodulatory agents** (e.g., JAK inhibitors) to maintain pigment after nongrafting procedures is underway, with the goal of developing maintenance therapies that prevent recurrence.

Lastly, the potential of **regenerative medicine** and **stem cell therapy** in vitiligo is a burgeoning field [21]. Future studies could explore how stem cells or their derivatives could be applied alongside or following nongrafting procedures to regenerate functional melanocytes in vitiligo-affected skin. Similarly, research into **bioengineered skin substitutes** or **melanocyte-enhancing scaffolds** that can be applied postprocedure may revolutionize how nongrafting techniques are performed, offering more consistent and durable repigmentation outcomes [22, 23]. These advancements suggest a future where nongrafting surgical techniques could achieve results comparable to more invasive options, with fewer risks and faster recovery times.

19.9 Conclusion

Nongrafting surgical techniques for vitiligo represent a significant advancement in the management of this challenging condition, offering patients effective alternatives to traditional surgical approaches. Techniques such as microneedling, dermabrasion, and laser therapy provide valuable options for inducing repigmentation by leveraging the skin's natural wound-healing responses and enhancing the delivery of adjunctive therapies. Microneedling and dermabrasion focus on creating controlled epidermal injuries to stimulate melanocyte migration and proliferation, while laser therapies, including ablative and nonablative lasers, offer targeted approaches to both remove and remodel skin layers or stimulate melanocyte activity directly.

Emerging technologies and innovations are poised to further enhance these nongrafting techniques. Advances such as automated microneedling devices, laser-assisted drug delivery, and photothermal therapy are set to refine current procedures, improving efficacy and patient outcomes. The integration of nanotechnology and the exploration of regenerative medicine hold promise for addressing the limitations of existing methods, potentially leading to more consistent and durable repigmentation.

Future research will be crucial in optimizing treatment protocols and addressing potential complications. By identifying biomarkers for treatment response, improving the long-term durability of repigmentation, and exploring novel therapies like stem cell treatments, the field of nongrafting vitiligo management is likely to achieve more personalized and effective solutions. Continued advancements in these areas will enhance the ability to provide stable and cosmetically satisfactory results for patients, making nongrafting techniques an increasingly valuable component of vitiligo care.

Acknowledgments None.

Conflicts of Interest None.

Source of Funding None.

Ethics Statement N/A.

References

1. Grochocka M, Wełniak A. Białczyk A, Marek-Jozefowicz L, Tadrowski T, Czajkowski R. Management of stable vitiligo-a review of the surgical approach. J Clin Med. 2023;12:1984.
2. Salloum A, Bazzi N, Maalouf D, Habre M. Microneedling in vitiligo: a systematic review. Dermatol Ther. 2020;33:e14297.
3. Chhabra S, Chahar YS, Singh A. A comparative study of microneedling combined with topical 5-fluorouracil versus microneedling alone in treatment of localized stable vitiligo. Indian J Dermatol. 2021;66:574.

4. Ebrahim HM, Elkot R, Albalate W. Combined microneedling with tacrolimus vs tacrolimus monotherapy for vitiligo treatment. J Dermatolog Treat. 2021;32:999–1004.
5. Kaur A, Barman KD, Sahoo B, Choudhary P. A comparative interventional study of narrowband ultraviolet B alone and narrowband ultraviolet B in combination with microneedling in patients with stable vitiligo. Photodermatol Photoimmunol Photomed. 2023;39:357–63.
6. Awad SS. Dermabrasion may repigment vitiligo through stimulation of melanocyte precursors and elimination of hyperkeratosis. J Cosmet Dermatol. 2012;11:318–22.
7. Kubelis-López DE, Zapata-Salazar NA, Said-Fernández SL, et al. Updates and new medical treatments for vitiligo (review). Exp Ther Med. 2021;22:797.
8. Bayoumi W, Fontas E, Sillard L, et al. Effect of a preceding laser dermabrasion on the outcome of combined therapy with narrowband ultraviolet B and potent topical steroids for treating nonsegmental vitiligo in resistant localizations. Br J Dermatol. 2012;166:208–11.
9. Mahajan BB, Sethi S, Tyagi S. Dermabrasion in vitiligo. In: Comprehensive textbook on vitiligo. Boca Raton: CRC Press; 2020. p. 273–6.
10. Sacchidanand S, Purohit V, Sujaya SN. Surgical excision and primary closure for the treatment of lip vitiligo. J Cutan Aesthet Surg. 2011;4:216–7.
11. van Geel N, Depaepe L, Speeckaert R. Laser (755 nm) and cryotherapy as depigmentation treatments for vitiligo: a comparative study. J Eur Acad Dermatol Venereol. 2015;29:1121–7.
12. Post NF, Ezekwe N, Narayan VS, et al. The use of lasers in vitiligo, an overview. J Eur Acad Dermatol Venereol. 2022;36:779–89.
13. Raizada A, Panda M, Singh BS, Kar BR. Fractional carbon dioxide laser versus fractional carbon dioxide laser with autologous intralesional platelet-rich plasma in the treatment of stable, non-segmental vitiligo: a randomized comparative study. J Cutan Aesthet Surg. 2021;14:55–63.
14. Doghaim NN, El-Tatawy RA, Ismail MA, Ali DAM, El Attar YA. Study the effect of erbium:YAG laser plus topical 5-flurouracil in stable vitiligo resistant to NB-UVB phototherapy. J Cosmet Dermatol. 2020;19:122–30.
15. Deshpande AJ. 308nm excimer lamp monotherapy for lip vitiligo-a short case series. J Cosmet Laser Ther. 2020;22:253–5.
16. Yu S, Lan CE, Yu HS. Mechanisms of repigmentation induced by photobiomodulation therapy in vitiligo. Exp Dermatol. 2019;28(Suppl 1):10–4.
17. Singh A, Yadav S. Microneedling: advances and widening horizons. Indian Dermatol Online J. 2016;7:244–54.
18. Ng WHS, Smith SD. Laser-assisted drug delivery: a systematic review of safety and adverse events. Pharmaceutics. 2022;14:2738.
19. Sun MC, Xu XL, Lou XF, Du YZ. Recent Progress and future directions: the Nano-drug delivery system for the treatment of vitiligo. Int J Nanomedicine. 2020;15:3267–79.
20. Yang Q, Zhang G, Su M, et al. Vitiligo skin biomarkers associated with Favorable therapeutic response. Front Immunol. 2021;12:613031.
21. Esquivel D, Mishra R, Srivastava A. Stem cell therapy offers a possible safe and promising alternative approach for treating vitiligo: a review. Curr Pharm Des. 2020;26:4815–21.
22. Anish S. Skin substitutes in dermatology. Indian J Dermatol Venereol Leprol. 2015;81:175–8.
23. Varshney N, Sahi AK, Vajanthri KY, et al. Culturing melanocytes and fibroblasts within three-dimensional macroporous PDMS scaffolds: towards skin dressing material. Cytotechnology. 2019;71:287–303.

Chapter 20
Complications in Vitiligo Surgery

Tanvi Dev and Somesh Gupta

Abstract The constant evolution of surgical procedures has resulted in multiple innovative techniques that can be utilized for repigmentation in vitiligo. All of these procedures are associated with some complications and limitations. Additionally, multiple novel techniques and pearls have been devised to improve the overall cosmetic result of each of these procedures. This chapter focuses on various complications of these procedures and practical ways and novel techniques to avoid or treat them.

Keywords Complications · Results · Vitiligo surgery · Cobblestoning · Polka dot appearance · Perigraft halo · Color mismatch · Achromic fissuring · Marginal halo · Scarring

20.1 Introduction

The results and complications of any surgical procedure depend upon several factors. Some of the common factors include appropriate patient selection, proper procedure selection, skill and expertise of the surgeon, following standard operating procedures for asepsis, and availability of appropriate instruments and machinery, among others. While most of the procedures for vitiligo surgery are simple with a small learning curve, the formula for perfection lies in taking cognizance of the minute details and intricacies of each step [1].

In a recent meta-analysis, among 117 studies and 8776 patients, the mean rate of repigmentation of more than 90% for surgical procedures overall was 52.69%. The occurrence of adverse events was reported in 56 studies. Common adverse events at

T. Dev
Department of Dermatology, Maulana Azad Medical College, New Delhi, India

S. Gupta (✉)
Department of Dermatology, All India Institute of Medical Sciences, New Delhi, India

R. Sarkar, V. Narayan R (eds.), *A Concise Guide to The Management of Vitiligo*,
https://doi.org/10.1007/978-981-95-3857-7_20

the recipient site included pain, hyperpigmentation, and hypopigmentation at the donor site, irrespective of the kind of procedure. Other complications in all the procedures included marginal halo, mottled pigmentation, and scarring. Koebner phenomenon at the donor site or disease progression has also been reported in several studies, signifying the importance of detailed evaluation regarding the stability of the disease before commencing surgery [2].

This chapter discusses various complications of different surgical procedures for vitiligo and innovative ways and novel techniques to avoid or treat them. The surgical procedures can be classified into tissue grafting methods and cellular grafting methods.

20.2 Tissue Grafting Methods

20.2.1 Punch Grafting

The complications at the recipient site include a cobblestone appearance, a polka dot appearance, a perigraft halo, a static graft, depigmentation of the graft, graft rejection, keloidal or hypertrophic scarring, and color mismatch [1, 3]. The common complications at the donor site include scarring (superficial, keloidal, or hypertrophic), depigmentation due to koebnerization, and secondary infection.

The cobblestone appearance is the commonest of these complications (Figs. 20.1 and 20.2). It can be minimized or avoided by adhering to certain simple techniques. The size of the punch should be small (1–1.2 mm on the face and neck and 1–1.5 mm on other sites), and the size of the graft should be equal to or slightly smaller than the pit. The excess adipose tissue can be trimmed from the grafts, and the depth of the recipient pit should be 1 mm deeper than the length of the graft so that the upper surface of the graft is at the level of the surrounding recipient skin. The punches should be sharp, and handling of the grafts should be gentle in order to minimize tissue trauma. These grafts should be placed at a distance of at least 5 mm from each

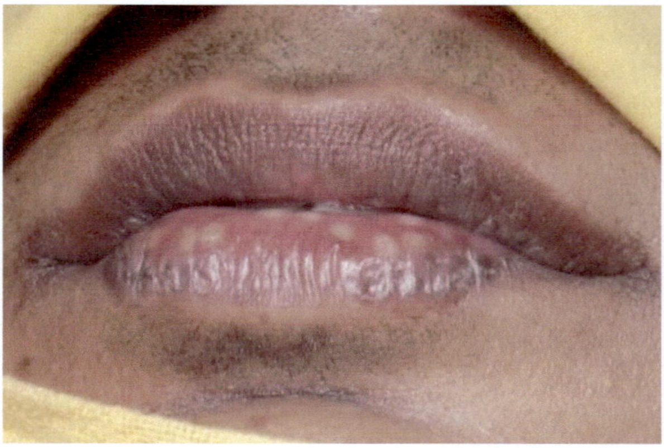

Fig. 20.1 Cobblestoning and residual depigmentation in the case of lip vitiligo after mini-punch grafting

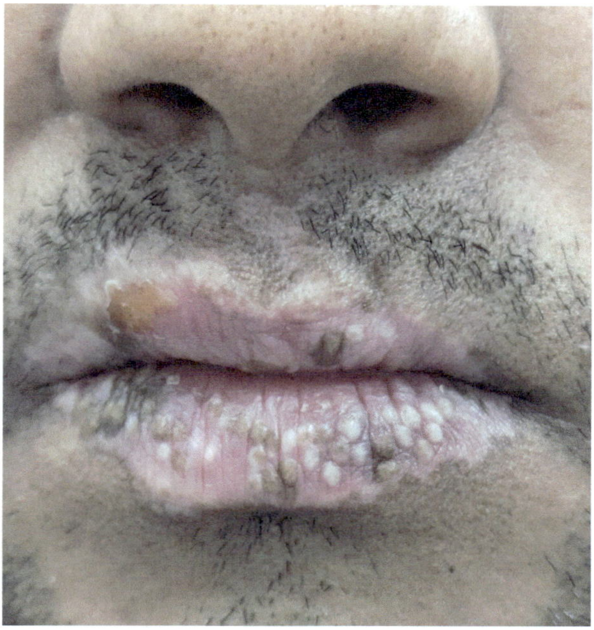

Fig. 20.2 Cobblestoning after mini-punch grafting on lip vitiligo

other to prevent overcrowding, hence reducing edema and inflammation. The use of silicone gel sheet for postoperative dressing has been reported to decrease the incidence of cobblestoning and graft dislodgement by virtue of the firm pressure provided by the sheet, which nullifies the forces that tend to lift the grafts and acts as a brace for the grafts [4]. Anbar et al. noted that silicone gel application after minigrating, although it improved the final response, had no significant effect on the occurrence of cobblestoning [5]. In established cases of cobblestoning, pinhole ablation using needle-assisted radiofrequency ablation and ablative lasers has been tried with satisfactory results [6].

The chances of developing a perigraft halo can be minimized by placing the grafts on or very close (1–2 mm) to the border of the lesion. The graft is expected to produce repigmentation at least 25 times the original size of the graft; hence, the grafts can be placed at a distance of 5–10 mm from each other or according to the result of test grafting [7].

Depigmentation of the grafts is a distressing complication. It is important to ensure the stability of the disease before commencement of the procedure [8]. Test grafting can be performed in doubtful cases [9]. Postoperative exposure to narrowband ultraviolet-B, excimer laser, PUVA, or PUVA-SOL has been reported to minimize the chances of graft depigmentation and improve the overall result [10].

In order to circumvent the chances of graft rejection, graft handling should be gentle, as mentioned above, and nontoothed forceps should be used. It is important to ensure that the graft edges are not folded or that the graft is not placed upside down in the recipient pit. The grafts can be placed directly from the donor site to the recipient site to speed up the procedure, minimize the "outside body time" of the grafts and reduce the risk of infection and hence graft rejection. The postoperative dressing can include a silicone gel sheet for bracing the grafts. The recipient site can be immobilized when necessary. After lip surgery, the patient can be advised a liquid diet using a straw for the first 18–24 h [1]. Graft dislodgement can also be prevented by using tissue glue.

Manual punch grafting can be time-consuming and fatigue-inducing for the surgeon when a larger area is targeted. Motorized punches can be used to increase the number of grafts harvested with ease without the surgeon's fatigability. The entire procedure can be performed in one session, hence saving time and consumables for the surgery and the overall cost of the procedure [11].

20.2.2 Suction Blister Epidermal Grafting

Suction blister epidermal grafting (SBEG) provides an excellent cosmetic appearance with good color match; however, the major disadvantages are that it is a time-consuming process and only small areas can be treated. It usually takes approximately 2 h to form a 2.2 cm blister; however, intradermal infiltration of anesthesia or saline can reduce the time significantly [12, 13]. Anbar et al. concluded that syringes or cups with smaller diameter and preheating of the donor area shortened the suction blister induction time (SBIT) significantly, while intrablister injection of normal saline increased the blister size and turned multilocular blisters into unilocular blisters [14].

Another technical difficulty is that the syringes used to create suction blisters usually come off during the procedure, or sometimes, the negative pressure generated is inadequate, hence needing frequent reapplication of the vacuum. To circumvent this, "Hijama" therapy cups can be used [15].

At the recipient site, the complications include wrinkling, folding, and displacement of the graft and graft rejection. To avoid this, the graft can be secured by using cyanoacrylate glue or stay sutures, especially at mobile recipient sites. To prevent perigraft halo, it is recommended to dermabrade the recipient area 1–2 mm beyond the margin of the lesion [1].

Complications are uncommon, although hyperpigmentation, incomplete pigmentation, a perigraft halo, and graft rejection may occur [16]. Batra et al. performed SBEG in 60 patients and reported that the overall success rate of the procedure was 91.7%, the common complications noted were perilesional hypopigmentation (15%) and hyperpigmentation (10%) at the recipient site, and hyperpigmentation (21.7%) and infection (8.3%) were observed at the donor site [17]. Laxmisha et al. noted that the immediate complications at the donor site included purpura at the margin of application of the suction syringe (52 cases) and pigmentation at the donor site (52 cases), which started 1 week after the procedure and lasted for around 2 months before it started subsiding. By the end of 3 months, imperceptible macular pigmentation remained in most of the cases (51 of 52 cases) [18].

20.2.3 *Split Thickness Skin Grafting*

In this technique, a split thickness graft is harvested from the donor site. This graft is relatively thicker as it contains dermal tissue, which leads to a stuck-on appearance, uneven and nonuniform texture, and color mismatch at the recipient site (Figs. 20.3 and 20.4). In thicker grafts, hypertrophy can develop [1]. The most important factor determining the cosmetic outcome is the thickness of the graft. It is advisable to harvest ultrathin graft with minimal to no dermal tissue; however, this requires surgical skill and expertise. The advent of electric dermatomes has made it easier to obtain uniform ultrathin grafts. It is recommended to use topical anesthetic creams or ring block and avoid infiltration anesthesia at the donor site, as it leads to an irregular surface that hinders the harvest of a uniform thin graft [1, 16].

Very often, perigraft halo and achromic fissures can develop between the grafts due to the shrinkage of the tissue. Hence, dermabrasion should be done 1–2 mm beyond the depigmented area, and the graft should extend even beyond the abraded area. Overlapping of graft edges is also useful [1, 16].

In a recent meta-analysis, it was noted that thin skin grafting was frequently associated with graft contracture, overhanging margin, wrinkles over the graft surface, and perigraft halo [2]. Similarly, curling of the graft can give rise to a beaded

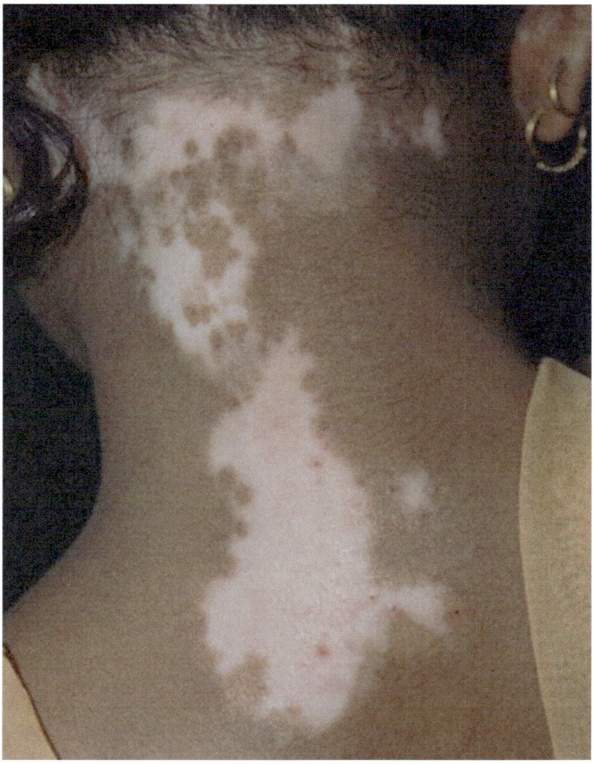

Fig. 20.3 Presurgery photograph showing localized vitiligo involving the posterior hair line extending to involve the neck and upper back in a linear pattern

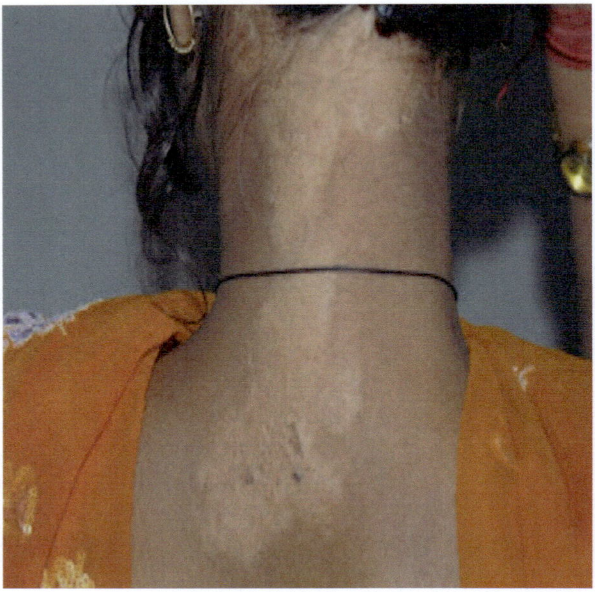

Fig. 20.4 Post ultra-thin split skin grafting, complete repigmentation was noted; however, there were textural alteration and color mismatch (hypopigmentation)

appearance (Fig. 20.4). The graft should be spread uniformly over the recipient area, and the margins should be secured using cyanoacrylate or surgical glue.

Milia formation and scarring are other complications at the donor and recipient sites. Milia resolve spontaneously or can be extirpated.

In dark-skinned patients, especially over sun-exposed areas, prolonged hyperpigmentation can occur. Hence, postprocedure NBUVB or PUVA therapy should be planned judiciously to avoid overexposure, which can lead to hyperpigmentation [1, 2].

Due to the limitation of the donor site area, multiple sessions can be required for treating larger areas of depigmentation [16].

20.2.4 Mesh Grafting

The size of the split thickness graft can be increased up to four times by meshing [19]. Complications at the recipient site include color mismatch, beading at margins and textural irregularity, and over the donor site, there is a risk of scarring [16].

20.2.5 Flip-Top Pigment Transplantation

In this technique, 1–2 mm sections of thin skin grafts obtained by shaving the donor area using a razor blade are placed between a flap of epidermis and dermis at the recipient site. It requires surgical expertise to obtain thin grafts. Thicker grafts can lead to irregular surface and beading at the recipient site [16, 20].

20.2.6 Transplantation of Hair Follicles

This procedure requires surgical expertise and specialized equipment and is often time-consuming. At the recipient site, cobblestoning, scarring, and graft rejection can occur. Scarring occurs at the occipital area from where the graft is taken [16]. The resultant area of repigmentation is small due to transplantation of intact hair follicles and the limited donor area. This drawback has been mitigated by the advent of a novel technique of using hair follicle outer root sheath cell suspension.

20.3 Cellular Grafting Methods

Cellular grafts include autologous noncultured epidermal cellular suspension (mixture of melanocytes and keratinocytes), noncultured hair follicle outer root sheath cell suspension, and cultured pure melanocytic cell suspension [21].

20.3.1 Autologous Noncultured Epidermal Cell Suspension

The harvesting of epidermal graft from the donor site requires skill and expertise. It requires experience to obtain a good suspension. Depending upon the thickness of the graft, the patient can develop scarring, which can be superficial or hypertrophic, and in some cases, a keloid can develop if the patient has a keloidal tendency. Gupta et al. described a minimally invasive and scarless novel technique of using epidermal brushings obtained by manual dermabrasion at the donor site for the preparation of epidermal cell suspension [22]. The depth of dermabrasion at the recipient site should be controlled and of adequate depth. Deeper or nonuniform dermabrasion leads to altered texture, color mismatch, and scarring at the recipient site, especially over acral areas where skin is thicker and slightly deeper dermabrasion is required (Fig. 20.5). Other adverse events include pain, secondary infection, and color mismatch (Fig. 20.6). Van Geel et al. described the presence of some color

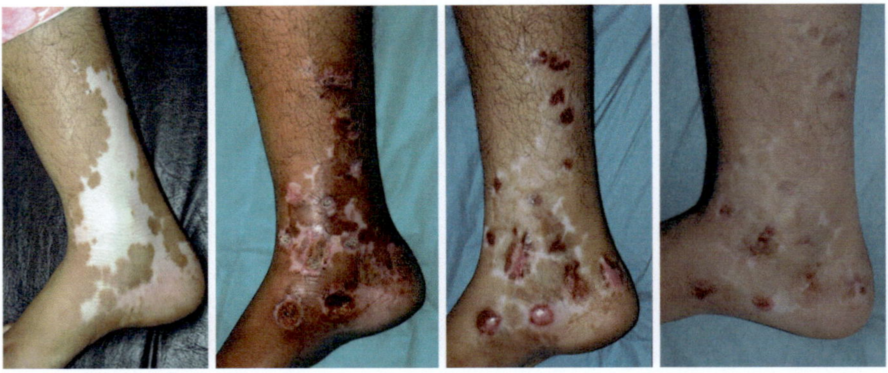

Fig. 20.5 Acral area showing hypertrophic scarring due to deeper dermabrasion

Fig. 20.6 Color mismatch and perigraft halo in a dark-skinned individual in a patch of vitiligo over the leg after NCES. (Courtesy: Dr. VK Sharma and Dr. Nimitha P)

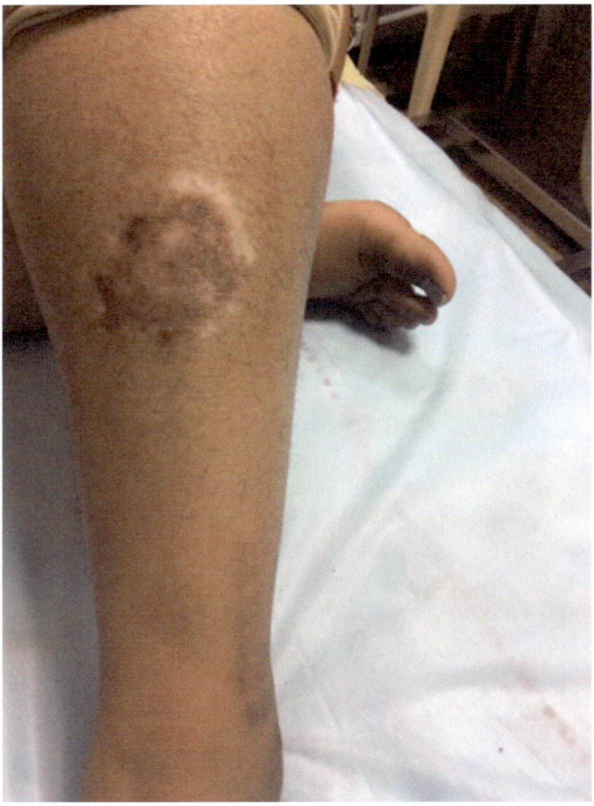

mismatch in the recipient area in 80.4% of the 54 evaluated patients. However, the patients were satisfied and did not bother about the color mismatch. At the donor site, minor textural skin changes were observed in 65% of the patients [23].

This is a multistep procedure, and each step needs to be performed appropriately; otherwise, it can lead to poor results. It requires cell culture-grade biochemicals, media, and equipment. The operating room needs to be equipped with a laboratory incubator, centrifuge machine, and sterile environment to prepare an uncontaminated cellular suspension. Besides being relatively expensive, it is more time-consuming and requires more manpower than tissue grafting methods [21].

Doolan et al. suggested the preparation of the recipient site using hyfrecation instead of using motorized or conventional manual dermabrader in order to prevent scarring and for better margin delineation. In order to improve the quality of the suspension before centrifugation, the authors also suggested using an intravenous giving set with a filter, which would allow the epidermal suspension (after enzymatic digestion and cleaning of the remaining trypsin using phosphate-buffered saline) to pass through but filter out the larger debris [24].

In order to shorten the cell preparation time, Goh et al. described a simplified technique using a “6-well plate” in the extraction of epidermal cells from donor skin. This technique also reduces the risk of contamination, the amount of reagents and equipment needed, and the overall cost of the procedure [25].

Gupta et al. suggested mixing the final keratinocyte-melanocyte suspension (obtained after centrifugation) with a few drops of methylcellulose ophthalmic solution to increase the viscosity of the suspension, which prevents it from flowing away when applied onto curved surfaces [26].

Gupta et al. described a new technique for the preparation of noncultured epidermal cell suspension, in which cell separation and harvesting are performed inside sterile blisters induced by suction on the patient’s thigh. This technique has the advantage of being simple, easy to learn, and inexpensive, and it requires minimal processing and handling of the tissue outside the body [27].

Recently, authors have described innovative ways to circumvent the use of a laboratory incubator for incubation of the suspension by using heat obtained from focused operation theatre lights or from the patient’s body itself by taping the Eppendorf tube containing the suspension to the medial wall of the axillary vault for 50 min [28, 29].

20.3.2 Autologous Noncultured Hair Follicle Outer Root Sheath Cell Suspension

This is a relatively simple, minimally invasive, scarless technique to target large areas of depigmentation. However, the limitation is that the extraction of intact hair follicular units requires skill and expertise to avoid the transection of the follicle during extraction [30]. Although repigmentation with this technique is excellent, complications like achromic fissures and incomplete pigmentation can be seen (Fig. 20.7).

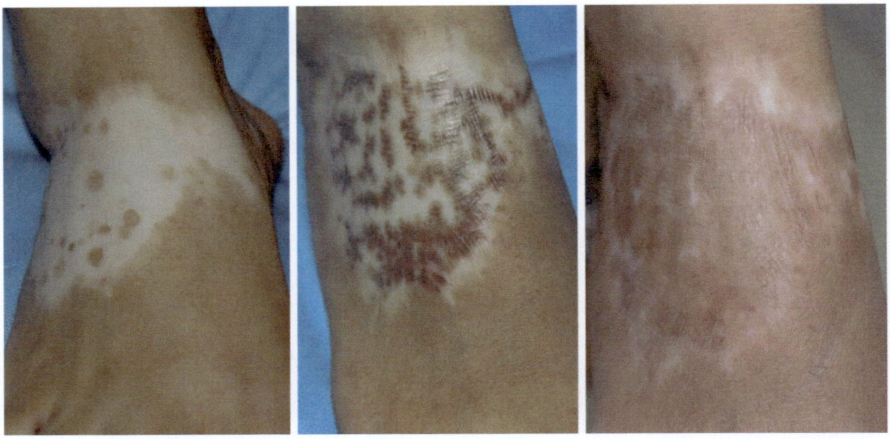

Fig. 20.7 Achromic fissures and marginal halo after hair follicle outer root sheath cell suspension surgery

20.3.3 Autologous Cultured Pure Melanocyte Transplantation

Although this procedure increases the yield of melanocytes by many folds, there are significant safety concerns regarding the use of cultured melanocytes due to the risk of mutagenicity and the development of malignancies. Previously, 12-tetradecanoylphorbol 13-acetate (TPA) was used in the culture medium. It is a tumor promoter; hence, its long-term safety is highly questionable. Nevertheless, the recent availability of TPA-free media is a possible solution to this problem. Beta-fibroblast growth factor (bFGF) has been used as a substitute with satisfactory results [21].

Conclusively, there is a dynamic armamentarium of constantly evolving surgical techniques for the treatment of refractory stable vitiligo. Each procedure has an inherent risk of complications. As mentioned before, although vitiligo surgery is minimally invasive with a smaller learning curve, the overall results depend upon the appropriate choice of procedure, patient selection, skill of the operating surgeon, and availability of necessary equipment, manpower, and aseptic environment.

References

1. Majid I. Grafting in vitiligo: how to get better results and how to avoid complications. J Cutan Aesthet Surg. 2013;6:83–9.
2. Ju HJ, Bae JM, Lee RW, Kim SH, Parsad D, Pourang A, Hamzavi I, Shourick J, Ezzedine K. Surgical interventions for patients with vitiligo: a systematic review and meta-analysis. JAMA Dermatol. 2021;157:307–16.

3. Lahiri K. Evolution and evaluation of autologous mini punch grafting in vitiligo. Indian J Dermatol. 2009;54:159–67.
4. Agarwal US, Jain D, Gulati R, Bhargava P, Mathur NK. Silicone gel sheet dressings for prevention of post-minigraft cobblestoning in vitiligo. Dermatol Surg. 1999;25:102–4.
5. Anbar T, Abd El Raheem T, Bassiouny DA, Fawzy MM, El Maadawi Z, Farouk N, Hassan M. Value of silicone gel in prevention of cobblestoning following punch minigrafting in vitiligo. J Dermatol Treat. 2022;33:306–13.
6. Bhingradia YM, Patel NK. Pinhole technique for cobblestoning in patients post mini-punch grafting for stable vitiligo. Indian J Dermatol Venereol Leprol. 2021;87:861–3.
7. Falabella R. Repeigmentation of stable leucoderma by autologous Minigrafting. J Dermatol Surg Oncol. 1986;12:172–9.
8. Parsad D, Gupta S. Standard guidelines of care for vitiligo surgery. Indian J Dermatol Venereol Leprol. 2008;74:37–45.
9. Falabella R, Arrunategui A, Barona MI, Alzate A. The minigrafting test for vitiligo: detection of stable lesions for melanocyte transplantation. J Am Acad Dermatol. 1995;32:228–32.
10. Linthorst Homan MW, Spuls PI, Nieuweboer-Krobotova L, de Korte J, Sprangers MA, Bos JD, et al. A randomized comparison of excimer laser versus narrow-band ultraviolet B phototherapy after punch grafting in stable vitiligo patients. J Eur Acad Dermatol Venereol. 2012;26:690–5.
11. Chandrashekar B, Madura C, Varsha D. Autologous mini punch grafting: an experience of using motorized power punch in 10 patients. J Cutan Aesthet Surg. 2014;7:42–5.
12. Kim T, Roh HJ, Kim JY, Noh S, Oh SH. Rapid formation of suction blister through intradermal injection of local anesthetics in epidermal graft for vitiligo. Dermatol Surg. 2010;36:1642–3.
13. Gupta S, Kumar B. Suction blister induction time: 15 minutes or 150 minutes? Dermatol Surg. 2000;26:754–6.
14. Anbar TS, El-Fakahany HM, El-Khayyat MA, Abdel-Rahman AT, Saad EK. Factors affecting the outcome of the suction blisters using two different harvesting techniques in vitiligo patients. J Cosmet Dermatol. 2020;19:1723–9.
15. Jain S, Patra S, Choudhary S, Kaur M. An easy way to make blisters in suction blister grafting of vitiligo with Hijama therapy cups. J Am Acad Dermatol. 2022;86:e149–50.
16. Khunger N, Kathuria SD, Ramesh V. Tissue grafts in vitiligo surgery—past, present, and future. Indian J Dermatol. 2009;54:150–8.
17. Batra R, Bhatija SC. Suction blister epidermal grafting: a novel technique for the treatment of stable vitiligo. Curr Med Res Pract. 2012;2:7–11.
18. Laxmisha C, Thappa DM. Reliable site for suction blister induction and harvesting. Indian J Dermatol Venereol Leprol. 2005;71:321–4.
19. Srinivas CR, Rai R, Uday Kumar P. Meshed split skin graft for extensive vitiligo. Indian J Dermatol Venereol Leprol. 2004;70:165–7.
20. McGovern TW, Bolognia J, Leffell DJ. Flip-top pigment transplantation: a novel transplantation procedure for the treatment of depigmentation. Arch Dermatol. 1999;135:1305–7.
21. Mysore V, Salim T. Cellular grafts in management of leucoderma. Indian J Dermatol. 2009;54:142–9.
22. Gupta S, Kumar A, Mahendra A, Gupta S. A minimally invasive, scarless technique of donor tissue harvesting for noncultured epidermal cell suspension transplantation in vitiligo. J Am Acad Dermatol. 2015;73:e213–5.
23. Van Geel N, Goh BK, Wallaeys E, De Keyser S, Lambert J. A review of non-cultured epidermal cellular grafting in vitiligo. J Cutan Aesthet Surg. 2011;4:17–22.
24. Doolan BJ, Weaich M, Mamo J, Gupta M. Autologous non-cultured epidermal cellular grafting in the surgical treatment of stable vitiligo: the skin hospital protocol. Dermatology. 2022;238:167–9.
25. Goh BK, Chua XM, Chong KL, de Mil M, van Geel NA. Simplified cellular grafting for treatment of vitiligo and piebaldism: the "6-well plate" technique. Dermatologic Surg. 2010;36:203–7.

26. Gupta V, Gupta S, Sahni K, Gupta S. Novel methods of preparing epidermal cell suspension for transplantation in vitiligo. In: Gupta S, Olsson MJ, Parsad D, Lim HW, Geel N, Pandya AG, editors. Vitiligo. Chichester: Wiley Blackwell; 2018. https://doi.org/10.1002/9781118937303.ch35.
27. Gupta S, Sahni K, Tembhre MK, Mathur S, Sharma VK. A novel point-of-care in vivo technique for preparation of epidermal cell suspension for transplantation in vitiligo. J Am Acad Dermatol. 2015;72:e65–6.
28. Sahni K, Dev T, Gupta S, Mehta N. Heat from operation theater light as a replacement for incubator in cellular grafting techniques for vitiligo. CosmoDerma. 2023;3:184.
29. Bhatia S, Rajput L, Gupta S. Axillary incubator for cell-based therapies in vitiligo. J Am Acad Dermatol. 2021;85:e279–80.
30. Kumar A, Mohanty S, Sahni K, Kumar R, Gupta S. Extracted hair follicle outer root sheath cell suspension for pigment cell restoration in vitiligo. J Cutan Aesthet Surg. 2013;6:121–5.

Part V
Special Topics

Chapter 21
Depigmentation Therapies in Vitiligo

Aseem Sharma, Neha Akhoon, and Madhulika Mhatre

Abstract Depigmentation therapy is a viable treatment option for patients with extensive vitiligo, particularly those with >50% body surface area involvement, in patients who fail to respond to repigmentation protocols, and those who have obvious cosmetic disfigurement due to patchy pigmentated areas seeking a uniform skin tone. Counseling of the patient holds utmost importance and should include detailed information regarding the permanency of this treatment; its cost, duration, and course; adverse effects; and the possibility of repigmentation. Monobenzyl ether of hydroquinone (MBEH) is the key therapy and the only agent approved by the FDA so far, while many other chemical agents and physical therapies have been explored. Other chemical agents include 4-methoxyphenol, 4-hydroxyanisole, phenol, imatinib, imiquimod, and diphencyprone. Physical therapies comprise cryotherapy and lasers like Q-switched ruby, Q-switched alexandrite, and Q-switched Nd:YAG laser. The efficacy of the combination of these therapies has also been demonstrated in the existing literature. In addition to the clinical efficacy, this chapter delves into the safety profiles of these modalities and also addresses their potential adverse effects. Emerging therapies and novel approaches have also been discussed, offering insights into the future of depigmentation in vitiligo management.

Keywords Depigmentation · Vitiligo · Monobenzyl ether of hydroquinone MBEH · 4-methoyphenol · Laser

---

A. Sharma (✉) · M. Mhatre
Skin Saga Centre for Dermatology, Mumbai, Maharashtra, India

N. Akhoon
Department of Dermatology, Government Medical College, Jammu, Jammu and Kashmir, India

R. Sarkar, V. Narayan R (eds.), *A Concise Guide to The Management of Vitiligo*,
https://doi.org/10.1007/978-981-95-3857-7_21

21.1 Introduction

Vitiligo does not discriminate. It affects people of all ages, races, skin types, and ethnicities. Given its disfiguring aspect, vitiligo can profoundly impact quality of life in children and adults, especially in people of darker racial and ethnic groups, who have a highly visible contrast between the constitutive skin color and vitiliginous patches [1–3]. Although many patients achieve successful repigmentation outcomes, some develop progressive disease affecting an extensive body surface area and fail to respond to repigmentation protocols.

Depigmentation therapy represents a unique and specialized approach to treating vitiligo, particularly for individuals with extensive involvement, thus providing a consistent skin tone and alleviating the psychological and aesthetic burden on patients. Repigmentation with conventional therapies like phototherapy, steroids, and topical immunomodulators occurs in a perifollicular pattern, reflecting melanocyte reservoirs around hair follicles containing immature melanocytes and melanocyte stem cells [4, 5]. In long-standing vitiligo, these melanocyte reservoirs may be exhausted, leading to an irreversible state of depigmentation. Hence, depigmentation therapy in extensive and refractory vitiligo can be an option. Also, in cases where repigmentation treatments cannot restore satisfactory results, depigmentation therapies offer an alternative path to visual consistency and psychological relief. Depigmentation therapies can be broadly studied under chemical and physical modalities of treatment. Various depigmenting therapies like depigmenting creams, lasers, cryotherapy, and systemic drugs have been used. Careful patient selection, education, and counseling are crucial for positive long-term outcomes.

21.2 Candidates for Depigmentation Therapy [6–9]

1. Patients with widespread and extensive vitiligo with a body surface area (BSA) > 50%, who desire permanent matching of skin color, and where the probability of achieving cosmetically significant repigmentation is low
2. Patients with less extensive disease (30–50% BSA) who have progressive disease or who have shown resistance to standard therapies for repigmentation
3. Vitiligo extensively involving cosmetically sensitive areas of the face and hands
4. Vitiligo involving areas known to be resistant to treatment, e.g., hands and malar areas

In addition to the above, the patient needs to be emotionally stable and willing to adhere to photoprotection. It is advised that the possibility of future and more successful therapies be discussed with patients and their families. Given the permanency of depigmentation therapies, patient selection is considered to be of paramount importance.

The broad gambit of depigmentary therapeutic modalities is given in Table 21.1.

Table 21.1 Depigmentation therapies in vitiligo [15]

Chemical modalities	Monobenzyl ether of hydroquinone Monomethyl ether of hydroquinone 88% phenol Imatinib Imiquimod Diphencyprone
Physical modalities	Laser Cryotherapy
Experimental agents	Hydroquinone 4 Ethoxyphenol 4 Methyl catechol Catechol IFN-gamma Busulfan Vaccines using melanoma-associated antigen

21.2.1 Chemical Depigmentation Therapies

1. Monobenzyl Ether of Hydroquinone (MBEH) In the late 1930s, a group of tannery workers began to develop patches of pigment loss in a distribution that corresponded primarily to areas of the skin that were in contact with new rubber gloves. In 1939, Oliver et al. discovered that monobenzone (monobenzone ether of hydroquinone or p-benzyloxyphenol) was present in rubber gloves of leather tannery workers, which was added to reduce the deterioration of rubber and induced progressive skin depigmentation [5].

Depigmentation at sites other than sites of application was earlier blamed on the patients for inadvertently touching those areas while MBEH was still on their hands. Later, reports of Leucomelanoderma began to appear where patients developed disfiguring dyschromatosis with areas of hyper/hypo/depigmentation predominantly at sites of application but also at distant sites [10–12].

This depigmentation was indistinguishable from vitiligo, spreading to nonexposed sites upon prolonged occupational exposure, suggesting a systemic reaction [13].

Mechanism of Action of MBEH [14, 15]

1. Reacts with tyrosinase → forms a reactive quinone product → binds covalently to cysteine residues in tyrosinase proteins through the -SH (sulfhydryl) group → forms carrier-hapten complexes → generation of neoantigen in the tyrosinase peptide chain → excites a systemic, melanocyte destructive inflammatory response.
2. Induction of cellular oxidative stress in exposed pigmented cells by the formation of ROS, e.g., peroxide leads to:
   (a) Lysosomal degradation of melanosomes by autophagy
   (b) Disruption of the melanosome membrane
   (c) Increase melanosomal antigen surface expression by MHC I/II
   (d) Initiation of melanocyte antigen-specific T cell responses

3. Reactive oxygen species lead to the release of tyrosinase- and MART-1-containing exosomes, which contribute to the immune response.
4. Innate immune activation in MBEH-exposed skin, as it acts as a contact sensitizer, inducing a type IV (delayed hypersensitivity) response and the production of proinflammatory cytokines, e.g., IL-1β and IL-18 by Langerhans cells or keratinocytes.

Treatment Procedure [16] An open-use test is first performed on the pigmented skin of the forearm. MBEH is applied topically as a 20% cream. A thin layer of cream should be applied uniformly and rubbed into the pigmented area two to three times daily. Prolonged sunlight exposure should be avoided during treatment, or sunscreen should be used, as exposure to sunlight reduces the depigmenting effect. Depigmentation is usually obtained after 1–4 months of treatment. After 4 months of treatment without success, the drug should be discontinued. When the desired degree of depigmentation is obtained, monobenzone should be applied as often as needed to maintain depigmentation [17]. Lightening of the skin usually occurs gradually over 4–12 months [9]. Histologically, a loss of melanosomes and melanocytes is observed [6]. MBEH can be quite toxic to epidermal melanocytes, but often does not destroy follicular melanocytes [18]. This can be explained by a lack of penetration to the level of hair matrices [18] and the population of melanocytes, which are more vulnerable to vitiligo residing in the epidermis. When vitiligo has been stable for years, a higher concentration of MBEH may be required. Different concentrations of MBEH are required according to the body site involved. For instance, 5% for neck, 10% for face, and 20% for arms and legs. If 20% is insufficient, especially for the arms and legs, we can increase the concentration to 30% or 40%. Similar to HQ, MBEH is redox sensitive; a loss of active ingredient is therefore expected within several weeks of opening the product. The shelf-life of the compounded product is 6 months, and it must be refrigerated [9].

Adverse Effects

1. Contact dermatitis: An irritant reaction is more commonly encountered than allergic contact dermatitis, mainly in pigmented rather than vitiliginous skin. If this happens, MBEH is withheld, topical steroids are applied, and the therapy is reinstated with reconstitution of MBEH at 5%, with a reduced frequency, and mixed with emollients [15]. There have been reports of irritant contact dermatitis developing in the area of contact, especially in darkly pigmented skin. If irritant contact dermatitis develops, control is achieved using topical corticosteroids, and then, gradually, the patient is started with 20% MBEH. If the patient experiences a problem with this concentration, it is decreased to 5%, and then the concentration is gradually increased to 10–15%.
2. Exogenous ochronosis, leucomelanoderma en confetti, the unmasking of telangiectasias and phlebectasias on the lower extremity [9], pruritus, xerosis, erythema, rash, edema, and distant depigmentation [8].

3. MBEH does not affect follicular melanocytes, but its application around the eyes is to be avoided, as conjunctival melanosis and corneal pigmentation deposits in patients have been reported.
4. The risk of carcinogenesis cannot be ruled out; therefore, it has been banned from the European Union since 2001 [7].

Important Considerations Before Starting MBEH Therapy

1. Counseling: Counseling of the patient and the guardians is of utmost importance, especially in younger patients and patients with less extensive involvement, as the nature of depigmentation is usually permanent, and this may prevent the patient from the possibility of exploring more successful therapies for vitiligo, which may be discovered in years to come.
2. Cost: Cost intensiveness has to be explained to the patient. The overall cost depends on the surface area still pigmented and the rate at which the remaining pigment is lost. Several concentrations of MBEH may be required for different parts of the body. Concentrate on cosmetically sensitive areas like the face, neck, and exposed arms to cut costs.
3. Time and course of treatment: Explaining the gradual depigmentation process, i.e., 10–12 months of therapy, may be required.
4. Adverse effects of therapy: Explaining the adverse drug reactions like contact dermatitis to MBEH and the duration of subsequent downtime when the skin is being treated with topical corticosteroids and avoidance of MBEH is required.
5. Potential for repigmentation: The concept of a follicular melanocyte reservoir is essential. Sun exposure can lead to perifollicular pigmentary macules; therefore, it must be limited.
6. Conjugal depigmentation: Avoiding contact of MBEH-applied skin with the skin of others is essential. Family members are strictly advised to follow instructions to prevent permanent depigmentation.
7. Social aspects: More issues with darker skin types (Fitzpatrick IV-V).

The same has been appended as a convenient instruction sheet that can be consumed by patients. (Fig. 21.1)

2. Monomethyl Ether of Hydroquinone (MMEH) Also known as mequinol/p-hydroxyanisole/4-methoxyphenol. Its mechanism of action is similar to MBEH. In a series of 16 patients with extensive vitiligo, depigmentation of the skin was observed in 11 (69%) of those who applied 20% 4-MP twice a day; the onset of depigmentation was noted at 4–12 months [9].

Combination Therapy with All-Trans Retinoic Acid (ATRA) ATRA, in combination with MBEH and Mequinol, has been shown to have a synergistic effect, as it increases the melanocytotoxic effect by inhibition of glutathione-S-transferase in melanocytes. ATRA causes hypopigmentation by decreasing the transport of melanin into keratinocytes while leaving melanocytes intact. In this manner, higher concentrations of MBEH or Mequinol can be avoided. Other less irritant retinoids, like retinaldehyde or retinol, have also been tried [19]. A 2% 4 MP with 0.01% ATRA has produced depigmentation in 7–12 weeks.

Dear Patient,

You have been prescribed topical depigmentation therapy using **Monobenzyl Ether of Hydroquinone (MBEH)** for your extensive vitiligo. Please carefully read and follow these instructions to ensure safe and effective use.

What is MBEH?

MBEH is a cream used to permanently lighten (depigment) the skin by selectively removing pigment-producing cells (melanocytes). It helps in achieving a uniform skin tone in cases of widespread vitiligo.

How to Apply MBEH:

1. **Percentage and Frequency**
    - You will typically be provided with an **MBEH cream of 20% concentration**
    - Start by applying a thin layer **once daily** to small test areas first, gradually increasing to **twice daily** application as directed by your dermatologist.
2. **Gradual Step-Up Approach**
    - **Week 1-2:** Apply a small amount once daily to assess tolerance.
    - **Week 3 onwards:** If no severe irritation, increase gradually to twice daily or as instructed.
    - Always follow your dermatologist's specific guidance for frequency adjustments.

Managing Possible Side Effects:

- **Skin Irritation and Itching:**
  Mild redness, itching, or irritation can occur initially. Usually, these side effects decrease after the first few weeks.
    - If irritation persists, **pause treatment** and contact your dermatologist.
    - You may use fragrance-free moisturizers or soothing creams (as recommended by your dermatologist) to manage mild irritation.
- **Avoid Sensitive Areas:**
    - **DO NOT apply** cream near your eyes, mouth, nostrils, genitals, or other mucosal areas, as these areas are sensitive and can easily get irritated.

Fig. 21.1 Patient instruction sheet

Sun Protection:

- **Sun protection is critical** during and after your depigmentation treatment.
- Use a high-quality, broad-spectrum sunscreen (**SPF 50+**) generously and reapply every 2-3 hours, especially after sweating, swimming, or toweling off.
- Wear protective clothing, hats, and sunglasses when outdoors.

Maintaining Results:

- Depigmentation is typically permanent, but occasionally repigmentation can occur, particularly with sun exposure.
- **Continued diligent sun protection** and occasional maintenance applications may be needed. Your dermatologist will advise you on the maintenance schedule.

Precautions & Contraindications:

- **Pregnancy and Lactation:** MBEH should not be used during pregnancy or breastfeeding.
- **Allergy:** Inform your dermatologist immediately if you experience signs of allergic reaction (severe itching, swelling, blistering).

Psychological Considerations:

- Please understand that depigmentation is permanent and irreversible.
- It's important to discuss any emotional or psychological impact this treatment may have on you with your dermatologist.

Always follow your dermatologist's personalized instructions, and do not hesitate to reach out to your healthcare provider if you have questions or concerns.

Dermatologist's Name:

Date:

Fig. 21.1 (continued)

Procedure A 20% concentration in an oil/water cream base is applied twice daily after the test dose until complete depigmentation.

Adverse Drug Reactions Mild burning/itching, leukoderma, contact dermatitis, ochronosis

MBEH v/s 4 MP: Equally efficacious and less irritation than MBEH but slower onset of action than MBEH. MBEH is the only FDA-approved agent, with results expected with 20% MBEH (61–92% depigmentation) at treated sites after 10 months [20, 21, 22].

3. Phenol Baker-Gordon's phenol formula (40–50% phenol) and 88% phenol have been used. A total of 88% phenol rapidly coagulates in the epidermis, thus stopping its further percutaneous penetration. Since it is more concentrated than Baker-Gordon's formula, which is more dilute, phenol does not coagulate the epidermis. Hence, it shows enhanced penetration and systemic absorption [23].

Mechanism of Action Phenol incapacitates melanocytes from synthesizing melanin normally; hence, the activity of melanocytes is compromised without destroying melanocytes, unlike other depigmenting agents like MBEH and hydroquinone.

Treatment Procedure A swab moistened with phenol is used to treat small areas; on application, frosting occurs, and a burning sensation is felt by the patient for 60 s, which increases in intensity and can last from minutes to hours. The session is repeated after 45 days, with no signs of repigmentation till 1–2 years after therapy [23].

Adverse Drug Reactions If an untrained professional does the procedure, it may lead to dyschromia and nonaesthetic scar formation. Suppose that a large surface area is involved; this modality is not recommended due to its toxic nature as being lipophilic. In that case, it can get systemically absorbed rapidly and may affect the liver, kidney, respiratory, and cardiovascular systems. Cardiovascular shock, cardiac arrhythmias, bradycardia, and metabolic acidosis have been reported within 6 h of skin peeling procedures with phenol. There is a theoretical risk of repigmentation, as with other depigmenting agents. Hence, protection from UV radiation is recommended [23].

4 Imatinib

Imatinib mesylate (IM), a tyrosine kinase inhibitor and standard of care for managing chronic myeloid leukemia, has been tried as a depigmenting agent in vitiligo.

Tsao et al., in a series of six patients, first reported the development of hypopigmentation in patients with CML who were treated with imatinib mesylate, which was reversible and dose-related [24]. The c-Kit receptor and its ligand, stem cell factor (SCF), play a critical role in human melanocyte development, homeostasis and survival, and prolonged kit inhibition leads to melanocyte apoptosis [25]. IM specifically inhibits autophosphorylation of tyrosine kinases, and this decrease in tyrosine kinase has been reported to be an early event in the pathogenesis of vitiligo. This may take 1–6 months to appear, primarily observed in exposed areas [26].

Leong et al. reported gradual skin depigmentation in 13 out of 20 patients with CML receiving IM, and in one patient, hyperpigmentation was reported upon discontinuation of IM and depigmentation upon reintroducing IM [27].

Adverse Drug Reactions Other than the systemic ADRs like nausea, vomiting, anorexia, blurred vision, and myalgia, dermatological ADRs like pruritus, xerosis, alopecia, facial edema, photosensitivity, and hair graying have been noted [28]. The proposed paradoxical stimulation of melanogenesis hyperpigmentation following cKIT inhibition and drug-melanin metabolite accumulation has also been reported [26].

5. Imiquimod

Commercially available as 2.5%, 3.75% and 5% low topical cream, it is US FDA-approved for treating superficial basal cell carcinoma, actinic keratosis, and external genital and perianal warts. Histological examination with MELAN A staining revealed the absence of melanocytes in the areas of application of imiquimod, which is consistent with vitiligo [29].

Mechanism of Action Imiquimod is proposed to cause depigmentation by the following mechanisms:

(i) Direct action on melanocytes à apoptosis due to decreased expression of anti-apoptotic Bcl-2 and increased in proapoptotic factors like cytotoxic T lymphocytes, granzyme B, and natural killer cells.
(ii) Induction of local melanocyte apoptosis [30], which was observed by the TUNEL assay for apoptosis [31].
(iii) Activation of TLR 7 leads to the activation of the Th1 pathway due to the stimulation of specific cytokines, such as IFN-α, IL-12, and IL-18.
(iv) Th1 pathway activation leads to predominantly cytotoxic CD8 + T cell infiltrates, which play a critical role in the onset and progression of vitiligo due to melanocyte destruction [32, 33].
(v) Downregulation of tyrosinase and MITF gene expression (master gene that regulates melanogenesis, melanocyte differentiation, and survival) in melanocytes [34].
(vi) Increases nitric oxide, which leads to the autodestruction of melanocytes [32].
(vii) Increases Langerhans cell activity, which leads to increased melanocyte destruction due to cytotoxic T cell activation [32].

Method of Application About 5% imiquimod application leads to erythema, which gradually turns into depigmentation over 3 months [15]; no repigmentation is seen till 6 months after depigmentation in areas limited to treatment with imiquimod.

Adverse Drug Reactions Burning, itching, pain, erythema, erosion, scabbing, and crusting at the target site.

6 Diphencyprone

Topical immunotherapy has been extensively tested in various dermatological disorders, especially those believed to have an immunologic basis [29, 35]. DPCP is a contact sensitizer that, when used to treat alopecia areata, was found to produce depigmentation over 6 weeks.

In 1990, Duhra and Foulds reported the first case of DPCP-induced depigmentation, in which marked erythema and edema on the forearm appeared after 3 days, which subsided after 2 weeks and was replaced by a depigmented patch 6 weeks later, which remained unchanged 2 years after discontinuing this therapy.

Mechanism of Action This hypo- or depigmentation may result from the Koebner phenomenon or a consequence of the direct cytotoxic effect on melanocytes [36, 37].

Adverse Drug Reactions Eczema with blistering and regional lymphadenopathy may also cause hyperpigmentation.

21.2.2 Physical Therapies

1. Cryotherapy

Physical modalities like cryotherapy have been recommended to achieve rapid results. Radmanesh [38] demonstrated that their use can lead to permanent depigmentation and excellent cosmetic results, but only over limited areas at a time.

A case study by Di Nuzzo et al. showed that a single cryotherapy session with two freeze-thaw cycles followed by twice-daily application of topical 4-hydroxyanisole (4-HA) cream over a 14-month duration achieved complete depigmentation in a patient. Five patients with residual pigmented patches were treated with one to three sessions of cryotherapy using a closed flat contact probe in one case series [38, 39].

Radmanesh demonstrated the effect of cryotherapy using a closed contact CO_2 cryogen in 5 patients with vitiligo universalis who achieved complete and permanent depigmentation with excellent cosmetic results and no complications after being treated with one to three sessions with 4- to 6-week intervals [38].

Mechanism of Action Intracellular ice formation leads to irreversible damage to melanocytes. Within 24 h, inflammation develops, further contributing to the destruction of the lesion through immunologically mediated mechanisms.

Procedure Both CO_2 and liquid nitrogen can be used. Spot testing by a single freeze-thaw cycle is done, and consequently, the patches are treated with cryotherapy 3–6 weeks later [15]. Within a week, a depigmented and unscarred area appears. In cases of partial depigmentation, another session after 4–6 weeks can be administered.

Advantages

1. If chemical agents like MBEH have failed, cryotherapy can be instituted.
2. It is an OPD procedure, which makes it simple, easy,and cost effective.
3. Permanent depigmentation without scarring can be achieved if performed by trained hands.
4. Outcomes are predictable and faster, as compared to treatment with depigmenting agents.

Disadvantage Permanent scarring may occur if treated aggressively.

2. Lasers

Laser therapy can be orchestrated in cases where:

1. Treatment with other depigmentation modalities has failed.
2. Rapid pigmentation is required (for instance, on the face).
3. Disadvantages of topical therapy include local redness, burning, itching, and a long duration of depigmentation.
4. Large areas need to be depigmented in a single setting.

Lasers target melanosomes in residual melanocytes using selective photothermolysis and photoacoustic effects [17, 40, 41]. Individuals who have an active disease at the time of therapy are more likely to have a satisfactory result than those whose disease is quiescent. Rapid depigmentation via irreversible tissue damage can be achieved, particularly in patients sensitive to Koebner's phenomenon, with the advantages of an excellent safety profile.

A wavelength ranging between 532 and 755 nanometers (nm), targeting pigmentation, is used for depigmentation. Q-switched (QS) nanosecond lasers with 532, 694, and 755 nm wavelengths have been used for depigmentation therapy. QS nanosecond lasers emit radiation with high absorption by melanin and a concise pulse duration within the nanosecond range to match the thermal relaxation time of melanosomes. This results in a photomechanical laser tissue interaction, leading to selective melanocyte damage.

Q-switched ruby (755 nm) Q-switched alexandrite laser has a faster pulse frequency than the Q-switched ruby. Hence, it permits more rapid therapy and emits light of greater wavelength, which may provide better tissue penetration. The Nd:YAG laser has also been used at a wavelength of 532 nm to target only epidermal pigmentation and to induce the Koebnerization of vitiliginous lesions.

QS Ruby Laser (QSRL) QSR selectively targets melanocytes and leads to their destruction, causing depigmentation by inducing selective photothermolysis of pigmented lesions because their wavelength is between 600 and 800 nm, which are absorbed by melanin. The energy pulse duration is shorter than melanosomes' thermal relaxation time. Therefore, no energy is transduced into the surrounding tissue [7].

Treatment Procedure With a wavelength of 694 nm, pulse duration of 25–28 ns, frequency of 1–1.2 Hz, and spot size of 5 mm, the laser can administer pulse with energy intensity between 0 and 10 J/cm^2. A eutectic mixture of lidocaine and prilocaine is administered topically for anesthesia. A test spot of 5 cm^2 is treated and evaluated after 8 weeks for clinical depigmentation; if present, total depigmentation is targeted with concurrent laser treatments at 2–4-week intervals. A maximum of 80 cm^2 can be treated in each session. Patients are advised to have sun protection for at least 6 weeks. Tanning of the skin prior to using QSR can induce the activation of melanocytes, which then become the target of selective photothermolysis, leading to permanent damage [15].

Njoo et al. demonstrated the use of a QSR laser for depigmentation in vitiligo. It was also demonstrated that combining hydroquinone and the QS ruby laser results in complete depigmentation in 69% of patients; however, 44% had repigmentation due to 18 months posttreatment [22]. It can also be used in combination with methoxyphenol [42, 43].

Thissen et al. [41] achieved complete depigmentation in eight patients after 1 QSRL session. However, five patients developed follicular repigmentation during the 9-month follow-up. The other three, all with initially positive Koebner phenomenon, remained depigmented in the treated areas. A retrospective study with 27 patients also evaluated the long-term efficacy of the QSRL after complete depigmentation was achieved. While only half of the patients showed > 75% depigmentation after a mean follow-up of 13 months, many patients (85%) were satisfied with the treatment [44].

Depigmentation can be achieved earlier with the help of combination therapy (1–2 weeks) of QSR with depigmenting agents.

QS Alexandrite Laser (QSAL) It has a faster pulse frequency than the Q-switched ruby laser, which permits more rapid therapy and emits light of a greater wavelength (755 nm), which ensures greater tissue penetration and improved results.

QS Neodymium-Doped Yttrium Aluminum Garnet (QS Nd:YAG) Laser
Majid et al. [45] investigated the efficacy of the 532-nm QS Nd:YAG laser in a prospective open-label study. In total, 15 patients with > 80% depigmentation were treated one to three times, of whom 13 achieved ≥ 90% depigmentation, and only one patient reported recurrence at 3 months follow-up. Moreover, an RCT with 40 patients showed better outcomes for the face in patients with active vitiligo for the QS Nd:YAG laser than TCA peeling [46]. Long-term depigmentation after QS Nd:YAG laser was evaluated in a retrospective study with 28 patients. After a follow-up period of 2–5 years, 85% of the patients were delighted, and 89.3% maintained depigmentation of > 90% [45].

Adverse Effects

1. Short-term side effects are common and include purpura, crusts, and oozing of the skin, although no long-term side effects or scarring have been reported.
2. It may be a painful procedure; hence, topical anesthesia is often necessary.
3. The therapy is also time-consuming, limiting the treatment area.
4. Laser therapy may not affect perifollicular melanocytes, leading to repigmentation after a few months.
5. Koebner phenomenon has been considered the basis for laser therapy. Hence, active vitiligo may respond better to laser therapy than those with stable disease, and patients with negative Koebner may relapse [17].

Comparison of Laser Therapy with Other Modalities

Laser therapy and cryotherapy are physical modalities that can be used to achieve faster depigmentation. Various studies have been conducted to compare their efficacy and safety [38]. Cryotherapy can lead to complete depigmentation after three sessions. Despite the inevitable side effects of cryotherapy, like edema, blistering, oozing, prolonged erythema, and longer downtime, no scarring or permanent sequelae have been noted.

Van Geel et al. [47] compared the efficacy of cryotherapy and 755-nm alexandrite laser in 22 patients and found no significant difference in the capacity to induce depigmentation (46.7% vs. 42.9%). However, side effects were predominantly observed with cryotherapy, such as mild burning, pain, and mild hyperpigmentation, especially on the face.

El Mofty et al. [46] conducted a study in which 40 patients were divided equally into facial and extrafacial groups. They compared the efficacy and tolerability of the TCA 25%, 50%, and Q-switched Nd:YAG laser (1064/532 nm) for facial depigmentation and cryotherapy, Phenol 88%, and Q-switched Nd:YAG laser (1064/532 nm) for extrafacial pigmentation. In the facial group, the Q-switched Nd:YAG laser yielded superior results when compared to TCA; at extra facial sites, the Q-switched Nd:YAG, cryotherapy, and phenol were equally effective.

In a retrospective study, six patients with 16 normally pigmented skin areas and a BSA of 5–15% were treated with either a 694 nm QS ruby laser, or 755 nm QS Alexandrite, or 532-nm QS Nd:YAG laser until complete depigmentation with a median of two sessions. Two-thirds of the patients had a relapse after a median follow-up of 36 months [48].

In a nutshell, laser-induced depigmentation therapy has proven to be a safe treatment with high patient satisfaction [41, 45, 47]. High depigmentation rates with QS lasers are best achieved when vitiligo is active in the presence of the Koebner phenomenon. Patients are delighted with the results, and severe side effects are uncommon. Laser treatments can be standardized, yielding highly reproducible effects. Nonetheless, all laser treatments are relatively expensive, only available in some hospitals, not home based, and only suited for small areas. Each type of laser has associated benefits and risks and should therefore be individually chosen based on location, extent, activity, and type of vitiligo.

21.2.3 Experimental Agents

Voluntary depigmentation is a widespread practice in sub-Saharan Africa. Plant extracts of *Brillantaisea cicatricosa* Lindau, *Chenopodium ugande*, *Dolichopentas longiflora*, *Protea madiensis*, and *Sesamum angolense* have been studied briefly, where in vitro experiments indicated the modulation of melanogenesis by these plant extracts [49].

For clarity and an "at-a-glance-therapeutic-wheel," all the modalities discussed above have been converted to a flowchart, which is appended below:

Depigmentation Therapies in Vitiligo: A Flowchart

- Chemical Modalities
  - Monobenzyl Ether of Hydroquinone (MBEH) [FDA Approved]
  - Monomethyl Ether of Hydroquinone (4-Methoxyphenol)
  - Phenol (88%)
  - Imatinib
  - Imiquimod
  - Diphencyprone (DPCP)
- Physical Modalities
  - Cryotherapy (CO_2, Liquid Nitrogen)
  - Laser Therapy

    Q-Switched Ruby (694 nm)
    Q-Switched Alexandrite (755 nm)
    Q-Switched Nd:YAG (532 nm/1064 nm)
- Experimental/Novel Therapies
  - Hydroquinone Derivatives (e.g., 4-Ethoxyphenol, Catechol)
  - Cytokines (e.g., IFN-gamma)
  - Busulfan
  - Melanoma-Associated Antigen Vaccines
  - Plant-Based Extracts (e.g., Brillantaisea, Chenopodium, Dolichopentas)

21.3 Conclusion

Depigmentation therapy offers a valuable therapeutic alternative for patients with extensive or refractory vitiligo, enabling them to achieve uniformity of skin tone and considerable psychological relief. Although MBEH remains the gold standard and FDA-approved treatment, the emergence of alternative chemical agents, physical modalities like lasers and cryotherapy, and experimental treatments continues to broaden the therapeutic horizon. Careful patient selection, meticulous counseling on permanence, side effects, and possible repigmentation are critical for long-term satisfaction. Future research and novel therapies promise to refine these approaches, potentially improving patient outcomes and overall quality of life.

References

1. Grimes PE. Vitiligo: pathogenesis, clinical features, and diagnosis. In: Tsao H, editor. UpToDate; 2016.
2. Kruger C, Schallreuter KU. Stigmatisation, avoidance behaviour and difficulties in coping are common among adult patients with vitiligo. Acta Derm Venerol. 2015;95:553.
3. Grimes PE, Nashawati R. Depigmentation therapies for vitiligo. Dermatol Clin. 2017;35(2):219–27.
4. van den Boorn JG, Melief CJ, Luiten RM. Monobenzone-induced depigmentation: from enzymatic blockade to autoimmunity. Pigment Cell Melanoma Res. 2011;24(4):673–9.
5. Oliver EA, Schwartz L, Warren LH. Occupational leukoderma. JAMA. 1939;113:927–8.
6. Alghamdi KM, Kumar A. Depigmentation therapies for normal skin in vitiligo universalis. J Eur Acad Dermatol Venereol. 2011;25:749–57.
7. Gawkrodger DJ, Ormerod AD, Shaw L, Mauri-Sole I, Whitton ME, Watts MJ, et al. Guideline for the diagnosis and management of vitiligo. Br J Dermatol. 2008;159:1051–76.
8. Drake LA, Dinehart SM, Farmer ER, Goltz RW, Graham GF, Hordinsky MK, et al. Guidelines of care for vitiligo. J Am Acad Dermatol. 1996;35:620–6.
9. Bolognia JL, Lapia BK, Somma S. Depigmentation therapy. Dermatol Ther. 2001;14:29–34.
10. Becker SW Jr, Spencer MC. Evaluation of monobenzone. JAMA. 1962;180:279–84.
11. Canizares O, Jaramillo FU, Kerdel Vegas F. Leukomelanoderma subsequent to the application of monobenzyl ether of hydroquinone. Arch Dermatol. 1958;77:220–3.
12. Dogliotti M, Caro I, Hartdegen RG, Whiting DA. Leuko- melanoderma in blacks. A recent epidemic. S Afr Med J. 1974;48:1555–8.
13. Forman L. A note on the depigmentary properties of mono- benzylether of hydroquinone. Br J Dermatol. 1953;65:406–9.
14. Van doon Boorn JG, Melief CJ, Luiten RM. Monobenzone induced depigmentation: from enzymatic blockade to autoimmunity. Pigment Cell Melanoma Res. 2011;24:673–9.
15. Gupta D, Kumari R, Thappa DM. Depigmentation therapies in vitiligo. Indian J Dermatol Venereol Leprol. 2012;78(1):49.
16. Taieb AV, Alomar A, Böhm M, Dell'Anna ML, De Pase A, Eleftheriadou V, Ezzedine K, Gauthier Y, Gawkrodger DJ, Jouary T, Leone G. Guidelines for the management of vitiligo: the European Dermatology Forum consensus. Br J Dermatol. 2013;168(1):5–19.
17. Rao J, Fitzpatrick RE. Use of the Q-switched 755-nm alexandrite laser to treat recalcitrant pigment after depigmentation therapy for vitiligo. Dermatol Surg. 2004;30:1043–5.
18. Peck SM, Sobotka H. Effect of monobenzyl hydroquinone on oxidase systems in vivo and in vitro. J Invest Dermatol. 1941;4:325–9.
19. Nair X, Parab P, Suhr L, Tramposch KM. Combination of 4-hydroxyanisole and all-trans retinoic acid produces synergistic skin depigmentation in swine. J Invest Dermatol. 1993;101:145–9.
20. Mosher DB, Parrish JA, Fitzpatrick TB. Monobenzylether of hydroquinone. A retrospective study of treatment of 18 vitiligo patients and a review of the literature. Br J Dermatol. 1977;97(6):669–79.
21. Riley PA. Hydroxyanisole depigmentation: in-vivo studies. J Pathol. 1969;97:185–91.
22. Njoo MD, Vodegel RM, Westerhof W. Depigmentation therapy in vitiligo universalis with topical 4-methoxyphenol and the Q-switched ruby laser. J Am Acad Dermatol. 2000;42(5):760–9.
23. Zanini M. Depigmentation therapy for generalized vitiligo with topical 88% phenol solution. An Bras Dermatol. 2005;80:415–6.
24. Tsao AS, Kantarjian H, Cortes J, O'Brien S, Talpaz M. Imatinib mesylate causes hypopigmentation in the skin. Cancer. 2003;98(11):2483–7.
25. Kitamura R, Tsukamoto K, Harada K, Shimizu A, Shimada S, Kobayashi T, Imokawa G. Mechanisms underlying the dysfunction of melanocytes in vitiligo epidermis: role of SCF/KIT protein interactions and the downstream effector, MITF-M. J Pathol. 2004;202(4):463–75.
26. Saraswat N, Neema S, Kumar S. Vitiligo-like lesions following imatinib mesylate therapy: a case series and review of literature. Pigment Int. 2024;11(1):42–5.

27. Leong KW, Lee TC, Goh AS. Imatinib mesylate causes hypopigmentation in the skin. Cancer. 2004;100(11):2486–7.
28. Sharma A, Vora A, Bhutani M. Generalized hypopigmentation due to imatinib: a fairness boon? Indian J Dermatol Venereol Leprol. 2005;71:45–6.
29. Happle R, Hausen BM, Wiesner-Menzel L. Diphencyprone in the treatment of alopecia areata. Acta Derm Venereol (Stockh). 1983;63:49–52.
30. Long FQ, Zhao LS, Qian YH. Vitiligo or vitiligo-like hypopigmentation associated with imiquimod treatment of condyloma acuminatum: not a causal event. Chin Med J (Engl). 2017;130(4):503–4.
31. Kim CH, Ahn JH, Kang SU, Hwang HS, Lee MH, Pyun JH, et al. Imiquimod induces apoptosis of human melanocytes. Arch Dermatol Res. 2010;302:301–6.
32. Sriprakash K, Godbolt A. Vitiligo-like depigmentation induced by imiquimod treatment of superficial basal cell carcinoma. Australas J Dermatol. 2009;50(3):211–3.
33. Ezzedine K, Harris J. Vitiligo. In: Kang S, Amagai M, Bruckner A, Enk A, Margolis D, McMichael A, et al., editors. Fitzpatrick's dermatology, vol. 1. 9th ed. New York: McGraw-Hill Education LLC; 2018. p. 1330–50.
34. Mori S, Akasaka T. Imiquimod-induced vitiligo-like hypopigmentation after treatment for radiation keratosis. Clin Exp Dermatol. 2016;41(8):930–2.
35. MacDonald-Hull S, Norris JF. Diphencyprone in the treatment of longstanding alopecia areata. Br J Dermatol. 1988;119:367–74.
36. Ganzetti G, Simonetti O, Campanati A, Giuliodori K, Offidani A. Phototherapy as a useful therapeutic option in the treatment of diphenylcyclopropenone-induced vitiligo. Acta Derm Venereol. 2010;90(6):642–3.
37. Mario CP. Vitiligo after diphencyprone for alopecia areata. Dermatol Res Pract. 2010;2010:2.
38. Radmanesh M. Depigmentation of the normally pigmented patches in universal vitiligo patients by cryotherapy. J Eur Acad Dermatol Venereol. 2000;14(3):149–52.
39. Hedges TR III, Kenyon KR, Hanninen LA, Mosher DB. Corneal and conjunctival effects of monobenzone in patients with vitiligo. Arch Ophthalmol. 1983;101:64–8.
40. Kim YJ, Chung BS, Choi KC. Depigmentation therapy with Q-switched ruby laser after tanning in vitiligo universalis. Dermatol Surg. 2001;27:969–70.
41. Thissen M, Westerhof W. Laser treatment for further depigmentation in vitiligo. Int J Dermatol. 1997;36:386–8.
42. Nordlund JJ. Depigmentation for the treatment of extensive vitiligo. In: Hann SK, Nordlund JJ, editors. Vitiligo. Oxford: Blackwell Science; 2000. p. 207–13.
43. Solano F, Briganti S, Picardo M, Ghanem G. Hypopigmenting agents: an updated review on biological, chemical and clinical aspects. Pigment Cell Res. 2006;19:550–71.
44. Komen L, Zwertbroek L, Burger SJ, et al. Q-switched laser depigmentation in vitiligo, most effective in active disease. Br J Dermatol. 2013;169:1246–51.
45. Majid I, Imran S. Depigmentation therapy with Q-Switched Nd:YAG laser in universal vitiligo. J Cutan Aesthet Surg. 2013;6:93–6.
46. El-Mofty M, Mostafa WZ, Esmat S, et al. Site-oriented depigmentation in vitiligo patients using Q-switched Nd:YAG laser(1,064/532 nm), cryotherapy and chemical peels: a comparative study. Dermatol Ther. 2019;32:e13052.
47. Van Geel N, Depaepe L, Speeckaert R. Laser(755nm) and cryotherapy as depigmentation treatments for vitiligo: a comparative study. J Eur Acad Dermatol Venereol. 2015;29:1121–7.
48. Boukari F, Lacour JP, Petal OJ. Laser-assisted depigmentation for resistant vitiligo: a retrospective case series with long-term follow-up. J Eur Acad Dermatol Venereol. 2014;28:374–7.
49. Mapunya MB, Nikolova RV, Lall N. Melanogenesis and antityrosinase activity of selected South African plants. Evid Based Complement Alternat Med. 2012;2012:374017.

Chapter 22
Camouflage in Vitiligo

Astha Arora and Mala Bhalla

Abstract Vitiligo, which is characterized by complete loss of pigment, results in visible disfigurement. The treatment for vitiligo is difficult, may result in partial pigmentation, and usually takes time to show results. The use of corrective makeup or camouflage to cover lesions till they show a clinical response has been shown to improve patients' quality of life. Camouflage is described as a system of techniques to conceal, diminish, and disguise visible disfigurements of skin using various methods and revolves around concepts of concealing, color correction, and contour correction. It may be temporary or permanent, determined by its duration of stay on the skin. Temporary techniques include indigenous clay or henna mixes, liquid dyes, spray tan, and foundation-based camouflage formulations. Permanent camouflage is achieved by the deposition of pigment in the skin, which is achieved either by micropigmentation or decorative tattooing. The evidence in the literature gives an insight into the positive effects of camouflage when offered to patients with vitiligo. It encourages us to provide supportive clinical care to patients beyond standard treatment protocols and explore the field of camouflage therapy in vitiligo while waiting for curative remedies to bring about repigmentation.

Keywords Cosmetic camouflage · Vitiligo · Cover-up makeup
Micropigmentation · Camouflage · Quality of life

Vitiligo, which is characterized by complete loss of pigment, results in visible disfigurement and is of great cosmetic concern, especially in Indian skin tone. The stigma associated with vitiligo often has a devastating effect on patients, resulting in hampered personal and social relationships and decreased quality of life (QOL)

A. Arora
Department of Dermatology, Sohana Hospital, Sector 77, Mohali, Punjab, India

M. Bhalla (✉)
Department of Dermatology & Venereology, Government Medical College & Hospital, Chandigarh, India

R. Sarkar, V. Narayan R (eds.), *A Concise Guide to The Management of Vitiligo*,
https://doi.org/10.1007/978-981-95-3857-7_22

[1, 2]. The treatment for vitiligo is difficult, may result in partial pigmentation, and usually takes time to show results. Patients invariably try to hide patches of vitiligo by clothing like wearing full sleeve shirts and gloves or even by modifying their hairstyles. The use of corrective makeup or camouflage to cover lesions that cannot be covered, especially over the face and hands, till they show a clinical response has been shown to improve patients' QOL.

22.1 Introduction and Brief History

Camouflage may simply be described as a system of techniques to conceal, diminish, and disguise visible disfigurements of skin, mainly over visible areas using various methods. The main purpose of this supportive modality is to help cope with psychological effects, as it helps normalize appearance and increases social acceptability. It was first introduced during World War II to help with the rehabilitation of burn victims. It was further integrated with medical management by Joyce Allsworth in the 1950s, who formed the British Association of Skin Camouflage [3–6].

Cosmetic camouflage revolves around concepts of concealing, color correction, and contour correction. Stated simply, concealing is covering the lesion with a product that matches the skin color and can be used for low-contrast skin discoloration. In lesions where high contrast is present between the lesion and normal skin or the hue of the lesion is different, then color correction needs to be done prior to the application of skin-matched color to provide good camouflage. It follows the principle of color theory, wherein colors falling on opposite sides of a complementary color wheel neutralize each other (Fig. 22.1). For example, red-colored lesions like

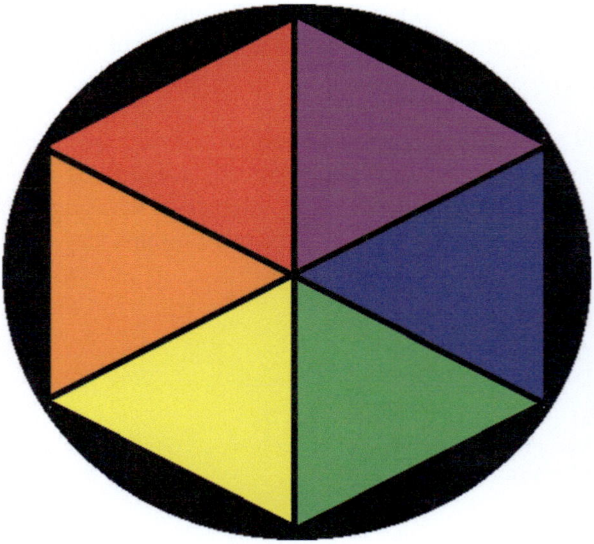

Fig. 22.1 Pictorial representation of a color wheel

vascular malformations and acne need color correction with a green color, and blue to purplish pigmented lesions need to be corrected using the color yellow-orange. Contour correction is needed for lesions that have a rough or uneven surface and works on the principle of creating an optical illusion. Deeper areas are covered with a lighter color, and the raised parts with a darker color. This creates the illusion of being above and deeper from the surface, thereby making the lesion, usually a scar, look flatter and uniform. When used correctly for patients with the right technique, camouflage can greatly modify the visual deformity, making it almost imperceptible [7].

22.2 Camouflage in Vitiligo

22.2.1 Rationale of Use in Vitiligo

Vitiligo causes significant deformity in the skin of color, as the color discrepancy is more evident, thereby proving to be an ideal dermatosis for camouflage therapy, as the skin texture is maintained and only the skin color needs to be corrected by a carefully matched skin shade. In addition, in vitiligo, there are no underlying hues that need to be neutralized, and in low-contrast lesion, color-matched camouflage product is adequate. Only in high-contrast lesions, black or dark brown color is needed to balance the whiteness of the vitiligo patch.

22.3 Types and Products Available

The camouflage may be temporary or permanent, defined by the duration of its stay on the skin.

22.3.1 Temporary

These techniques provide temporary, short-term cover of the lesions and can be removed.

Indigenous Methods Clay mixture with henna and oils and iron fillings have been used in the past in our culture to hide lesions, but attaining a good color match is difficult.

Liquid Ddyes Dyes made from indigo carmine, Bismarck brown, henna paste, and potassium permanganate may be used, but they easily get washed away, and achieving color match is difficult [8, 9].

Fig. 22.2 Dermacolor camouflage crème color palette for demonstration in patients

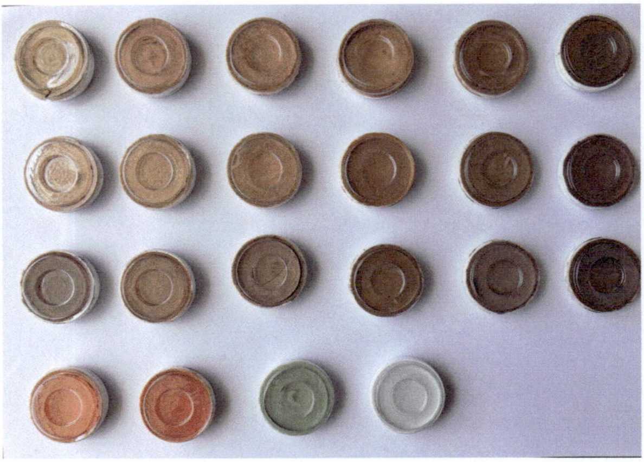

Spray Tan/Dihydroxyacetone (DHA)-Based Camouflage DHA is an ingredient of self-tanning preparations that, through the oxidation of tryptophan and histidine in the stratum corneum, causes staining of skin brown. It usually lasts for several days and is not washed or rubbed off easily, and a darker color can be achieved by increasing the number of applications. It can be used in both spray and cream formulations. Various reports in the literature have shown its successful use in patients with vitiligo [10–13].

Foundation-Based Preparations A wide variety of options are available which can be used as camouflage cosmetics. The features common to all are that they should be opaque, waterproof, provide a good color match, be easy to apply, and have good adherence to the skin, allowing long wear. The formulations of the camouflage cosmetics include creams, creamy and alcohol-based liquids, sticks, and roll-ons. They usually have a higher pigment content (25% more) and fillers with optical properties, thereby making them more opaque and more efficacious than commonly used makeup. Various companies provide commercially available camouflage cosmetics in multiple colors, common ones being Dermacolor, Microskin, Zanderm wide and precision applicators, Veil Cover Cream, and Dermablend Cover Creme Foundation (Fig. 22.2) [14, 15].

22.3.2 Cosmetic Camouflage Therapy

22.3.2.1 Products

A wide array of products is marketed for camouflage, but an ideal product should have these characteristics [15, 16]:

- Color: It should be available in multiple shades with varying hue, intensity, and value so that it matches the skin of the patient perfectly.

- Opaque: Though camouflage products have fillers and a larger quantity of pigment, they should have the opacity to hide the blemish to give a normal appearance.
- Sun protecting ability: Usually, camouflage products provide some sun protection due to their opacity and pigments like iron oxide and titanium dioxide.
- Waterproof and sweat resistant: The product should not be easily washed off by water and should not move due to sweating.
- Long wear: The product should have good holding power so that it adheres to the skin for a long duration, ideally for a full day without smudging or fading, and should feel comfortable on the skin.
- Inert: The pigments and other adjuvants of the camouflage product should not have allergenic potential, nor should they cause photosensitivity or cause/worsen acne.
- Easy application and removal: Camouflage product should go on the skin easily without needing any special tools or technique and, similarly, should be easy to remove at the end of the day without the need for specialty removers.
- Cost effectiveness and easy availability: These form an important factor in influencing the regular use of cosmetic camouflage products.

Formulations The camouflage products are available as creams, creamy and alcohol-based liquids, sticks, and roll-ons.

Composition The foundations are emulsions of either oil or water in which pigments, fillers, preservatives, stabilizers, etc., are suspended. They can be of four types, as shown in Table 22.1 [15, 16].

Table 22.1 Various compositions of camouflage foundations

Formulation	Type of emulsion	Suspending medium	Skin type/ indication
Oil-based foundations	Water-in-oil emulsions	Mineral oil or lanolin alcohol—pigments suspended in oil	For dry skin as it leaves a moist feeling
Water-based facial foundations	Oil-in-water emulsions	Water—small amount of pigment	Minimally dry to normal skin
Oil-free facial foundations	Dimethicone, cyclomethicone, or silicon-in--water emulsion	Water	Oily skinned individuals
Water-free or anhydrous	Oil phase: high concentration of pigment suspended	Vegetable oil, mineral oil, lanoline, alcohol, synthetic esters, or waxes	Ideal facial camouflaging product Waterproof

22.3.2.2 Patient Selection and Counselling

Patients with lesions in visible areas are ideal candidates for cosmetic camouflage therapy. Before prescribing the same, the patient should be assessed about their knowledge of camouflage, their willingness to use it, and provided with a demonstration before they make a decision. It should be emphasized that camouflage therapy is just a supportive treatment and a means to hide the apparent deformity and not a therapeutic modality. The patient's ability to understand and execute the instructions of the application also needs to be assessed so that the patient can get the maximal benefit from camouflage. Additionally, the patient also needs to be informed about the cost of camouflage products like Dermacolor (cost varies from 550 to 2200 INR), which can be bought online from various websites and through select representatives.

22.3.2.3 Technique

Cosmetic camouflage therapy should be properly demonstrated and taught in a stepwise manner to the patient so that the patient can reap the full benefit of camouflage (Fig. 22.3a–d) [4, 17, 18]:

- The area where camouflage is to be used should be cleaned with soap and water, adequately moisturized, and free from any erosions, active infection, or dermatitis.
- A small amount of product is taken, warmed over the back of the hand, and should be applied on the lesion in a tapping or dabbing motion. Rubbing should be avoided. Patients can use sponges or finger tips for applying the camouflage while taking care to merge it with the surrounding normal skin.
- In a few patients, where high contrast exists between the vitiligo patch and surrounding normal skin, color-matched camouflage cream may not be adequate to provide complete coverage, and color correction may be needed. Color correction in vitiligo patches is done with dark brown to black color camouflage cream, which is then layered with skin-matched shade.
- The final step is the application of a fixing spray or powder. This is a translucent powder which sets the product, makes it waterproof and smudges proof, and gives a matte and natural look. Apply a generous amount of powder on the area, let it sit for 5–10 min, and then dust off the excess.
- The correct removal of camouflage is as important as a flawless application. Water-soluble cream-based remover, oil-based melting balms, and biphasic removers are all suitable. They should be applied generously; the foundation should be emulsified and then wiped off with a cotton pad or rinsed with warm

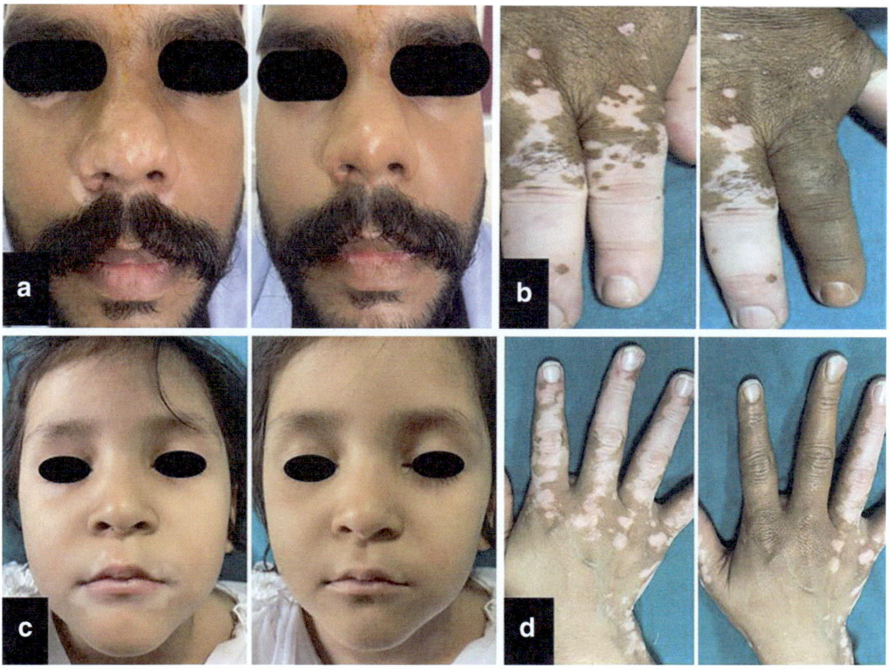

Fig. 22.3 (**a–d**) Demonstration of camouflage in a patient with vitiligo

water. This should be followed by washing with gentle soap or a cleanser and moisturization.

22.3.2.4 Practical Tips and Tricks

- Advise the patient to apply the topicals being used for treatment before the application of the camouflage foundation. Sun protection can be supplemented by layering the camouflage cream with sunscreen.
- All closest possible shades should be tried directly on the patient's skin, as it may look different on the skin than in the container.
- The demonstration should be done in a well-lit room with natural light, as artificial lights can alter color perception.
- Cream formulations are preferred for small and cosmetically important areas, and lotion formulations for larger surface areas like limbs.
- Airbrush may be used as it results in a thinner and more uniform distribution of the product over the skin.

- Patients may apply a thin layer of skin-matched camouflage cream or a layer of their regular makeup foundation over the whole area, including the normal skin, to give a more seamless and uniform appearance.
- Barrier film sprays, commonly used at stoma sites, may be used as a sealant to prevent smudging of camouflage, especially over the lips and fingertips, as has been demonstrated by Tanioka et al. [19]
- Black mascara may be advised for the camouflage of leukotrichia, especially of eyebrows, eyelashes, and along the frontal hair line.
- Lip colors are an ideal camouflaging product for lips. They may be matched with the color of the lips in males, and in females, the choice of color may be influenced by attire, mood, or personal choice.

22.3.3 *Permanent*

Permanent camouflage is achieved by the deposition of color-matched pigment in the skin, which is achieved by tattooing, also called micropigmentation. Alternatively, the patch of vitiligo may be covered with a decorative tattoo. Permanent camouflage is ideal for patients with localized, stable vitiligo patches which are not responding to treatment.

Decorative Tattooing Patches of vitiligo can also be camouflaged by elaborate decorative tattoos using various colors, patterns, and designs; fashioned and placed to cover or obscure the underlying patch. Tattoos, though fascinating, are only suitable for certain areas and may not be acceptable over areas like the face. Also, the underlying depigmentation may not be covered entirely.

Micropigmentation The procedure of micropigmentation involves using minute, inert, nontoxic, nonallergenic pigments in creamy paste form composed mainly of iron oxide to camouflage lesions of vitiligo (Table 22.2). It can be used ideally for

Table 22.2 Pigments used for micropigmentation

Color	Pigment used
Black	Iron oxide
Brown	Iron oxide
Yellow	Cadmium sulfate
Camel yellow	Iron oxide
Red	Cinnabar, mercuric sulfate
White	Titanium dioxide

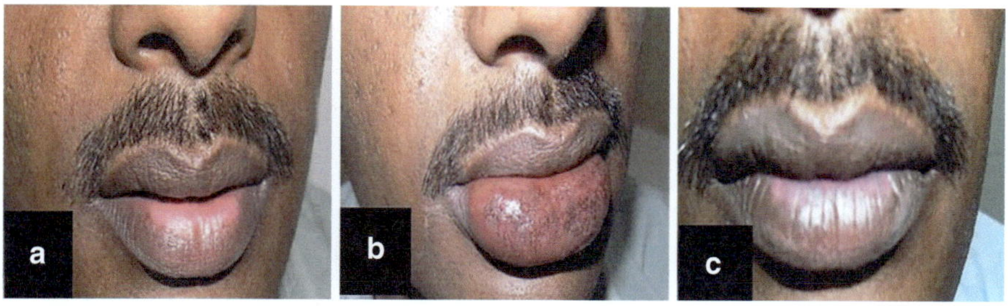

Fig. 22.4 (**a**–**c**) Preprocedure, immediately after, and postprocedure images of a patient with lip tattooing

distal digits, lips, genital mucosa, areolae, and mucocutaneous junctions, as these areas are difficult to treat and also show resistance to treatment (Fig. 22.4a–c). Sterile pigments are deposited in the upper and mid-papillary dermis using either manual tattoo needles or a mechanized tattoo gun uniformly in circular motion, preferably in a single sitting.

The procedure is followed by crust and scab formation, which falls off in 7–10 days. Touch-up session for skip areas or inadequate pigment deposition is analyzed at 4 weeks, and corrective micropigmentation is done accordingly. The procedure of micropigmentation holds several advantages: simple office procedure, rapid instant results, relatively inexpensive, and can be used in areas where vitiligo surgeries are difficult. Despite these advantages, the procedure faces various challenges, such as getting a perfect color match is difficult, color tends to fade over time, deeper pigment deposition can result in the Tyndall effect, and rarely few patients may develop contact allergy to pigment. Being an invasive procedure, the risk of infection is always present and can be prevented by adequate systemic and topical antibiotic cover postprocedure [20–29].

22.4 Benefits and Limitations

Vitiligo patients may not suffer physically distressing symptoms but face social stigma and suffer emotionally and psychologically, which affects their personal and professional lives. Thus, camouflage provides an instantaneous result by safeguarding patients from prying eyes.

Despite the ample evidence in the literature of the efficacy of camouflage in improving DLQI, the widespread use is riddled with limitations. The biggest drawback is that camouflage does not have a therapeutic role, and this raises a question in the mind of patients about the treatability of their disease. The product may smudge or wear off with sweating and over friction-prone areas.

22.5 Patient Knowledge and Acceptance

In order to help patients learn the subtleties of camouflage makeup, the British Red Cross Society provides education services in the United Kingdom in Skin Camouflage clinics free of cost. "*Changing Faces*" is a charity organization which provides patients with medical makeup free of charge and provides training with trained practitioners of camouflage. In the United States, state-licensed medically trained therapists are available, who not only have the knowledge to demonstrate but also educate patients on how to use makeup correctly [30, 31].

The authors performed a questionnaire-based study on 25 patients attending the dermatology clinic eligible for cosmetic camouflage about their existing knowledge and willingness to try camouflage. Those willing were provided with a demonstration of the technique, and a correct color match for their skin was provided. Patients were further interviewed about their satisfaction with the results and if they were willing to use them regularly. Of the 25 patients recruited, 16 patients had vitiligo. Only four patients with vitiligo had previous knowledge of camouflage, and of these two patients used it regularly. However, after demonstration of camouflage, patients showed satisfaction with the results but had hesitancy toward its use due to various reasons, like cost, lack of easy availability, and distortion of self-image, and showed preference toward curative modalities.

22.6 Evidence-Based Exploration of QOL Effect of Camouflage in Vitiligo

The QOL of an individual is a major determinant of mental and social health, with ill health usually resulting in deterioration of the same. Vitiligo results in a decline in QOL and has been well substantiated in the literature. Various studies have proven that the use of camouflage improves QOL. Ongenae et al. in 2005 performed an open-label study in 62 patients with vitiligo who were advised to use cosmetic camouflage for 1 month, and the Dermatology Life Quality Index (DLQI) and adapted stigmatization questionnaire were used, both showing improvement. In a prospective control group study, Tanioka et al. (2010) enrolled 32 patients, 21 of whom were given camouflage lessons and were advised to apply camouflage for 4 weeks. The DLQI showed improvement in the intervention group with maximum improvement in the symptoms and feelings item. In 2020, Bassioumy et al. recruited 100 patients with vitiligo in a prospective randomized study conducted over 4 weeks, and DLQI improvement was observed in the camouflage group ($p < 0.05$). Morales et al. in 2022 performed an uncontrolled quasiexperimental study in 45 patients with vitiligo over 16 weeks and used various parameters for QOL improvement assessment, including the DLQI, EuroQol-5 Dimension questionnaire, Short Form Health Survey, and Vitiligo Quality-of-Life Index, and all showed improvement. Some authors believe that camouflage therapy may hamper the treatment of vitiligo, but Li et al. in 2020 demonstrated that there was no difference in repigmentation and transepidermal water loss in patients using dihydroxyacetone (DHA)-containing camouflage as compared to controls [32–37].

This mounting evidence in the literature gives us an insight into the positive effects of camouflage/cover-up makeup when offered to patients with vitiligo. It encourages us to provide supportive clinical care for patients beyond standard treatment protocols and explore the field of camouflage therapy in vitiligo.

22.7 Conclusion

Camouflage seems to have the ability to provide some relief to vitiligo patients with patches in areas that are resistant to treatment or when the lag between the onset of treatment and adequate clinical response is long. Despite evidence in the literature of the efficacy of camouflage in improving QOL, there is still hesitancy in the acceptance of its use as part of mainstream vitiligo management by dermatologists and patients alike. It is time that a change is set afoot in our approach toward managing vitiligo by educating patients and providing supportive therapy like camouflage while waiting for curative remedies to bring about repigmentation.

References

1. Talsania N, Lamb B, Bewley A. Vitiligo is more than skin deep: a survey of members of the vitiligo society. Clin Exp Dermatol. 2010;35:736–9.
2. Kent G, Al'Abadie M. Psychologic effects of vitiligo: a critical incident analysis. J Am Acad Dermatol. 1996;35:895–8.
3. Rayner VL. Camouflage therapy. Dermatol Clin. 1995;13:467–72.
4. Westmore MG. Make-up as an adjunct and aid to the practice of dermatology. Dermatol Clin. 1991;9:81–8.
5. Allsworth J. Skin camouflage-a guides to remedial techniques: cover creams. Cheltenham: Stanley Thornes Ppublishers; 1985. p. 18–33.
6. History of Skin Camouflage—the British Association of Skin Camouflage. n.d. https://skin-camouflage.net/scwp/index.php/history-of-skin-camouflage/?cn-reloaded=1
7. Sandhu JK, Sharma P. Skin camouflage therapy. Indian J Dermatol Venereol Leprol. 2022;88:717–23.
8. Sarveswari KN. Cosmetic camouflage in vitiligo. Indian J Dermatol. 2010;55:211–4.
9. Sugathan P, Nejeeba R. A new camouflage for vitiligo. Indian J Dermatol Venerol Leprol. 1991;57:45–6.
10. Hsu S. Camouflaging vitiligo with dihydroxyacetone. Dermatol Online J. 2008;14:23.
11. Suga Y, Ikejima A, Matsuba S, Ogawa H. Medical pearl: DHA application for camouflaging segmental vitiligo and piebald lesions. J Am Acad Dermatol. 2002;47:436–8.
12. Rajatanavin N, Suwanachote S, Kulkollakarn S. Dihydroxyacetone: a safe camouflaging option in vitiligo. Int J Dermatol. 2008;47:402–6.
13. Steuer AB, Zampella JG. Camouflaging vitiligo using a spray tan. Dermatol Online J. 2020;26:13030/qt63j996qx.
14. Westmore MG. Camouflage and make-up preparations. Dermatol Clin. 2001;19:406–12.

15. Draelos ZD. Colored facial cosmetics. Dermatol Clin. 2000;18:621–31.
16. Antoniou C, Stefanaki C. Cosmetic camouflage. J Cosmet Dermatol. 2006;5:297–301.
17. Bouloc A. Camouflage techniques. In: Draelos ZD, editor. Cosmetic dermatology: products and procedures. 2nd ed. Oxford: Wiley-Blackwell; 2016. p. 186–92.
18. Draelos ZD. Cosmetic camouflaging techniques. Cutis. 1993;52:362–4.
19. Tanioka M, Miyachi Y. Waterproof camouflage age for vitiligo of the face using Cavilon 3M as a spray. Eur J Dermatol. 2008;18:93–4.
20. Vassileva S, Hristakieva E. Medical applications of tattooing. Clin Dermatol. 2007;25:367–74.
21. Mazza JF Jr, Rager C. Advances in cosmetic micropigmentation. Plast Reconstr Surg. 1993;92:750–1.
22. Halder RM, Pham HN, Breadon JY, Johnson BA. Micropigmentation for treatment of vitiligo. J Dermatol Surg Oncol. 1989;15:1092–8.
23. Wolfley DE, Flynn KJ, Cartwright J, Tschen A. Eyelid pigment implantation: early and late histopathology. Plast Reconstr Surg. 1988;82:770–4.
24. Garg G, Thami GP. Micropigmentation: tattooing for medical purposes. Dermatol Surg. 2005;31:928–31.
25. Singal A, Thami GP, Bhalla M. Watchmaker's pin-vise for manual tattooing of vitiligo. Dermatol Surg. 2004;30:203–4.
26. Savant SS. Tattooing. In: Savant SS, editor. Textbook of dermatosurgery and cosmetology. 2nd ed. Mumbai: ASCAD; 2005. p. 337–44.
27. Epstein E. Therapeutic tattooing. In: Epstein E, editor. Skin surgery. 2nd ed. Philadelphia: Lea and Febiger; 1962. p. 308–15.
28. Tazelaar DJ. Hypersensitivity to chromium in a light-blue tattoo. Dermatologica. 1970;141:282–7.
29. Kerure AS, Marwah M, Wagh ND, Udare S. Micropigmentation. Indian Dermatol Online J. 2023;14:605–10.
30. Ekwegh U. The contribution of skin camouflage volunteers in the management of vitiligo. Case Rep. 2011;2011:bcr0920114783.
31. Skin Camouflage Services For Disfigurement | Changing Faces. Changing Faces. n.d. https://www.changingfaces.org.uk/services-support/skin-camouflage-service/
32. Amer AA, Gao XH. Quality of life in patients with vitiligo: an analysis of the dermatology life quality index outcome over the past two decades. Int J Dermatol. 2016;55:608–14.
33. Ongenae K, Dierckxsens L, Brochez L, Van Geel N, Naeyaert JM. Quality of life and stigmatization profile in a cohort of vitiligo patients and effect of the use of camouflage. Dermatology. 2005;210:279–85.
34. Tanioka M, Yosuke Y, Mayumi K, Yoshiki M. Camouflage for patients with vitiligo vulgaris improved their quality of life. J Cosmet Dermatol. 2010;9:72–5.
35. Bassiouny D, Hegazy R, Esmat S, Gawdat HI, Ahmed Ezzat M, Tawfik HA, et al. Cosmetic camouflage as an adjuvant to vitiligo therapies: effect on quality of life. J Cosmet Dermatol. 2020;00:1–7.
36. Morales-Sánchez MA, Laguna-Meraz JP, Peralta-Pedrero ML, Jurado-Santa CF. Effect of cosmetic camouflage in adults with vitiligo. Actas Dermosifiliogr. 2022;113:316–8.
37. Li M, Wang F, Ding X, Xu Q, Du J. Evaluation of the potential interference of camouflage on the treatment of vitiligo: an observer-blinded self-controlled study. Dermatol Ther. 2021;34(1):e14545.

Chapter 23
Childhood Vitiligo and Late-Onset Vitiligo

Rashmi Sarkar and Damini Verma

Abstract Vitiligo is a chronic, acquired cutaneous disorder characterized by the loss of melanocytes, leading to depigmented skin and hair. It affects 0.1–2% of the population worldwide, without gender or racial predisposition. Childhood vitiligo, typically presenting before the age of 12 years, tends to be more progressive, with generalized and segmented subtypes being common. Childhood vitiligo is often associated with atopy and a positive family history. In contrast, late-onset vitiligo, which occurs after the age of 40 years, progresses more slowly and is more likely to be associated with autoimmune disorders. Treatment strategies differ by age, with early intervention crucial in children to prevent psychological distress, while adults also require the management of associated autoimmune disorders. This chapter discusses the epidemiology, clinical features, and management strategies for both childhood and late-onset vitiligo.

Keywords Childhood vitiligo · Late-onset vitiligo · Autoimmune disorders

23.1 Introduction

Vitiligo is an acquired, chronic skin disorder characterized by the loss of pigmentation due to the destruction of melanocytes of the skin and hair. Its prevalence ranges from 0.1% to 2% of the population worldwide, without any sexual, regional, or racial predominance [1]. This condition can manifest at any age but is generally categorized into early and late onset based on the age of onset. Early-onset vitiligo typically occurs in children and young adults, while late-onset vitiligo is diagnosed in older adults. Understanding the differences between these two forms of vitiligo is crucial for appropriate clinical management and treatment strategies (Table 23.1).

R. Sarkar (✉) · D. Verma
Department of Dermatology, Lady Hardinge Medical College and Hospitals, New Delhi, Delhi, India

R. Sarkar, V. Narayan R (eds.), *A Concise Guide to The Management of Vitiligo*,
https://doi.org/10.1007/978-981-95-3857-7_23

Table 23.1 Key differences between early- and late-onset vitiligo

Characteristic	Early-onset vitiligo	Late-onset vitiligo
Age of onset	Typically before 12 years of age	After 50 years of age
Clinical presentation	Often generalized or segmental; rapid progression	Usually focal or generalized; rarely segmental; slower progression
Commonly affected areas	Face, especially around eyes and mouth; trunk and extremities	Face and extremities
Prevalence of leukotrichia	High	Lower than in early onset
Koebner phenomenon	Frequently observed	Less common
Associated autoimmune diseases	Lower association	Strongly associated with thyroid disease, diabetes mellitus
Association with atopy	Higher association	Lower as compared to early-onset vitiligo
Psychosocial impact	Significant, especially in children due to cosmetic concerns	Variable, depending on extent and location of lesions
Response to treatment	Generally responds well to early, aggressive treatment	Slower response; combination therapy often required Phototherapy is a good option
Audiological abnormalities	Rarely studied; not a common feature	No significant association; hypoacusis can occur
Surgical interventions	Less commonly needed; focus on early medical therapy	Considered for stable, unresponsive lesions
Progression and stability	More aggressive with potential for widespread involvement	Often stable with localized depigmentation

23.2 Childhood Vitiligo

23.2.1 Epidemiology

Childhood vitiligo accounts for a significant proportion of cases, with onset typically occurring before the age of 12. Around 50% of patients usually present with symptoms before the age of 20 years [2]. The mean age of disease onset ranges from 5 to 9.1 years, as reported by most Indian studies [3].

23.2.2 Pathogenesis

The pathogenesis of childhood vitiligo is believed to involve a combination of genetic predisposition, environmental triggers, and immune system dysfunction. Genetic susceptibility in vitiligo is evidenced by frequent clustering in families and occurrence in monozygotic twins. Various susceptibility loci for vitiligo are AIS1 (chromosome 1), AIS2 (chromosome 7), AIS3 (chromosome 8), and SLEV1 (chromosome 17) [4]. The immune system in children is still developing, and dysregulation can lead to the autoimmune destruction of melanocytes. Several other hypotheses exist regarding the pathogenesis of NSV, including autoimmune mechanisms, melanocyte destruction due to cellular immunity abnormalities, the autocytotoxic hypothesis, the inhibition of melanogenesis, and altered vitamin D3 metabolism [5].

23.2.3 *Clinical Characteristics*

Childhood vitiligo is generally defined as vitiligo that begins before the age of 12. Studies have shown that the clinical presentation in childhood differs significantly from that in adults. Early-onset vitiligo is associated with a more extensive, progressive course and a higher likelihood of affecting multiple body areas [6]. Generalized and segmental vitiligo are usually found to be the most common type, followed by acrofacial types, with a very small percentage of focal vitiligo [7, 8]. The oral mucosa is considered to be less affected. The majority of patients who present with early-onset vitiligo are females [9].

Children with early-onset vitiligo often present with lesions on the head and neck area, especially around the eyes and mouth (Figs. 23.1a, b). The trunk and extremities are also commonly affected [9]. Leukotrichia has been frequently reported in childhood vitiligo, with incidence varying from 4.4% to 41.8% [10]. The Koebner phenomenon is reported more frequently in early-onset disease, is more common in nonsegmental vitiligo (NSV) than in segmental vitiligo (SV), and is associated mostly with unstable disease [4].

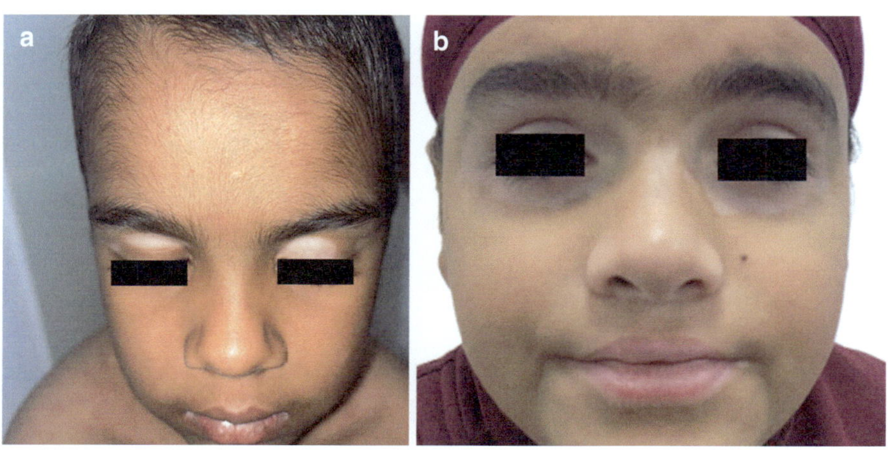

Fig. 23.1 (**a**) Periorbital pigmentation in a 5-year-old boy. (**b**) A 10-year-old boy presenting with depigmented macules present around the eyes and lips

23.2.4 Associations

Children with early-onset vitiligo have a greater association with atopy and allergic disorders. They are more associated with positive family history as compared with those with late-onset vitiligo. They may have a lower incidence of autoimmune disorders compared to their adult counterparts [9]. They are associated with anemia and premature canities [11].

23.2.5 Management

The treatment of vitiligo has primarily two main objectives: halting the progression of the disease and inducing the repigmentation of affected areas to restore a cosmetically pleasing result. The selection of the most appropriate treatment for childhood vitiligo depends on various factors, including the child's age, psychological well-being and expectations, the extent and distribution of skin lesions, whether the vitiligo is stable or progressive, and the availability and cost of treatment options. It involves a combination of topical therapies such as topical corticosteroids and calcineurin inhibitors, phototherapy, and, in some cases, systemic treatments. Early and aggressive treatment is often recommended to prevent the psychological impact of the disease on children [12].

23.3 Late-Onset Vitiligo

23.3.1 Epidemiology

Late-onset vitiligo is less common than childhood vitiligo is, with studies showing that only about 5–10% of vitiligo cases begin after the age of 40. The epidemiology of late-onset vitiligo is not well characterized. No standard definition for late-onset vitiligo exists, but the majority of studies have defined it as being aged 50 years and above at the time of clinical onset [13].

23.3.2 Pathogenesis

The pathogenesis of late-onset vitiligo is believed to be similar to that of other age groups, involving a complex interplay of genetic, autoimmune, and environmental factors. The age of vitiligo onset is influenced primarily by nongenetic environmental factors, with susceptibility governed by major genes. The disease begins when genetically predisposed individuals encounter specific environmental triggers. It is

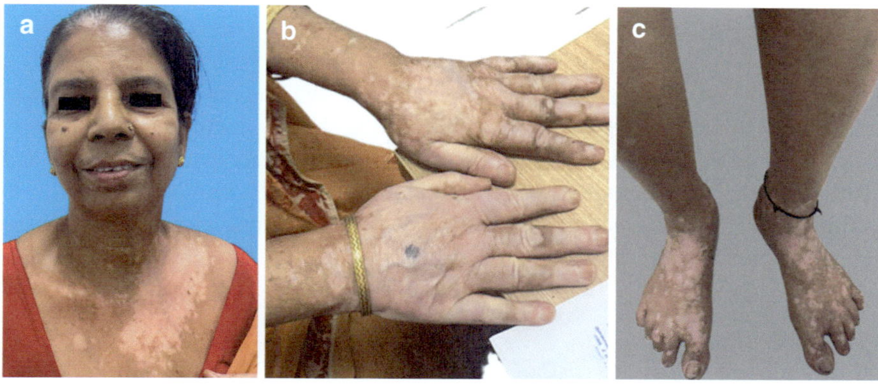

Fig. 23.2 A 65-year-old woman presenting with depigmented macules over the upper part of the forehead, along the frontal hair line, neck, and upper chest (**a**), bilateral hands (**b**), and bilateral lower legs (**c**)

suggested that vitiligo may have two inheritance patterns: early onset typically follows a dominant mode with incomplete penetrance, while late onset is linked to a recessive genotype triggered by environmental factors [14].

23.3.3 Clinical Characteristics

Generalized vitiligo is more commonly seen in patients with late-onset vitiligo, followed by focal vitiligo, primarily on the face and extremities (Fig. 23.2a–c). Segmental vitiligo is uncommon. Unlike childhood vitiligo, disease progression is usually slower, and lesions may remain stable for extended periods. The presence of leukotrichia and the Koebner phenomenon is less common in late-onset vitiligo compared to early-onset vitiligo [15].

23.3.4 Associations

Late-onset vitiligo is strongly associated with a number of autoimmune disorders, particularly alopecia areata, Addison's disease, pernicious anemia, Hashimoto's thyroiditis and Grave's disease. Diabetes mellitus is also commonly observed in these patients [16]. Unlike in early-onset vitiligo, the association with audiological abnormalities is not statistically significant, although hypoacusis can still be present in some patients [15].

23.3.5 Management

The treatment of late-onset vitiligo is often more challenging due to the slower response to therapy in older patients. Combination therapy, including topical treatments and phototherapy, is typically recommended. Phototherapy is efficacious and well tolerated in the treatment of patients with late-onset vitiligo. However, it is essential to screen for and manage associated autoimmune conditions in these patients to improve overall treatment outcomes [13].

23.4 Conclusion

Both early- and late-onset vitiligo present unique challenges in terms of clinical management and treatment. Early-onset vitiligo tends to be more aggressive, with a higher likelihood of progression and involvement of multiple body areas. In contrast, late-onset vitiligo is often more localized and slower to progress. Segmental vitiligo is more common in early-onset vitiligo. Early-onset vitiligo is more associated with atopy, a more positive family history, and a lower probability of autoimmune disorders as compared to their adult counterparts. While the underlying pathophysiology may share common features across age groups, the clinical presentation, psychosocial impact, and treatment strategies differ significantly between childhood and late-onset vitiligo. Understanding these differences is crucial for tailoring treatment strategies and improving patient outcomes across different age groups.

References

1. Premkumar M, Bhaskar Kalarani I, Mohammed V, Veerabathiran R. An extensive review of vitiligo-associated conditions. Int J Dermatol Venereol. 2024;7(1):44–51.
2. Handa S, Dogra S. Epidemiology of childhood vitiligo: a study of 625 patients from North India. Pediatr Dermatol. 2003;20(3):207–10.
3. Gupta M. Childhood vitiligo: a clinicoepidemiological study. Indian J Paediatr Dermatol. 2018;19(3):212–4.
4. Palit A, Inamadar AC. Childhood vitiligo. Indian J Dermatol Venereol Leprol. 2012;78:30.
5. Singh M. Cellular and molecular basis of autoimmunity in vitiligo pathogenesis [Internet] [PhD Thesis]. Maharaja Sayajirao University of Baroda (India); 2017 [cited 2024 Sep 5]. Available from: https://search.proquest.com/openview/15d018232540442f835719d7431dc77c/1?pq-origsite=gscholar&cbl=18750&diss=y
6. Mu EW, Cohen BE, Orlow SJ. Early-onset childhood vitiligo is associated with a more extensive and progressive course. J Am Acad Dermatol. 2015;73(3):467–70.
7. Hafi NB, Thokchom NS, Singh SC, Bachaspatimayum R. Childhood vitiligo: a hospital-based study on 200 patients in Northeast India. Indian J Paediatr Dermatol. 2019;20(2):128–33.
8. Kambil SM. Clinical profile of childhood vitiligo at a tertiary hospital in North Kerala. Int J Res Dermatol. 2018;4(2):115–7.

9. Mokhtarpour Neilagh A, Alizadeh F, Aghazadeh Barenji M, Behrouz Sharif S, Sedokani A. Different characteristics of early-onset vitiligo versus lateonset vitiligo. Iran J Dermatol. 2020;23(4):132–6.
10. Agarwal S, Gupta S, Ojha A, Sinha R. Childhood vitiligo: clinicoepidemiologic profile of 268 children from the Kumaun Region of Uttarakhand. India Pediatr Dermatol. 2013;30(3):348–53.
11. Zahra FT, Amin SS, Adil M, Sarshar F, Pathak P. Clinico-epidemiological study of childhood vitiligo and its associations: a hospital-based cross-sectional study. Indian J Paediatr Dermatol. 2022;23(2):116–22.
12. Augustine M, John V. Childhood onset vitiligo- clinical profile and impact on quality of life of family members. Pigment Int. 2023;10(1):30–6.
13. Kong YL, Ching VHL, Chuah SY, Thng TG. Retrospective study on the characteristics and treatment of late-onset vitiligo. Indian J Dermatol Venereol Leprol. 2017;83:625.
14. Arcos-Burgos M, Parodi E, Salgar M, Bedoya E, Builes J, Jaramillo D, et al. Vitiligo: complex segregation and linkage disequilibrium analyses with respect to microsatellite loci spanning the HLA. Hum Genet. 2002;110:334–42.
15. Al-Mutairi N, Al-Sebeih KH. Late onset vitiligo and audiological abnormalities: is there any association? Indian J Dermatol Venereol Leprol. 2011;77:571.
16. Fan KC, Yang TH, Huang YC. Vitiligo and thyroid disease: a systematic review and meta-analysis. Eur J Dermatol. 2018;28(6):750–63.

Chapter 24
Animal and In Vitro Vitiligo Models

Vinod Kumar, Laveena Kaushal, Mohinder Kaur, and Davinder Parsad

Abstract Vitiligo pathogenesis is complex, involving genetic, environmental, and immunological factors. Various experimental models, including in vitro and animal models, have been established to elucidate disease mechanisms, immune responses, and potential therapeutic interventions. These models facilitate the study of cellular interactions, oxidative stress, cytokine involvement, and immune-mediated melanocyte destruction.

Animal models play a crucial role in vitiligo research by replicating various aspects of the disease, which are difficult to incorporate into in vitro cultures. However, no single model fully represents human vitiligo, and the results must be interpreted cautiously. The most commonly used animal models are mice, which are developed through chemical induction (monobenzone and hydroquinone), immunization (recombinant melanocyte-specific antigens), or genetic modifications (involving antigen presentation). However, in vitro models are more precise and provide a controlled environment for studying melanocyte biology, immune interactions, and drug responses. These models are cost-effective, ethically favorable, and offer high reproducibility. Melanocytes, keratinocytes, and fibroblasts can be isolated from skin biopsies and cultured in specific growth medium in dishes in the laboratory. Altogether, both these models are indispensable in vitiligo research. While animal models provide a holistic view of disease progression, in vitro models enable mechanistic studies of melanocyte-immune interactions. Monobenzone- and interferon-induced models remain extensively used due to their relevance in studying vitiligo pathogenesis and therapeutic responses. Future research should be more focused on refining the existing models to enhance reproducibility and translational relevance. Advancements in vitiligo modeling will improve our understanding of disease mechanisms and accelerate the development of effective treatments.

Keywords Vitiligo pathogenesis · Melanocytes · Depigmentation · Oxidative stress · Immune response · In vitro and animal models

V. Kumar (✉) · L. Kaushal · M. Kaur · D. Parsad
Department of Dermatology, Venerology, and Leprology, PGIMER, Chandigarh, India

R. Sarkar, V. Narayan R (eds.), *A Concise Guide to The Management of Vitiligo*,
https://doi.org/10.1007/978-981-95-3857-7_24

Abbreviations

4-TBP	4-Tertiary butylphenol
Apaf-1	Apoptotic protease activating factor-1
APCs	Antigen-presenting cells
BAX	BCL-2-associated X protein
bFGF	Basic fibroblast growth factor
CCR5	C-C chemokine receptor type 5
CD8+ T cells	Cluster of differentiation 8 positive T cells
CXCR3	CXC chemokine receptor 3
ECM	Extracellular matrix
gp100	Glycoprotein 100 (melanoma antigen)
GSH	Glutathione
H2O2	Hydrogen peroxide
HMGB1	High mobility group box 1
HSP70i	Heat shock protein 70 inducible
IFN-γ	Interferon gamma
IL-13	Interleukin-13
IL-17	Interleukin-17
IL-6	Interleukin-6
Krt14-Kitl Pmel-1	Krt14-Kit ligand Pmel-1
LAMP-1	Lysosome-activated membrane protein-1
MART-1	Melanoma antigen-recognized by T cells 1
MITF	Microphthalmia-associated transcription factor
RAG-deficient mice	Recombination-activating gene-deficient mice
SCF	Stem cell factor
TBC	4-Tertiary butyl catechol
TCR	T cell receptor
THP-1	Human monocytic cell line
TRP1/2	Tyrosinase-related protein 1/2
TYR	Tyrosinase
UPR	Unfolded protein response
VEGF	Vascular endothelial growth factor

24.1 Introduction

Vitiligo is a chronic, multifactorial skin condition characterized by the loss of skin melanocytes and the subsequent appearance of white patches. While the exact cause of vitiligo is unknown, it is believed to be a combination of genetic, environmental, and immunological factors. In order to understand the cellular and molecular mechanisms of vitiligo pathogenesis, researchers have used in vitro models as well as animal models that mimic the vitiligo microenvironment. These models allow studying the precise effect of a single molecule, cell, or combination of cell type and cytokine on vitiligo severity, pathogenesis, and symptoms in a controlled setting. This helps in establishing the current understanding of vitiligo disease. The identification of oxidative stress, cytokines (like IFN-γ), and immune cells (like CD8-T cells) that impact the survival of melanocytes and the immunological response is the result of such models. Furthermore, models that focus on different aspects of the disease mechanism, cell types (melanocytes, keratinocytes, etc.), immune response (TCR, etc.), and unique epitope expressions (like tyrosinase) unravel the vitiligo pathogenesis to the extent we know at present. This chapter delves into the few models that researchers have created, showcasing their valuable contributions to the discovery of vitiligo.

24.2 Animal Models

Animal models are valuable for studying vitiligo, though no single model can capture all aspects of vitiligo. Different models simulate specific elements of vitiligo, such as immune involvement, genetics, and potential treatments. Each model has strengths and limitations, so the choice should align with the research focus. However, the results from these models must be interpreted cautiously, as they may not fully represent the complexity of human vitiligo [9, 10].

Mouse models are the most convenient and explored animal to study the pathogenesis of a variety of diseases [40]. Vitiligo mouse models can be developed by inducing melanocyte stress using chemicals, immunizing with culprit pathogenic immune cells, pathogenic melanocyte antigen activation, and genetic alterations [25, 27, 28].

24.2.1 Chemically Induced

Topical application, or localized injection of substances like monobenzone and hydroquinone, results in vitiligo-type depigmentation [16, 41]. Monobenzone-induced vitiligo is clinically more relevant, as it causes cellular stress in melanocytes, as observed in vitiligo. Topical application of 40% monobenzone cream [41] on the shaved abdomens of 4-week-old mice showed hair depigmentation at the site, which later spread to distant areas like the ears and tail. Histopathological analysis revealed that CD8+ T cells infiltrated the affected skin. In contrast, in RAG-deficient mice, monobenzone application showed depigmentation only at the treatment site. This suggests that monobenzone causes localized depigmentation through direct toxicity, whereas an adaptive immune response is necessary for depigmentation to spread. Hydrogen peroxide (H_2O_2) also damages the localized melanocytes by inhibiting tyrosinase and generating ROS [15]. It also causes the apoptosis of skin cell through BAX and Caspase-3 activation.

24.2.2 Immunization-Induced Vitiligo Model

Injection of recombinant melanocyte antigens is also utilized to induce an autoimmune response toward the melanocyte to cause their damage. Overwijk et al. [25] injected TRP1 able to induce skin depigmentation in 80% of C57B16 mice. Histological analysis showed that this depigmentation was driven by CD4+ T cell and myelocyte-specific autoantibodies anti-melan-A (MART-1). In another similar study, DNA plasmids encoding human TRP2 were reported to cause depigmentation of new hair in mouse skin, involving CD8+ T cells and perforins. Studies have also found that simultaneous injection of TRP2 and HSP70i also induces depigmentation, mainly by dysregulation of immune responses and attack of melanocytes. Mutated HSP70i lost its potential to induce depigmentation, further support the importance of HSP70i in vitiligo [9, 24].

24.2.3 Transgenic Mice

A genetically modified mouse model was also developed that mimics the melanocyte-specific antigen and elicits an immune response.

24.2.3.1 AAD+ Transgenic Mouse

This transgenic mice has induced expression of tyrosinase epitope, which stimulates a specific T cell clone for Tyr369 and causes depigmentation. Immunohistology analysis revealed infiltration of CD8 and CD4 T cells, along with increased expression of CXCR3, CCR5, and IFN-γ in the hair follicle [27, 28, 40].

24.2.3.2 H3TA2 Mouse Model

Similarly, Mehrotra et al. developed TCR transgenic mice for tyrosinase 368–376 presented on HLA-A2, a specific feature of melanoma-infiltrated CD8 T cells. Exhibits early-onset depigmentation and eye disorder due to disruptions in the retinal pigment epithelium by transgenic T cells [6, 8].

24.2.3.3 TrpHEL Mouse Model

Lambe et al. developed a hen egg lysozyme (HEL) peptide expression under the TRP-2 promoter in melanocyte. Depigmentation started at 21 days of age in these mice. The pathomechanism highlights the Fas-Fas ligand involvement in this; however, human melanocytes are not well known for Fas-mediated damage, and its relevance in humans is unsure [19].

24.2.3.4 Pmel-1 Mouse Model

It is genetically developed to express T cell receptors specific to the gp100 antigen of melanocytes. This elicits CD8 T cell immune response against melanocytes and causes depigmentation [9, 27].

24.2.3.5 Krt14-Kitl Pmel-1 Mouse Model

It involves the expression of the Kit ligand under the influence of the KRT14 promoter. This helps stabilize melanocyte growth and stability in the epidermis. This model provides the detailing of the mechanism that CD8 T cell evokes through Pmel-1 expression attack and damage the melanocytes to cause depigmentation [11].

24.3 In Vitro Models

In vitro models are always more accessible and workable because of their ease and low infrastructure demands compared to mouse studies. These studies are also cost effective and involve less ethical concerns than mouse studies. For in vitro studies, first, there is a need for melanocytes, which can be isolated directly from skin biopsies as a primary culture or can be purchased from commercially available sources. There are a few immortal cell lines, but their relevance in vitiligo is still minimal.

24.3.1 Primary Melanocyte Cell Culture

For isolating primary melanocytes, fresh skin biopsy is collected under aseptic conditions in phosphate buffer saline (PBS) with antibiotics (penicillin and streptomycin). After PBS removal, digest the biopsy overnight with trypsin-EDTA (0.025% trypsin and 0.02% EDTA) solution at 4 °C. The following day, add fetal bovine serum (FBS) in 1:1 ratio to neutralize the activity of trypsin. Peel the epidermis off the dermis with sterile forceps. Remove solid wastes of the tissue and centrifuge the suspension at 1500 rpm for 5 min. Discard the supernatant, avoiding disturbance to the pellet, and then wash with PBS. Add melanocyte-specific media to the pellet and put it in a culture plate after being thoroughly mixed. Maintain the culture at 37 °C in a humidified, 95% air, and 5% CO_2 atmosphere. Change the media at 3–4 day intervals and check for viability using trypan blue staining, and cell number by hemocytometer.

24.3.2 Chemically Induced Vitiligo In Vitro Models

To investigate the mechanisms of melanocyte death, various chemicals that induce cellular stress and mimic the vitiligo-like conditions have been utilized. These agents are useful in uncovering the key molecules in vitiligo research. We have listed the chemicals commonly used in in vitro vitiligo models.

24.3.2.1 Monobenzone-Induced Vitiligo

Monobenzone (monobenzyl ether of hydroquinone) is an FDA-approved depigmenting agent typically used to achieve an even skin tone in cases of universal vitiligo where depigmentation covers approx. 90% of the body surface area. In addition to the process of depigmentation, it has also been reported to increase melanocytes' immunogenicity by the formation of quinone haptens. Monobenzone affects tyrosinase and melanin production by inhibiting tyrosinase activity and disrupting the melanin synthesis pathway, resulting in reduced melanin production by melanocytes. The concentrations of monobenzone used in various in vitro studies range from 10 μM to 120 μM to study the effect on melanin production, inhibition and apoptosis. Low concentrations of monobenzone are used to examine the effect on melanin synthesis without causing significant cell death. The mechanism of action of monobenzone on melanocytes includes several processes, such as:

Tyrosinase Haptenation Tyrosinase is the key enzyme in the melanin biosynthesis pathway where it catalyzes the conversion of L-tyrosine to L-DOPA and further into dopaquinone, which are essential steps in melanin production. Monobenzone acts as a competitive substrate for tyrosinase due to the structural similarity of both hydroquinone and L-tyrosine, which is a phenolic compound. When monobenzone is oxidized by tyrosinase, it forms highly reactive quinones (also termed as benzoquinones) instead of progressing through the normal melanin synthesis pathway [33, 34]. The quinone haptens generated by monobenzone bind to the active site of tyrosinase, thereby reducing its ability to catalyze the conversion of L-tyrosine to precursors of the melanin pathway, leading to decreased melanin production. Furthermore, these quinone-haptens also increase the immunogenicity of melanocytes and increase MALT-1 expression after monobenzone treatment, thereby triggering an immune response against pigment-producing melanocytes [22].

Melanocyte Cytotoxicity and Death Along with directly inhibiting melanin synthesis, monobenzone also promotes the apoptosis of melanocytes. The mechanism of melanocyte death by monobenzone is derived by multiple pathways, such as oxidative stress, apoptotic pathway activation, and mitochondrial dysfunction. The quinone derivatives formed by monobenzone are highly reactive and can generate ROS that overpowers the protective system of melanocytes (e.g., glutathione and catalase), making cells vulnerable to oxidative damage. ROS damages the mitochondrial membrane, triggering the release of proapoptotic factors from mitochondria into the cytosol, such as cytochrome c. Once released into the cytosol, cytochrome c binds apoptotic protease activating factor-1 (Apaf-1), forming the apoptosome, which activates Caspase9 and initiates the apoptotic pathway. However, a contrasting in vitro study by Hariharan et al. [13] reported that the melanocyte death pathway by monobenzone is nonapoptotic. They demonstrated the release of HMGB1 and no caspase activation, reflecting necrosis as the method of melanocyte death by monobenzone [13]. Though both of these pathways have been reported, more research is required to rule out apoptosis as the mechanism of melanocyte destruction by monobenzone. Along with depigmentation, monobenzone induces the release of exosomes containing melanosomal proteins, which further leads to dendritic cells and other innate immune cells activation.

Melanosome Autophagy Monobenzone induces melanosome autophagy. When exposed to 20 μM monobenzone for 3 h, in the first hour of monobenzone treatment to melanoma cells, there were fewer stage IV melanosomes and stage II and III melanosomes were disorganized. After 3 h, there were no stage IV melanosomes, and melanin-containing autophagosomes were seen in electron microscopy. Lysosome-activated membrane protein-1 (LAMP-1) expression was seen upregulated, thereby suggesting lysosome-dependent melanosome degradation [34].

24.3.2.2 Hydrogen Peroxide (H_2O_2)

H_2O_2-induced depigmentation is a well-established in vitro model of vitiligo-like pathogenesis, mimicking oxidative stress-mediated melanocyte damage. H_2O_2 is reportedly an endogenous ROS found in vitiligo skin and is a common ex vivo approach to induce oxidative stress in melanocytes. Schallreuter et al. showed that vitiligo melanocytes exhibited significantly higher levels of ROS after H_2O_2 exposure, leading to significant damage via lipid peroxidation and tyrosinase inhibition [29]. It also extends damage to DNA, activating apoptotic pathways and possessing stress to the endoplasmic reticulum in melanocytes. This activates the unfolded protein response (UPR). H_2O_2 hampers the activity of antioxidant mechanisms by hitting glutathione (GSH), which is a major antioxidant that neutralizes ROS. Low glutathione levels leave cells vulnerable to oxidative damage.

24.3.2.3 4-Tertiary Butylphenol (4-TBP)

4-TBP is known to be a causative agent for occupational vitiligo. It is structurally similar to L-tyrosine and hydroquinone, both of which are crucial mediators of the melanin synthesis pathway. 4-TBP acts as a competitive inhibitor of tyrosinase; thus, instead of producing melanin, tyrosinase oxidizes 4-TBP to quinone haptens, thereby disrupting melanin synthesis. It also generates ROS during its metabolism that damages melanocytes. Similar to other chemically induced models, treatment of 4-TBP to primary melanocyte culture induced their destruction and disruption of the melanogenesis process, resembling depigmentation in vitiligo. Hariharan et al., in a study of ultrastructure changes, noticed the formation of apoptotic bodies, including plasma membrane blebbing, in contrast to monobenzone that involved necrosis [13, 35]. Therefore, 4-TBP mimics the apoptotic melanocyte destruction model in vitiligo. Since oxidative stress, immunization of melanocytes, and depigmentation are observed that mimic in vitro vitiligo conditions, this is an efficient in vitro vitiligo model that can be used for various drug response and repigmentation studies to move forward in vitiligo research [21].

24.3.2.4 4-Tertiary Butyl Catechol (TBC) and Other Phenolic Compounds

TBC was used in early vitiligo studies, wherein 15–30% of cultured melanocytes from adult guinea pig were observed to get detached from the plate after 6 h of TBC treatment. Mansur et al. observed unusual premelanosomes and melanosomes by ultrastructural studies, but did not cause lightening of the remaining melanocytes [23]. The findings suggested that TBC caused skin depigmentation by targeting melanocyte death but does not interfere with melanogenesis. Other phenolic compounds, majorly those that are causative of occupational vitiligo or used in the rubber and dye industries, are also studied in the context of in vitro depigmentation model generation to effectively study the pathogenesis, repigmentation strategies, and toxic effects in a shorter period of time [14, 32].

Both in vitro and in vivo monobenzone-treated mouse models are widely used as vitiligo research models for various purposes, such as vitiligo pathogenesis studies, pharmaceutical drug response, etc. Though animal models are considered superior to in vitro models, as they can mimic the entire in vivo microenvironment, in vitro vitiligo models have proved to be of greater importance when functional studies and the role and effect on a particular cell type are investigated. Monobenzone models for vitiligo have been extensively used in vitiligo research wherein primary melanocytes from the pigmented site of patients are cultured using melanocyte growth medium in a 37 °C CO_2 incubator. Once differentiated into melanocytes, these melanocytes are treated with different concentrations of monobenzone, followed by melanin content assay, apoptosis assay, and pigmentation marker study (MITF, TYR, and TRP1).

24.3.3 Cytokine-Based Vitiligo Models

Vitiligo pathogenesis is majorly regulated by IFN-γ and other inflammatory cytokines that drive the process of T cell activation and melanocyte destruction. Mimicking the inflammatory cytokine profile of vitiligo patients in vitro is another

Table 24.1 List of cytokines based on in vitro vitiligo models and their key contributions in understanding vitiligo pathogenesis

Sno.	Cytokines	Role in vitiligo	Key findings/effect on melanocytes/keratinocytes	References
1	IFN-γ	IFN-γ is the key driver of CD8+ T cell-mediated melanocyte apoptosis. It is critical for the progression of vitiligo	Inhibits melanogenesis in primary culture melanocytes	[36, 39]
		Induced chemokines CXCR3, CXCL9/CXCL10 for cytotoxic T cell skin homing	It directly induces melanocyte apoptosis as IFN-γ treatment increased the expression of BAX, BAK, and cleaved caspase 3 and reduced Bcl2	
			IFN-Y stimulates the JAK-1/STAT-1 signaling pathway	
2	TNF-α	1 Melanocyte and keratinocyte apoptosis	In response to elevated TNF-α, keratinocyte apoptosis was induced due to impaired P13/Akt and NF-kb activation	[17, 30]
		2. Promotes oxidative stress through inflammatory responses		
3	IL-17	1 Produced by Th17 cells and involved in chronic inflammation	Enhanced the melanocyte death along when given in combination with TNF-α and IFN-γ	[2]
		2 Impairs cellular functions and triggers inflammation	IL-17A receptor blocking resulted in increased melanin content	
4	IFN-γ, IL-17 combination model	Triggers the melanocyte destruction and activation	IFN-γ and IL-17 downregulate the keratinocyte GPNMB	[3]

mechanism markedly used for investigating their influence on melanocytes. Various cytokine-based models have been used in previous studies to dissect the pathways involved in depigmentation and immune activation in vitiligo. Some of these models and the associated studies conducted are summarized in Table 24.1.

24.3.3.1 Melanocyte Coculture and 3D Skin Models

To study the interactions between melanocytes and other cell types, such as keratinocytes, immune cells (T cells, macrophages, and dendritic cells), and fibroblasts, coculture models are widely used in vitiligo research. These models have proven crucial for understanding the complex cell-cell interactions that lead to melanocyte destruction in vitiligo.

24.3.3.2 Coculture with Keratinocytes

The interactions between melanocytes and keratinocytes are central to the process of melanogenesis. Melanocytes synthesize melanin within specialized organelles known as melanosomes. These melanosomes are transported to the tips of melanocyte dendrites and engulfed by keratinocytes. In response, keratinocytes also secrete various factors, such as endothelin-1, stem cell factor (SCF), and bFGF, that stimulate melanocyte to produce more melanin. Therefore, keratinocyte-melanocyte coculture models are used to explore pigmentation disorders, including vitiligo, under conditions like inflammation, oxidative stress, inflammation, and UV exposure [18, 20]. Similar to primary melanocyte culture, keratinocytes can be cultured in vitro using keratinocyte-specific growth medium by maintaining at 37 °C in a humidified, 95% air, and 5% CO_2 atmosphere. Once both the cultures get differentiated, they can be cultured together at a 1:10 cell ratio (melanocyte:keratinocyte) [26]. These Mel-Ker coculture models are well established and have been used to elucidate the role of keratinocytes, such as caveolae formation [7, 38], at the epidermis during pigmentation in melanogenesis regulation and to decipher the crosstalk between both of them under stress or drug treatment.

24.3.3.3 Coculture with T Cells

These models involve coculturing melanocytes with T cells to study immune interactions and responses in a vitiliginous microenvironment. For vitiligo research, T cells can be isolated from a patient's blood and sorted into specific T cell subtype. CD8+ T cells can be utilized to understand the cytotoxic pathways possessed by them to destroy melanocytes or Tregs to study impaired regulatory actions under inflammation. In one study, CD8+ T cells isolated from vitiligo perilesional margins and autologous melanocytes were cocultured at 1:1, 1:2, and 1:5 ratios and incubated for 3 days [37], showing an increased secretion of IL-6, IL-17, and IL-13. CD8+ T cells showed higher activation levels and melanocyte apoptosis [37].

24.3.3.4 Coculture with Macrophages and Dendritic Cells

Macrophages and dendritic cells are critical in immune surveillance, tissue repair, efferocytosis, and clearance of inflammation. To investigate the influence of macrophages on the process of melanin production, understanding melanocyte-macrophage cell crosstalk is critical. Macrophages exist in different functional states: M1 proinflammatory) and M2 macrophages (anti-inflammatory). Melanocyte-macrophage (THP-1 cell line) coculture studies revealed the role of M2 macrophages in stimulating melanogenesis through VEGF [12]. Like macrophages, dendritic cells play crucial roles in autoimmune diseases. As antigen-presenting cells, dendritic cells are involved in activating T cells, which can lead to melanocyte death and vitiligo. Srivastava et al. [31] revealed the role of proinflammatory dendritic cells in inflammatory cytokine production and their contribution to increased depigmentation in progressive vitiligo [31]. All cells, including immune cells, melanocytes, and keratinocytes, play a role in maintaining skin pigmentary homeostasis. Disruptions of this through oxidative stress or injury, can cause these cells to become self-destructive.

24.3.3.5 3D Skin Culture

Primary cell monolayer cultures do not completely reflect the complex skin structure; therefore, 3D skin equivalent models are the next generation of in vitro models to generate a replica of the skin microenvironment. In the past two decades, 3D-skin models have evolved from the development of a fully differentiated epidermis from keratinocytes using an air-liquid interface to reconstructed skin models with skin cells, T cells, and endothelial cells. In order to grow skin cells in layers, a matrix or support structure is required in culture plates. Various types of matrices are used, such as hydrogels (including collagen-based matrices like EpiSkin), polycarbonate inserts, and dead deepidermized dermis (DDD) [5]. Polycarbonate inserts are used to grow both keratinocyte and fibroblast layers. Type I collagen is typically used as it is the most abundant protein in human skin. Commercially available collagen solutions (EpiSkin) are kept on ice to prevent premature gelation. Collagen is mixed with a neutralizing solution (e.g., NaOH, pH= 7.0), kept cold during preparation, and then transferred into molds or culture plates. Gelation occurs when the collagen solution is warmed to 37 °C, allowing it to form a stable 3D gel matrix. The final gel should have a thickness of around 1–2 mm to simulate the dermal layer. Similar to collagen gels, DDD is used as a base, with fibroblasts cultured on top and subjected to adhesion and proliferation for ECM generation [1].

24.3.3.6 3D Culture Establishment

Fibroblasts provide an extracellular matrix and support the structural integrity of the model. These fibroblasts are suspended in a collagen gel. After fibroblasts are embedded, the collagen-cell mixture is cast into a mold or plate, and gelation occurs at 37 °C. It is cultured for several days to allow fibroblasts to proliferate and secrete ECM. Keratinocytes and melanocytes are then seeded on top of the gelled collagen matrix. The keratinocytes proliferate and differentiate to form a stratified epidermal layer.

24.3.3.7 Air-Liquid Interface Culture

After keratinocytes form a confluent monolayer, the 3D skin model is exposed to the air-liquid interface by removing some of the culture medium [1, 4]. This stimulates keratinocyte differentiation and stratification, mimicking the natural development

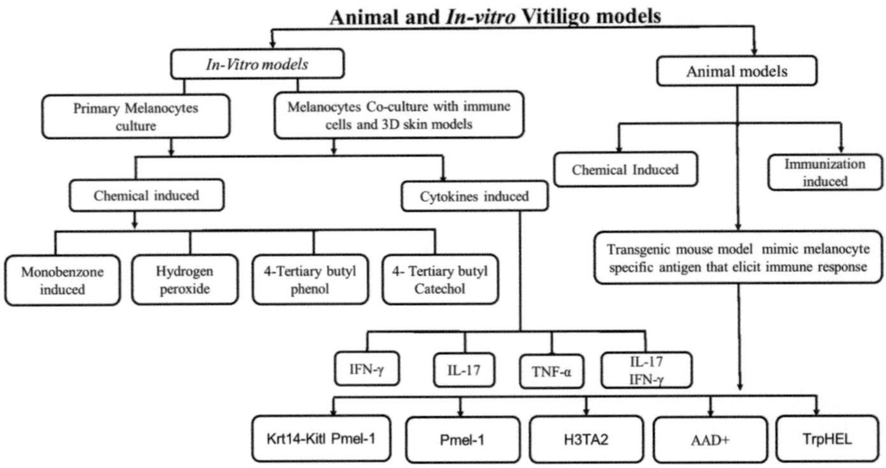

Fig. 24.1 Comprehensive overview of the cell culture and animal-based models used for vitiligo research

of the epidermis. After 7–14 days, the epidermis becomes fully developed, forming distinct layers (basal, spinous, granular, and stratum corneum). These 3D structures, after exposure to various triggering factors, form a compact vitiligo model for in vitro studies investigating vitiligo pathogenesis and the responses of particular cell type under different inflammatory and depigmentation conditions.

In conclusion, both in vitro and animal models play an important role in unveiling the mechanisms of vitiligo pathophysiology (Fig. 24.1). Monocultures, cocultures, and 3D models provide insights into the molecular and cellular interactions involved in melanocyte dysfunction and immune responses in vitiligo. These models have a crucial role in screening potential therapeutic agents. In contrast, animal models can mimic the in vivo microenvironment, including immune responses and depigmentation patterns, and real-time responses to drug treatments can be registered phenotypically. However, challenges such as species-specific differences and the complexity of immune regulation are still there. Together, these models complement each other, and further advancements and refinements in these models are essential to ensure the reproducibility, safety, and efficacy of potential treatments.

References

1. Bauer M, Metzger M, Corea M, Schädl B, Grillari J, Dungel P. Novel 3D-printed cell culture inserts for air-liquid Interface cell culture. Life (Basel, Switzerland). 2022;12(8):1216. https://doi.org/10.3390/LIFE12081216.
2. Bhardwaj S, Rani S, Srivastava N, Kumar R, Parsad D. Increased systemic and epidermal levels of IL-17A and IL-1β promotes progression of non-segmental vitiligo. Cytokine. 2017;91:153–61. https://doi.org/10.1016/J.CYTO.2016.12.014.

3. Biswas KB, Takahashi A, Mizutani Y, Takayama S, Ishitsuka A, Yang L, Yang F, Iddamalgoda A, Katayama I, Inoue S. GPNMB is expressed in human epidermal keratinocytes but disappears in the vitiligo lesional skin. Sci Rep. 2020;10(1):1–11. https://doi.org/10.1038/s41598-020-61931-1.
4. Cario-André M, Boniface K, Bernard FX, Taieb A, Dell'Anna ML, Seneschal J. In vitro models of vitiligo. In: Skin tissue models. London: Academic; 2018. p. 129–49. https://doi.org/10.1016/B978-0-12-810545-0.00006-1.
5. Chaturvedi D, Paranjape S, Jain R, Dandekar P. Disease-related biomarkers as experimental endpoints in 3D skin culture models. Cytotechnology. 2023;75(3):165–93. https://doi.org/10.1007/S10616-023-00574-2.
6. Chatterjee S, Eby J, Al-Khami AA, Soloshchenko M, Kang H-K, Kaur N, Naga O, Murali A, Nishimura MI, Le Poole IC, Mehrotra S. A quantitative increase in regulatory T cells controls development of vitiligo. J Invest Dermatol. 2014;134(5):1285–94. https://doi.org/10.1038/jid.2013.540.
7. Domingues L, Hurbain I, Gilles-Marsens F, Sirés-Campos J, André N, Dewulf M, Romao M, Viaris de Lesegno C, Macé AS, Blouin C, Guéré C, Vié K, Raposo G, Lamaze C, Delevoye C. Coupling of melanocyte signaling and mechanics by caveolae is required for human skin pigmentation. Nat Commun. 2020;11(1):1–14. https://doi.org/10.1038/s41467-020-16738-z.
8. Eby J, Kang H-K, Klarquist J, Chatterjee S, Mosenson J, Nishimura M, Garrett-Mayer E, Longley B, Engelhard V, Mehrotra S, Le Poole I. Immune responses in a mouse model of vitiligo with spontaneous epidermal De- and repigmentation. Pigment Cell Melanoma Res. 2014;27:1075–85. https://doi.org/10.1111/pcmr.12284.
9. Essien KI, Harris JE. Animal models of vitiligo: matching the model to the question. Dermatol Sin. 2014;32(4):240–7. https://doi.org/10.1016/j.dsi.2014.09.008.
10. Giri P, Desai D, Dwivedi M. Animal models unraveling the complexity of vitiligo pathogenesis. Autoimmun Rev. 2024;23(4):103515. https://doi.org/10.1016/j.autrev.2024.103515.
11. Harris J, Harris T, Weninger W, Wherry EJ, Hunter C, Turka L. A mouse model of vitiligo with focused epidermal depigmentation requires IFN-γ for autoreactive CD8+ T-cell accumulation in the skin. J Invest Dermatol. 2012;132:1869–76. https://doi.org/10.1038/jid.2011.463.
12. Han H, Kim Y, Mo H, Choi SH, Lee K, Rim YA, Ju JH. Preferential stimulation of melanocytes by M2 macrophages to produce melanin through vascular endothelial growth factor. Sci Rep. 2022;12(1):6416. https://doi.org/10.1038/S41598-022-08163-7.
13. Hariharan V, Klarquist J, Reust MJ, Koshoffer A, McKee MD, Boissy RE, Le Poole IC. Monobenzyl ether of hydroquinone and 4-tertiary butyl phenol activate markedly different physiological responses in melanocytes: relevance to skin depigmentation. J Invest Dermatol. 2010;130(1):211–20. https://doi.org/10.1038/JID.2009.214.
14. Hoshino S, Nishimura M, Fukuyama K, Gellin GA, Epstein JH. Effects of 4-tertiary butyl catechol on melanocytes of hairless mice. J Invest Dermatol. 1981;76(4):231–8. https://doi.org/10.1111/1523-1747.EP12526042.
15. Hu Z-M, Zhou Q, Lei T-C, Ding S-F, Xu S-Z. Effects of hydroquinone and its glucoside derivatives on melanogenesis and antioxidation: biosafety as skin whitening agents. J Dermatol Sci. 2009;55(3):179–84. https://doi.org/10.1016/j.jdermsci.2009.06.003.
16. Kaushik H, Kaul D, Kumaran MS, Parsad D. Chemical induced pathognomonic features observed in human vitiligo are mediated through miR-2909 RNomics pathway. J Dermatol Sci. 2020;100(2):92–8. https://doi.org/10.1016/j.jdermsci.2020.06.004.
17. Kim NH, Jeon S, Lee HJ, Lee AY. Impaired PI3K/Akt activation-mediated NF-kappaB inactivation under elevated TNF-alpha is more vulnerable to apoptosis in vitiliginous keratinocytes. J Invest Dermatol. 2007;127(11):2612–7. https://doi.org/10.1038/SJ.JID.5700900.
18. Kumar R, Parsad D, Kanwar A, Kaul D. Development of melanocyte-keratinocyte co-culture model for controls and vitiligo to assess regulators of pigmentation and melanocytes. Indian J Dermatol Venereol Leprol. 2012;78(5):599–604. https://doi.org/10.4103/0378-6323.100567.
19. Lambe T, Leung JCH, Bouriez-Jones T, Silver K, Makinen K, Crockford TL, Ferry H, Forrester JV, Cornall RJ. CD4 T cell-dependent autoimmunity against a melanocyte neoantigen induces

spontaneous vitiligo and depends upon Fas-Fas ligand interactions. J Immunol (Baltimore, Md: 1950). 2006;177(5):3055–62. https://doi.org/10.4049/jimmunol.177.5.3055.
20. Lei TC, Virador VM, Vieira WD, Hearing VJ. A melanocyte-keratinocyte coculture model to assess regulators of pigmentation in vitro. Anal Biochem. 2002;305(2):260–8. https://doi.org/10.1006/abio.2002.5665.
21. Manga P, Sheyn D, Yang F, Sarangarajan R, Boissy RE. A role for tyrosinase-related protein 1 in 4-tert-butylphenol-induced toxicity in melanocytes: implications for vitiligo. Am J Pathol. 2006;169(5):1652–62. https://doi.org/10.2353/ajpath.2006.050769.
22. Manini P, Napolitano A, Westerhof W, Riley PA, D'Ischia M. A reactive ortho-quinone generated by tyrosinase-catalyzed oxidation of the skin depigmenting agent monobenzone: self-coupling and thiol-conjugation reactions and possible implications for melanocyte toxicity. Chem Res Toxicol. 2009;22(8):1398–405. https://doi.org/10.1021/tx900018q.
23. Mansur JD, Fukuyama K, Gellin GA, Epstein WL. Effects of 4-tertiary butyl catechol on tissue cultured melanocytes. J Invest Dermatol. 1978;70(5):275–9. https://doi.org/10.1111/1523-1747.ep12541510. PMID: 641378.
24. Mosenson JA, Zloza A, Klarquist J, Barfuss AJ, Guevara-Patino JA, Poole ICL. HSP70i is a critical component of the immune response leading to vitiligo. Pigment Cell Melanoma Res. 2012;25(1):88–98. https://doi.org/10.1111/j.1755-148X.2011.00916.x.
25. Overwijk WW, Lee DS, Surman DR, Irvine KR, Touloukian CE, Chan CC, Carroll MW, Moss B, Rosenberg SA, Restifo NP. Vaccination with a recombinant vaccinia virus encoding a "self" antigen induces autoimmune vitiligo and tumor cell destruction in mice: requirement for CD4+ T lymphocytes. Proc Natl Acad Sci USA. 1999;96(6):2982–7. https://doi.org/10.1073/pnas.96.6.2982.
26. Phua R, Tien TZ, Goh G, Pantelireis N, Sim KSH, Lim J, Clavel C. In vitro quantification of pigment production and transfer in 2D co-cultures and 3D skin organotypic. STAR Protocols. 2023;4(2):102334. https://doi.org/10.1016/J.XPRO.2023.102334.
27. Riding RL, Richmond JM, Harris JE. Mouse model for human vitiligo. Curr Protoc Immunol. 2019;124(1):e63. https://doi.org/10.1002/cpim.63.
28. Gregg RK, Nichols L, Chen Y, Lu B, Engelhard VH. Mechanisms of spatial and temporal development of autoimmune vitiligo in tyrosinase-specific TCR transgenic mice. J Immunol (Baltimore, Md. : 1950). 2010;184(4):1909–17. https://doi.org/10.4049/jimmunol.0902778.
29. Schallreuter KU, Moore J, Wood JM, Beazley WD, Gaze DC, Tobin DJ, Marshall HS, Panske A, Panzig E, Hibberts NA. In vivo and in vitro evidence for hydrogen peroxide (H2O2) accumulation in the epidermis of patients with vitiligo and its successful removal by a UVB-activated pseudocatalase. J Invest Dermatol Symp Proc. 1999;4(1):91–6. https://doi.org/10.1038/SJ.JIDSP.5640189.
30. Singh M, Mansuri MS, Kadam A, Palit SP, Dwivedi M, Laddha NC, Begum R. Tumor Necrosis Factor-alpha affects melanocyte survival and melanin synthesis via multiple pathways in vitiligo. Cytokine. 2021;140:155432. https://doi.org/10.1016/J.CYTO.2021.155432.
31. Srivastava N, Bishnoi A, Parsad D, Kumaran MS, Vinay K, Gupta S. Dendritic cells sub-sets are associated with inflammatory cytokine production in progressive vitiligo disease. Arch Dermatol Res. 2021;313(9):759–67. https://doi.org/10.1007/S00403-020-02168-W.
32. Usami Y, Landau AB, Fukuyama K, Gellin GA. Inhibition of tyrosinase activity by 4-tert-butylcatechol and other depigmenting agents. J Toxicol Environ Health. 1980;6(3):559–67. https://doi.org/10.1080/15287398009529873.
33. Van Den Boorn JG, Melief CJ, Luiten RM. Monobenzone-induced depigmentation: from enzymatic blockade to autoimmunity. Pigm Cell Melanoma Res. 2011a;24(4):673–9. https://doi.org/10.1111/j.1755-148X.2011.00878.x.
34. Van Den Boorn JG, Picavet DI, Van Swieten PF, Van Veen HA, Konijnenberg D, Van Veelen PA, Van Capel T, Jong ECD, Reits EA, Drijfhout JW, Bos JD, Melief CJM, Luiten RM. Skin-depigmenting agent monobenzone induces potent T-cell autoimmunity toward

pigmented cells by tyrosinase haptenation and melanosome autophagy. J Invest Dermatol. 2011b;131(6):1240–51. https://doi.org/10.1038/JID.2011.16.
35. Vrijman C, Willemsen KJ, Tjin EPM, Kammeyer A, van den Boorn JG, van der Veen JPW, Jungbauer FHW, Kardaun SH, Luiten RM. T-cell responses against 4-tert-butylphenol-exposed pigmented cells in a patient with occupational vitiligo. Br J Dermatol. 2019;181(2):387. https://doi.org/10.1111/BJD.17713.
36. Wang S, Zhou M, Lin F, Liu D, Hong W, Lu L, Zhu Y, Xu A. Interferon-γ induces senescence in normal human melanocytes. PLoS One. 2014;9(3):e93232. https://doi.org/10.1371/JOURNAL.PONE.0093232.
37. Wu J, Zhou M, Wan Y, Xu A. CD8+ T cells from vitiligo perilesional margins induce autologous melanocyte apoptosis. Mol Med Rep. 2013;7(1):237–41. https://doi.org/10.3892/MMR.2012.1117.
38. Wu X, Hammer JA. Melanosome transfer: it is best to give and receive. Curr Opin Cell Biol. 2014;29(1):1–7. https://doi.org/10.1016/j.ceb.2014.02.003.
39. Yang L, Wei Y, Sun Y, Shi W, Yang J, Zhu L, Li M. Interferon-gamma inhibits melanogenesis and induces apoptosis in melanocytes: a pivotal role of CD8+ cytotoxic T lymphocytes in vitiligo. Acta Derm Venereol. 2015;95(6):664–70. https://doi.org/10.2340/00015555-2080.
40. Zhao Y, Kang G, Zhang R. Research status of vitiligo models. J Clin Images Med Case Rep. 2022;3. https://doi.org/10.52768/2766-7820/2001.
41. Zhu Y, Wang S, Xu A. A mouse model of vitiligo induced by monobenzone. Exp Dermatol. 2013;22:499–501. https://doi.org/10.1111/exd.12184.

Chapter 25
Further Directions in Vitiligo

Ayesha Kothari, Mohsen Mokhtari, Rebecca Quinonez, Jasira Ziglar, and Iltefat Hamzavi

Abstract The future of vitiligo research and treatment holds immense promise, with groundbreaking advancements shaping the path ahead. This chapter explores cutting-edge developments across multiple domains, from understanding disease pathogenesis to enhancing patient care. In Sect. 25.1, genetic advances, immune mechanisms, and environmental triggers offer deeper insights into vitiligo's complex etiology, paving the way for personalized medicine. Section 25.2 highlights innovative diagnostic techniques, with novel biomarkers and advanced imaging technologies revolutionizing early detection. Breakthrough treatments in Sect. 25.3, such as targeted immunotherapies and nanotechnology, aim to improve outcomes, while Sect. 25.4 focuses on optimizing existing therapies through combination approaches and enhanced efficacy. The psychosocial aspects addressed in Sect. 25.5 emphasize the importance of holistic patient care, including support and advocacy. Finally, Sect. 25.6 looks toward future research and global collaboration, ensuring sustained progress in vitiligo management.

Keywords Vitiligo · JAK inhibitors · Phototherapy · Biomarkers · Diagnostic techniques · Psychosocial vitiligo

---

A. Kothari
Department of Medicine, College of Human Medicine, Michigan State University, East Lansing, MI, USA

M. Mokhtari
The Henry W Lim Division of Photobiology and Photomedicine, Department of Dermatology, Henry Ford Health, Detroit, MI, USA

Department of Medicine, Oakland University William Beaumont School of Medicine, Rochester Hills, MI, USA

R. Quinonez · J. Ziglar · I. Hamzavi (✉)
The Henry W Lim Division of Photobiology and Photomedicine, Department of Dermatology, Henry Ford Health, Detroit, MI, USA
e-mail: iltefat@hamzavi.com

R. Sarkar, V. Narayan R (eds.), *A Concise Guide to The Management of Vitiligo*,
https://doi.org/10.1007/978-981-95-3857-7_25

25.1 Future Research in Pathogenesis

25.1.1 Epidemiology of Vitiligo

Vitiligo is the most common depigmenting disorder, with prevalence rates typically cited between 0.5% and 1% of the global population, though regional variations exist. The largest study, conducted in 1977 on the island of Bornholm, Denmark, reported a prevalence of 0.38%. Prevalence rates as high as 8.8% have been reported in India, possibly due to chemically induced depigmentation or clinic-specific data. In contrast, the prevalence in the French West Indies' Black population aligns with rates observed in white populations. The highest incidence rates occur in India, Mexico, and Japan, with disparities in data, likely due to social and cultural factors that influence reporting. Vitiligo affects both sexes equally, though women may seek treatment more frequently due to greater social stigma. The disorder can develop at any age, but nonsegmental vitiligo typically appears between ages 10 and 30, while segmental vitiligo is common in younger individuals, particularly before age 10. Studies have shown that nearly 70–80% of cases present before age 30, with childhood onset affecting 32–37% of patients [1–4].

25.1.2 Genetic Advances

25.1.2.1 Emerging Genetic Insights and Predispositions

Individuals predisposed to oxidative stress and immune-mediated destruction of melanocytes are also predisposed to developing vitiligo. Vitiligo has a strongly reported polygenic risk [5]. Certain human leukocyte antigen (HLA) alleles with either increased or decreased risk of vitiligo have been identified and vary among different ethnic groups [6]. Vitiligo's risk attributed to genetics is estimated to be about 80%, while the remaining 20% of the risk is attributed to environmental factors [7]. There appear to be many ethnic differences in relevant gene loci associated with vitiligo risk; however, there are seven non-major histocompatibility complex (MHC) loci associated with vitiligo risk found across different ethnicities. PTPN22, IKZF4, and FOXP3 are genes involved in the disruption of T cell signaling in the pathogenesis of vitiligo. A protein tyrosine phosphatase encoded by the PTPN22 gene is one of these risk factors. This phosphatase is involved in T cell signaling and is a common risk factor for vitiligo and other autoimmune diseases among different ethnicities. FOXP3 is a known gene silencer of T regulatory cells. The IKZF4 gene is a multiethnic risk factor that also exerts this silencing effect [8]. Downregulated DDR1 genes coding for melanocyte adhesion proteins are associated with vitiligo due to their destabilizing effect on epithelial structure.

Other risk factors for vitiligo include HLA-A*33, HLA-Aw*31, HLA-DR4, HLA-DR7, and HLA-DQB1*0303. Meanwhile, HLA-A*09 and HLA-Aw*19 are associated with a lower risk of vitiligo and may serve as protective factors [8]. Recently, the expression of the circadian gene (BMAL1) was found to be significantly elevated in patients with nonsegmental vitiligo compared to controls [9]. Studies suggest that the circadian gene may be a useful marker for the early detection of nonsegmental vitiligo. BMAL1 is also associated with metabolic syndrome. Vitiligo patients have a higher prevalence of metabolic syndrome compared to patients without vitiligo [10].

25.1.2.2 Potential for Personalized Medicine Based on Genetic Profiling

Understanding the unique genetic circumstances underlying different patients' vitiligo through transcriptomics, phosphoproteomics, and metabolomics shows promising potential for reducing treatment side effects and enhancing treatment outcomes. Vitiligo is not a uniformly presenting disease; patients vary in disease site, spread, total body surface area, age of onset, recurrence, and response to treatment.

Scientists have started utilizing metabolomics to identify potential metabolic pathways involved in vitiligo pathogenesis. Elevated pyruvate and decreased histidine are strongly associated with increased vitiligo disease risk [11]. These two blood metabolites suggest that impairment of the ammonia recycling pathway is a potential mediator of disease progression in vitiligo. Caffeine metabolites were also identified as potential mediators in this study.

A single-nucleotide polymorphism in lymphoid protein tyrosine phosphatase, encoded by the PTPN22 gene, is associated with vitiligo [12]. This phosphatase was first identified in other autoimmune diseases and then studied to determine its involvement in vitiligo. Comparing phosphorylation site activity between vitiligo patients, patients with other autoimmune diseases, patients with both, and control patients may identify unsuspecting therapeutic targets. Utilizing phosphoproteomics may serve to elucidate the true etiopathogenesis of vitiligo, identify different pathway disruptions in different patient populations, and target treatment accordingly. Transcriptomics can identify varying transcription factors involved in the vitiligo disease process. Transcriptomics was used to create ViCEKb [13].

25.1.3 Immune Mechanisms

25.1.3.1 Latest Findings on Autoimmune Processes in Vitiligo

Vitiligo is commonly comorbid with autoimmune diseases, namely, autoimmune hypothyroidism [14]. Understanding the pathogenesis of autoimmune hypothyroidism may be insightful for researching vitiligo. A targeted genome analysis comparing people with vitiligo, autoimmune hypothyroidism, both diseases, and neither may reveal genes previously unassociated with vitiligo. Heat Shock Protein 70 (HSP70) remains a key player at the forefront of mapping out the pathogenesis of vitiligo. HSP70 is a damage-associated molecular pattern (DAMP) that is secreted by cells under stress. HSP70 is known to activate mature inflammatory dendritic cells, leading to depigmentation in vitiligo [8]. Serum and lesion levels of a DAMP called high mobility group box protein 1 (HMGB1) are also increased in vitiligo patients [15]. HMGB1 is released from keratinocytes and melanocytes under oxidative stress and is suspected to be involved in the pathogenesis of vitiligo. In type 1 diabetes, an autoimmune process comorbid with vitiligo, HMGB1 impairs Treg function through the regulation of receptor for glycation end products/toll-like receptor 4 (RAGE/TLR4)-dependent phosphoinositide 3-kinase-Akt-mammalian target of rapamycin (PI3K–Akt–mTOR) signaling [16]. Understanding the pathogenesis of similar autoimmune disorders can help us target the treatment of vitiligo. Reinstating functional Treg in vitiligo patients may promote repigmentation in vitiligo skin lesions [17]. Catecholamines are released in response to physical or psychosocial stress (vitiligo triggers) via the hypothalamic/pituitary axis, which leads to altered immune system regulation. Lipids have been suspected to mediate vitiligo for decades. Neuropeptide Y is increased in vitiligo lesions compared to unaffected skin [18]. Lipids, composing the cell membrane, are among the cellular components damaged by free radicals and oxidative stress. Fatty acids and sphingomyelin are proposed to be contributing factors to the disruption of melanin production, considering the link between metabolic syndrome, oxidative stress, and vitiligo. High-fat diets increase vitiligo risk, and studies have reported that vitiligo regression upon high-dose simvastatin treatment, likely due to their anti-inflammatory and immunomodulatory effects [19].

Nuclear erythroid 2-related factor 2 (Nrf2) plays a downregulatory role in melanogenesis but is also the first functional antioxidant to respond to oxidative stress [20]. Nrf2 is a transcription factor that binds to antioxidant-response elements (AREs) to promote the transcription of antioxidants. The Nrf2/ARE pathway is a therapeutic target for vitiligo treatment, with ginsenoside and Rk1 having a protective effect on melanocytes under oxidative stress [21]. Nonapoptotic-regulated cell death mechanisms, including ferroptosis, pyroptosis, necroptosis, oxeiptosis, and parthanatos, are being studied for their potential involvement in vitiligo melanocyte destruction, but the mechanistic pathways are unclear [22].

25.1.3.2 Future Targets for Immunomodulation

Current immunosuppressive therapies indicated in the treatment of vitiligo include topical steroids, calcineurin inhibitors, and oral pulse steroids; however, these treatments are expensive and limited in efficacy and durability. Richmond et al. found that the use of CD122 inhibitors depletes tissue-resident memory T cells (TRM) through the blockade of IL-15 signaling, which repigmented vitiligo skin lesions in mice, and called for trials of intradermal administration of CD122 inhibitors in human subjects [23]. Interestingly, TRM are a unique type of T cell in that they require free fatty acid uptake to remain in the skin; thus, targeting mitochondrial beta-oxidation of free fatty acids may deplete TRM in the skin and induce repigmentation [24, 25]. Exploiting exosomes unique to vitiligo patients may help us better diagnose and treat this disease. Exosome-targeted treatment is clinically effective in wound repair and scar healing, but its use in autoimmune skin diseases has yet to be studied. Future research might consider halting the secretion of exosomes, facilitating autoimmune dysfunction [26].

Fibroblasts, the most prominent cells of the dermis layer of the skin, maintain the skin's structural integrity, secrete signaling molecules, and regulate tissue metabolism. Recent studies utilizing single-cell RNA sequencing of different fibroblast subtypes revealed unexpected involvement in immune cell function, suggesting that fibroblast dysfunction may be involved in the pathogenesis of inflammatory skin disorders [27]. Research has shown that interferon gamma (IFN-γ) stimulation in vitiligo-specific fibroblasts triggers the cytokines CCL2 and CCL8 (known modulators of the vitiligo inflammatory response) via the Janus kinase-signal transducers and activators of transcription (JAK-STAT) pathway [28, 29]. Further, Peng et al. demonstrated a protective effect on fibroblasts and keratinocytes from oxidative stress through the administration of Lycium barbarum polysaccharide (LBP) in vitiligo mice by targeting the previously mentioned pathway [30].

25.1.4 Environmental Factors

25.1.4.1 New Research on Environmental Triggers

Vitiligo-linked Chemical Exposome Knowledgebase (https://cb.imsc.res.in/vicekb/) is a new tool launched in 2024 that is the first database to detail vitiligo's environmental triggers. This knowledge base includes chemicals found in agriculture and farming, consumer products, industry, intermediates, medicine and healthcare, natural sources, and pollutants [13]. A systematic flowchart of the goals of understanding pathogenesis is shown in Fig. 25.1.

25.2 Innovative Diagnostic Techniques

25.2.1 Biomarkers for Early Detection

There has been much work on different biomarkers in the blood, where changes can lead to a predisposition to vitiligo, primarily focusing on immune system dysfunction and oxidative stress pathways. While there have been established studies providing diagnostic impact of these markers, newer transcriptomics and gene sequencing data have further associated these claims. CXCL10 is a chemokine that plays a crucial role in the recruitment of T cells to the skin, promoting the autoimmune response that leads to melanocyte destruction in vitiligo [31, 32].

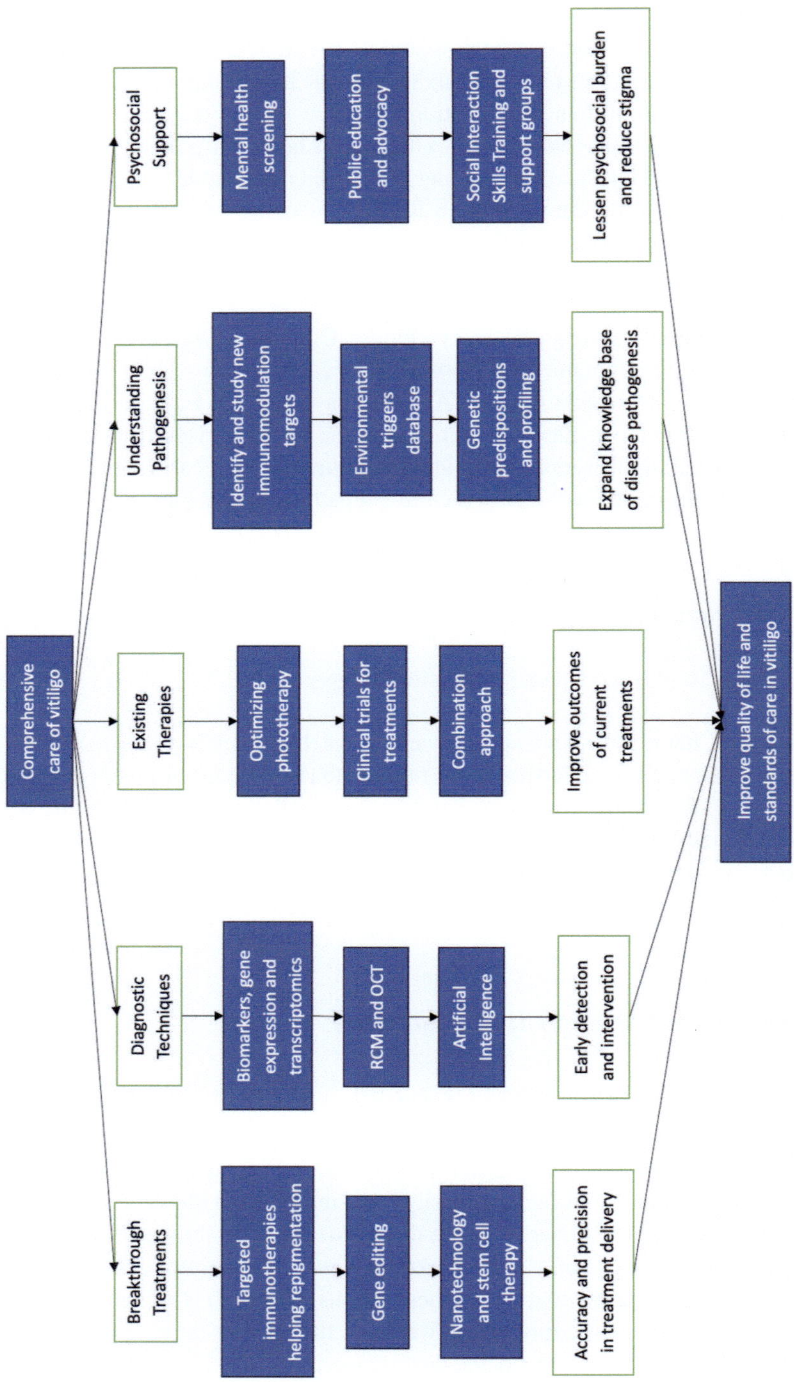

Fig. 25.1 Flow chart depicting a holistic approach to improving the quality of life and standards of care for patients with vitiligo

In 2024, research into vitiligo biomarkers advanced, with several showing promising potential for early detection and monitoring of disease progression. CXCL10, a chemokine responsible for recruiting T cells to the skin, has consistently demonstrated elevated levels in patients with active vitiligo. Recent studies reinforce its role not only in the autoimmune destruction of melanocytes but also as an indicator of disease activity, with potential for use as an early diagnostic marker. Clinical trials are exploring CXCL10's ability to predict flare-ups and guide immunomodulatory therapies [33, 34]. Furthermore, heat shock protein 70 (HSP70), known for its role in the melanocyte stress response, has been linked to the early stages of vitiligo development. Elevated levels of HSP70 in the skin and serum have been found to correlate with disease onset, and new research supports its potential as a target for early therapeutic interventions [35, 36].

Another biomarker gaining attention in 2024 is S100B, a calcium-binding protein that has shown elevated levels in vitiligo patients. This biomarker is closely associated with melanocyte damage and disease activity, and studies are evaluating its use in tracking disease progression. HMGB1 (High Mobility Group Box 1), involved in the inflammatory response, has also shown potential in identifying early melanocyte stress and apoptosis. Together with advanced gene expression panels like Fc receptor-like protein 3 (FCRL3) and T cell receptor (TCR), which can distinguish between different stages of vitiligo, these biomarkers are laying the groundwork for personalized treatment strategies that aim to intervene before extensive depigmentation occurs [34, 35].

25.2.2 Potential for Early Diagnosis and Intervention

Biomarkers in vitiligo hold significant promise for early diagnosis and intervention, especially as research continues to reveal more about the immune and molecular mechanisms underlying the disease. CXCL10, a chemokine involved in the recruitment of T cells, has been identified as a key player in the autoimmune response that leads to melanocyte destruction. Elevated levels of CXCL10 are frequently found in both the skin and blood of vitiligo patients, suggesting its potential as an early diagnostic marker that can identify active disease before widespread depigmentation occurs [33, 34]. Additionally, heat shock proteins like HSP70, which are secreted by stressed melanocytes, can serve as early indicators of cellular damage, signaling the onset of vitiligo and offering a window for early therapeutic intervention [35].

Recent transcriptomic analyses have also identified panels of genes associated with immune activation, such as FCRL3 and TCR, which differentiate responsive and nonresponsive vitiligo lesions. These genetic markers not only help in detecting early disease but also have the potential to guide personalized treatment strategies by identifying patients who may benefit from specific therapies [34, 35]. Furthermore, markers like S100B and HMGB1, which are associated with melanocyte damage and apoptosis, continue to show promise in monitoring disease activity and progression, making them valuable tools for both diagnosis and timely intervention [35]. These advances in biomarker research could lead to earlier and more targeted therapies, improving patient outcomes.

25.2.3 Advanced Imaging

In 2024, noninvasive imaging techniques made significant strides in the diagnosis and monitoring of vitiligo. Reflectance confocal microscopy (RCM) is gaining popularity for its ability to visualize the skin at the cellular level without the need for invasive biopsies. RCM allows for detailed examination of melanocyte density, providing valuable insight into disease progression and response to therapy. Studies have demonstrated that this imaging technique can effectively identify the loss of melanocytes in lesional skin, aiding in the early detection of vitiligo before it becomes clinically visible [37]. Additionally, RCM's high resolution enables clinicians to monitor melanocyte repigmentation during treatment, making it a useful tool for tracking therapeutic outcomes.

Another promising technique is optical coherence tomography (OCT), which provides real-time, cross-sectional images of the skin, allowing for the evaluation of both epidermal and dermal structures. OCT is being studied for its potential to assess the thickness of the epidermis and the integrity of melanocytes in vitiligo lesions. This noninvasive method can detect subtle changes in the skin's microarchitecture, potentially identifying early stages of the disease or predicting therapeutic responses [38]. The use of dermoscopy, which magnifies skin lesions, continues to be a widely used tool for assessing vitiligo, providing a clearer view of depigmentation patterns and perifollicular repigmentation. Together, these imaging modalities enhance the clinician's ability to diagnose vitiligo, monitor progression, and personalize treatment plans.

25.2.4 Use of Artificial Intelligence for Diagnostic Accuracy

Artificial intelligence (AI) is revolutionizing the diagnostic approach to vitiligo by enhancing accuracy and speeding up assessments. In 2024, AI-powered imaging tools were integrated with noninvasive techniques like dermoscopy, OCT, and RCM to automate the identification of melanocyte loss and disease progression. AI algorithms trained on large datasets of vitiligo images are capable of distinguishing subtle changes in skin pigmentation patterns, allowing for earlier detection of the condition. These tools not only reduce diagnostic subjectivity but also enable clinicians to predict how the disease will evolve over time, facilitating more personalized treatment plans [39–41]. Machine learning models are also being developed to analyze clinical data alongside imaging results to improve diagnostic accuracy. AI algorithms can process complex datasets, including patient demographics, disease history, and genetic information, to identify patterns associated with vitiligo onset and progression. This approach allows for the development of predictive models that can help determine which patients are at a higher risk of disease flares or non-response to treatment. Additionally, AI-based diagnostic systems enhance patient follow-up by providing more consistent and objective evaluations of therapeutic outcomes, improving the overall management of the disease [39–41]. This integration of AI into vitiligo diagnostics helps to streamline care, reduce costs, and improve patient outcomes through early, precise interventions. An upper-level breakdown of diagnostic methodologies is shown in Fig. 25.1.

25.3 Breakthrough Treatments

25.3.1 Targeted Immunotherapies

JAK-STAT inhibitors enhance Sonic Hedgehog and Wnt pathways crucial for pigmentation in the epidermis. Sonic Hedgehog signaling is key in the migration, proliferation, and differentiation of melanocytes. Janus kinase (JAK) inhibitors, such as upadacitinib, have demonstrated encouraging outcomes in trials. Upadacitinib notably led to substantial repigmentation in vitiligo patients, with a safety profile that supports its use for extended periods [42]. A notable initial case study reported successful treatment of vitiligo in a patient with atopic dermatitis and rapidly advancing vitiligo, achieving 90% pigmentation restoration on his face and neck within 4 months [43]. Since then, more studies have demonstrated that upadacitinib could offer a new therapeutic option for those affected by vitiligo, particularly at dosages that balance efficacy with minimized side effects [44].

Tofacitinib is a JAK 1/3 inhibitor that suppresses the autoimmune CD8+ and IFN-γ-dependent responses which attack melanocytes and lead to depigmentation [45]. Two percent tofacitinib cream twice a day in conjunction with narrowband ultraviolet B (NB-UVB) therapy thrice weekly demonstrated a mean improvement of 70% in facial Vitiligo Area Scoring Index (VASI). There was also a significant difference between facial and nonfacial lesions ($p = 0.022$). Ruxolitinib, a JAK 1/2 inhibitor approved by the Food and Drug Administration (FDA) for treating polycythemia vera and myelofibrosis, has been found to boost CD8+ cytotoxic T cell responses. A double-blind study using ruxolitinib cream at 1.5% BID showed the highest improvement rates, particularly noting that facial vitiligo responds better than nonfacial regions. A meta-analysis of individual patient data from case reports, series, and clinical trials revealed a positive repigmentation response in 57.8% of cases, which increased to 88.9% when JAK inhibitors were used alongside phototherapy [46].

Baricitinib, commonly used for rheumatoid arthritis, was noted to repigment vitiligo on the hands and forearms of a 67-year-old male who switched from toracitinib to baricitinib for arthritis treatment [47]. In a 36-week randomized trial, patients with active nonsegmental vitiligo were treated with either baricitinib or placebo in combination with NB-UVB. Baricitinib showed superior efficacy compared to placebo, with significant improvements in the total and facial VASI, including a −44.8% reduction in the T-VASI and a−65.2% in the F-VASI for the baricitinib group versus −9.2% and +4.2%, respectively, for the placebo group [48]. Lastly, while there are no studies directly linking anifrolumab with vitiligo treatment, the theoretical basis suggests that by blocking the type I interferon receptor, anifrolumab could help modulate the abnormal immune responses that lead to melanocyte destruction in vitiligo.

25.3.2 Gene-Based and Cell-Based Therapies

25.3.2.1 Advances in Gene Editing for Vitiligo

Gene therapy aims to directly alter the genetic makeup of cells to treat or prevent disease. In the context of vitiligo, gene therapy focuses on delivering genes that promote the growth and function of melanocytes, which are the cells responsible for producing melanin, the pigment that gives the skin its color.

25.3.2.2 Prospects for Stem Cell Therapy and Regenerative Medicine

The transplantation of healthy melanocytes has yielded encouraging outcomes for patients with stable vitiligo. Melanocyte-keratinocyte transplantation procedure (MKTP) is a grafting technique that involves the extraction of the epithelium from a donor site, preparation of the recipient area, and application of a cell mixture followed by wound dressing [49]. Various methods like cryotherapy, dermabrasion, and fractional lasers are employed to prepare the site, but carbon dioxide (CO2) fractional lasers have been recognized for providing a more consistent and controlled way to create the microinjuries necessary for the application of harvested melanocyte-keratinocyte cells [50]. The speed and extent of repigmentation vary, and not all treatments yield uniform results. MKTP has been well tolerated and effective, highlighting the need for more dermatologists trained in this specialized procedure [51].

Regenerative therapies for treating vitiligo have expanded to include stem cell therapy and cell-free modalities. A primary focus of stem cell therapy is the utilization of mesenchymal stem cells, specifically adipose-derived stem cells (ADSCs), and multilineage differentiating stress-enduring (MUSE) cells. ADSCs, explored in animal models, are notable for their antioxidant capabilities and their potential to modulate immune system responses, attributes crucial in managing vitiligo [52]. These cells have demonstrated properties that scavenge reactive oxygen species, offering a therapeutic advantage in vitiligo, where oxidative stress contributes to pathogenesis. Moreover, ADSCs can modulate the immune system by influencing the INF-gamma/STAT1 pathway, which in turn suppresses T cell proliferation—a primary driver of vitiligo activity.

Similarly, MUSE cells, which can be sourced from dermis and adipose tissue, have shown promise in ex vivo studies where they differentiate into fully functional melanocytes [53]. These advancements suggest a potential shift in how vitiligo can be effectively treated through innovative regenerative approaches.

Platelet-rich plasma is (PRP) a concentration of platelets in plasma that is known to be rich in growth factors such as platelet-derived growth factor, transforming growth factor, vascular endothelial growth factor, and epidermal growth factor. In the use of vitiligo, PRP can help promote the proliferation of existing melanocytes and enhance the migration of melanocytes from hair follicles to depigmented areas [54]. Furthermore, PRP may help in reducing oxidative stress in the skin. For enhanced therapeutic efficacy, PRP is often employed synergistically with ultraviolet (UV) light therapy, microneedling, and laser treatments, which augment the dermal penetration and biological activity of the infused growth factors [52].

25.3.3 Nanotechnology in Treatment

The prospective utility of nanotechnology in targeted drug delivery for vitiligo treatment encompasses enhanced dermal penetration, controlled release mechanisms, and precise targeting capabilities [52]. Nanoparticles have deeper skin penetration compared to conventional formulations, facilitating the delivery of therapeutic agents such as immunomodulators, growth factors, and antioxidants directly to the affected areas [55]. Extensive research has been conducted on liposomes, which serve as drug reservoirs, enabling the sustained release of medications and potentially reducing the frequency of administration. Additional nanotechnological strategies include microemulsions, ethosomes, lipid emulsions, lecithin organogels, and transferosomes [55].

Despite the promising potential of nanodrug delivery systems, concerns remain regarding their long-term safety and potential toxicity. These challenges underscore the need for continued research aimed at optimizing these delivery systems to enhance both their safety and efficacy [55]. Ongoing advancements in nanotechnology hold promise for revolutionizing dermatological treatments, with the goal of achieving more personalized and effective therapeutic interventions for vitiligo. A systematic breakdown of newer breakthrough treatments is shown in Fig. 25.1.

25.4 Enhancing Existing Therapies

25.4.1 Optimizing Phototherapy

In 2024, light-based therapies for vitiligo have seen notable advancements, particularly in the precision and efficacy of NB-UVB phototherapy. Innovations in targeted NB-UVB devices have allowed for more localized treatment of vitiligo patches, reducing the exposure of unaffected skin to ultraviolet light. This targeted therapy minimizes the risk of side effects while maximizing repigmentation, especially when used in combination with other therapies such as topical corticosteroids or calcineurin inhibitors [56]. Moreover, newer devices with enhanced precision are now equipped with dosimetry sensors that automatically adjust the intensity of ultraviolet B (UVB) light based on real-time feedback from the skin, ensuring that the optimal dose is delivered to achieve effective results.

Another innovation is the increasing use of excimer laser therapy, a form of light-based treatment that delivers highly focused UVB light directly to depigmented areas. In 2024, advancements in excimer laser technology improved both the accuracy and speed of treatment. This allows for more efficient sessions, especially for smaller, resistant vitiligo patches, while reducing treatment time compared to traditional NB-UVB therapy. Recent studies have shown that combining excimer laser therapy with cellular grafting techniques enhances repigmentation outcomes, making it a promising option for more localized vitiligo lesions [57, 58]. These advancements in light-based therapy are improving the efficacy of vitiligo treatment, offering patients faster and more targeted solutions with fewer side effects.

In 2024, combination therapies were increasingly utilized alongside phototherapy for vitiligo patients to enhance treatment outcomes. NB-UVB phototherapy remains the cornerstone of light-based treatments, but its efficacy is significantly boosted when combined with other therapies. For instance, topical agents such as calcineurin inhibitors (tacrolimus or pimecrolimus) or corticosteroids are frequently used with NB-UVB. This combination helps reduce inflammation and modulates the immune response, improving repigmentation rates compared to phototherapy alone. Studies have shown that adding these topicals to phototherapy enhances melanocyte migration and survival, leading to quicker and more sustained repigmentation in patients [57, 59].

Another promising combination is NB-UVB with systemic therapies, such as JAK inhibitors, which target the autoimmune aspect of vitiligo. JAK inhibitors like tofacitinib or ruxolitinib, when used alongside phototherapy, have shown enhanced repigmentation by interrupting the signaling pathways responsible for melanocyte destruction. Additionally, the combination of phototherapy with antioxidants such as *Polypodium leucotomos* extract is gaining attention. This combination helps reduce oxidative stress in melanocytes during phototherapy, thus preventing further damage and promoting repigmentation [60, 61]. These synergistic therapies not only accelerate treatment results but also improve long-term outcomes, offering more comprehensive approaches for managing vitiligo.

25.4.2 *Topical and Systemic Treatments*

In 2024, new clinical trials explored innovative topical treatments for vitiligo aimed at enhancing repigmentation and reducing depigmentation. One promising area of research involves JAK inhibitors, particularly ruxolitinib cream, which has shown encouraging results in clinical trials. This topical JAK inhibitor works by targeting the immune pathways responsible for melanocyte destruction, thus reducing the autoimmune response that causes vitiligo. Phase III trials have demonstrated that ruxolitinib cream can lead to significant repigmentation, especially on the face, making it a potential game changer for localized vitiligo treatment [60]. Early results suggest that JAK inhibitors may be more effective in combination with phototherapy, enhancing repigmentation outcomes when used as part of a comprehensive treatment plan. There are also promising results coming up for oral JAK inhibitors, which have been successful in phase 2 trials and are now in phase 3 trials. These are using the drugs ritlecitinib and upadacitinib. In the ritlecitinib trials, 364 patients treated with ritlecitinib, significant improvements in facial vitiligo were observed in the 50 and 30 mg groups compared to the placebo, with accelerated improvement in the 200/50 mg group during the extension period. No dose-dependent trends in treatment-emergent or serious adverse events were noted over 48 weeks [62]. In the upadacitinib trial, in 185 patients treated with upadacitinib (UPA) or placebo, upadacitinib 11 mg and upadacitinib 22 mg significantly improved skin repigmentation at week 24, with ongoing repigmentation observed through week 52. Serious treatment-emergent adverse events were more frequent in the upadacitinib 22 mg group, though most were unrelated to the study drug, and no new safety concerns were identified [63].

In addition to JAK inhibitors, clinical trials are investigating the use of topical antioxidants to protect melanocytes from oxidative stress, which is a key factor in vitiligo progression. One topical treatment under investigation is liposomal catalase, which targets oxidative damage in melanocytes. Early studies indicate that this antioxidant may slow disease progression and, when used alongside other treatments such as phototherapy, may promote faster repigmentation [31]. Moreover, new formulations of topical calcineurin inhibitors like tacrolimus are being studied for enhanced penetration and efficacy in treating vitiligo. These ongoing trials highlight the potential of combining immunomodulatory and antioxidant approaches in the topical management of vitiligo, offering hope for more effective and patient-friendly treatments. Lastly, a randomized placebo-controlled trial evaluated the efficacy of gliadin-protected superoxide dismutase (GP-SOD) combined with NB-UVB therapy for treating nonsegmental vitiligo. The study included 50 patients, and those receiving GP-SOD showed a significantly higher improvement in repigmentation (19.85%) compared to the placebo group (8.83%) [64].

25.4.3 Combination Therapies

In 2024, several new drugs beyond ruxolitinib were tested for the treatment of vitiligo, focusing on both immune modulation and melanocyte protection. One notable drug in clinical trials is adalimumab, an anti-tumor necrosis alpha (TNF-α) biologic commonly used in psoriasis. Adalimumab has been explored for its ability to modulate the immune response involved in vitiligo, with early trials showing the potential for reducing depigmentation by targeting inflammation, which leads to melanocyte destruction [65].

Another emerging treatment is afamelanotide, a synthetic analog of alpha-melanocyte-stimulating hormone (α-MSH). Afamelanotide works by stimulating melanogenesis, encouraging the production of melanin in the skin. This drug is being tested in combination with phototherapy to enhance repigmentation, particularly in difficult-to-treat areas like the hands and feet [59, 66]. Tofacitinib, another JAK inhibitor, is also under investigation for its systemic and topical applications, showing promise in improving repigmentation rates similar to ruxolitinib [67]. These new drugs are expanding the therapeutic landscape for vitiligo, offering hope for more effective, targeted treatments.

In 2024, several oral drugs were tested in clinical trials for vitiligo treatment, beyond topical agents like ruxolitinib. One promising class of drugs under investigation is JAK inhibitors, particularly tofacitinib and baricitinib, both of which are being studied for their oral formulations. These drugs work by targeting the JAK-STAT pathway, a key signaling pathway involved in the autoimmune attack of melanocytes. Clinical trials have shown that oral JAK inhibitors may improve repigmentation, especially when used in conjunction with phototherapy [68].

Another drug being studied for its potential in vitiligo treatment is nimodipine, a calcium channel blocker traditionally used for managing neurological conditions. Nimodipine has been found to have the potential to promote melanocyte survival and repigmentation in vitiligo patients. Early trials are examining its efficacy and safety as an oral treatment option [35]. Additionally, methotrexate, an immunosuppressive agent commonly used in autoimmune diseases, is also being evaluated at low doses for its ability to slow vitiligo progression, with studies focusing on its use in combination with other therapies like phototherapy or topical agents [69]. These oral drugs could offer systemic options for patients with widespread or treatment-resistant vitiligo. A layout for optimizing existing therapies is shown in Fig. 25.1.

25.5 Psychological and Social Support

25.5.1 Future Approaches to Addressing the Psychosocial Impact of Vitiligo

Vitiligo patients have varying and unique perceptions of their disease. Patients have different goals for their treatment based on their perceptions [70]. Providers have a duty to investigate patients' specific perceptions of the disease and treatment goals to assist patients in making informed decisions about their healthcare and treating them efficiently. For instance, a patient who views their vitiligo as a gift in making them unique and beautiful may not desire repigmentation therapy but rather choose to focus on comorbid mental health symptoms, whereas a patient who avoids social situations and feels shame/embarrassment due to their vitiligo may benefit more from repigmentation therapy in addition to mental health services [71]. Researchers highlighted the need for informed shared decision making and identifying treatment goals between disease stabilization and repigmentation, and the goal of mental health and self-acceptance may be a part of the patients' goals [72]. Evaluating both patient quality of life and percent skin repigmentation during vitiligo treatment may help providers address the psychological impact of vitiligo on their patients [73]. The vitiligo shared decision-making tool may assist providers in having these conversations with patients [74].

Vitiligo is significantly associated with depression, anxiety, low self-esteem, relationship and sexual dysfunction, and other mental health disorders [75]. Stigma largely contributes to the psychosocial burden of vitiligo. Ezzedine et al. suggest that educating the unaffected population may help destigmatize vitiligo because people who are educated on vitiligo are more likely to have positive attitudes toward people with the disease than those not as educated on the subject [75]. Educating the public, psychotherapy, and counseling for vitiligo are the current approaches to address the psychosocial needs of patients with vitiligo [75]. The concealment of vitiligo lesions through clothing, camouflage, and altered body movements is the most common coping mechanism reported by patients [75]. Perhaps if patients feel less of a stigma, they may have less of a psychosocial burden and feel less of a need to conceal their vitiligo.

The social interaction skills training (SIST) workshop was implemented in a group of vitiligo patients as a workshop opportunity aimed at helping people with visible differences improve their self-confidence and reduce social anxiety by reframing social interactions. Through cognitive behavioral therapy, lessons on coping mechanisms, role playing, and general self-help techniques, SIST helped improve social avoidance and distress up to 8 weeks after the workshop, providing participants with a sense of empowerment, new coping techniques, a sense of community, and increased social confidence [76]. These results are promising; however, the small sample size is limiting, and larger randomized controlled trials are needed to validate the findings.

25.5.2 Innovations in Patient Support and Counseling

Providers must be able to identify which demographics of vitiligo patients have the greatest risk of psychosocial burden: greater than 5% total body surface area, darker skin, and those with facial or hand lesions [77]. The VALIANT study found that more than half of the reported symptoms were consistent with depression, suggesting that depression is underdiagnosed in patients with vitiligo [77]. Research calls for efforts in reducing the psychosocial burden of vitiligo.

A longer disease duration is associated with worse quality of life reports. Early detection and referral to mental health services and support groups may intervene in exacerbating comorbid conditions [71, 75]. Providers should assess their patients' mental health in addition to their physical health to coordinate appropriate treatment of all symptoms, physical and mental. Studies have shown that while anxiety and depression are both common in patients with vitiligo, children with vitiligo have higher rates of anxiety than depression [78]. Providers should consider screening all vitiligo patients with the Patient Health Questionnaire-9 (PHQ-9) and General Anxiety Disorder-7 (GAD-7) to prevent underdiagnosing and undertreating comorbid mental health conditions, considering that early detection is crucial in many cases [71, 75, 79]. Providers may help their patients by recommending support groups for vitiligo and offering treatment beyond repigmentation therapies to include maintenance of mental health.

Patients who experienced vitiligo in childhood and who had adverse experiences related to the disease were more likely to have a worse quality of life in adulthood. Those patients suggested that more psychological support and interaction with other vitiligo patients may have attenuated the poorer quality of life outcomes [71, 80].

More research on support groups for managing the psychosocial burden of vitiligo is needed to further understand their efficacy and fill in gaps in care. In the meantime, Mahama et al. organized a list of support groups for physicians to share with their patients: Vitiligo Support International, Vitiligo Strong, VitFriends, Vitiligo National Foundation, Global Vitiligo Foundation, Speaking of Vitiligo! Blog, and MyVitiligoTeam [81–87].

Patients with vitiligo also report quality of life impairment due to sexual impairment and trouble with relationships [88]. Because sex is a sensitive subject for many patients, providers should initiate conversations to elucidate any sexual problems a patient may not be comfortable addressing on their own. This may allow patients to receive help regarding sexual dysfunction and improve their quality of life.

25.5.3 Education and Advocacy

25.5.3.1 Role of Patient Education in Future Management Strategies

Patient education can be utilized to help patients understand their vitiligo, triggers, treatment options, comorbidities and accompanying symptoms, and disease progression. Educating vitiligo patients on comorbid conditions, such as depression or autoimmune hypothyroidism, can aid in early detection and treatment. Physicians are typically able to detect symptoms on thorough physical exams, but depending on how frequent their visits are, patients should be aware of alarming symptoms and when to contact their physician.

Patients should have realistic expectations of the disease, and physicians can utilize shared decision making to determine a treatment plan that meets the patient's specific goals [72]. Providers should be aware of current treatment options for vitiligo patients' specific goals to help make treatment efficient.

25.5.3.2 Increasing Advocacy and Awareness to Improve Patient Outcomes

Insurance companies tend to view vitiligo as a purely cosmetic disease, creating financial barriers to treatment. This misconception further stigmatizes vitiligo and overlooks comorbid mental health conditions such as depression and anxiety. Vitiligo patients also have more prerequisites for insurance companies to assist them. Providers should be aware of these barriers and advocate for their patients [71]. Improving accessibility to treatment would improve patient outcomes.

Social media is increasingly serving as a medical information resource, undeniably influencing the population. Both dermatologists and nondermatologist social media influencers produce a range of content about different skin conditions. Videos with the hashtag "#vitiligo" have an average of 655,988 likes on TikTok and an average of 4330 on Instagram. Chandy et al. found that dermatologists produced primarily educational content, while nondermatologist social media influencers produced primarily promotional content; however, some overlap between the categories has the potential for the dissemination of misleading and false medical information [89, 90].

Social media health information reportedly influences almost half of American consumers' decisions to seek health care [91]. While many consumers continue to learn about skin conditions on social media, dermatologists can take advantage of this shift in consumerism and produce educational content on these platforms [92]. This would promote vitiligo awareness and the dissemination of accurate medical information [89]. Skincare and aesthetic dermatology are trending, and dermatologists could take advantage of this interest and partner with popular influencers to educate their followers on different skin conditions, worrisome symptoms, and preventative measures [92].

25.5.3.3 Mental Health Education with Vitiligo

Stigma is a significant mediator of discrimination and psychosocial burden in vitiligo patients. Assessing disease severity and visibility in visible skin conditions is not enough to measure the full emotional and psychosocial impact on the patient [93]. Asking about the patient's personal experience with stigmatization and discrimination is important to fully understand their condition [93]. Stigma around vitiligo has even been reported to be a barrier to employment, which can significantly decrease one's quality of life [79].

To ease the mental health burden of vitiligo, efforts must be made to destigmatize the disease and raise awareness. Effective destigmatizing strategies include education, contact, social activism, and increasing access to services and support [94]. Google trends showed an increased volume of searches containing the word "vitiligo" after Michael Jackson's death and, more recently, any time public figures with vitiligo make a public appearance [95]. Representation in the media increases awareness of vitiligo and is an important tool in destigmatizing. Populations with higher education on the nature of vitiligo tend to have more positive attitudes toward people with vitiligo, supporting the importance of public education of vitiligo [96]. The importance of psychosocial support is emphasized at a broader level in Fig. 25.1.

25.6 Research and Development Trends

25.6.1 Integrative Medicine

Vitiligo can be difficult to treat, requiring a long duration of therapy and follow-up to assess the clinical response. The therapeutic challenge of vitiligo can spark interest in pursuing alternative therapies. Patients may also perceive alternative therapies to be more natural and with less side effects than conventional therapies [97]. There have been studies that have assessed the efficacy of various alternative medicine treatments in the management of vitiligo, a few of which are mentioned here.

L-phenylalanine is an essential amino acid and precursor to tyrosine in the melanin synthesis pathway. Its uptake and turnover are important components in melanogenesis. [98] In several studies, its use was assessed in augmenting the repigmentation effects of phototherapy. Siddiqui et al. found higher repigmentation rates in patients treated with L-phenylalanine (L-phe) in conjunction with ultraviolet A (UVA) radiation in comparison to those treated with L-phe alone or without treatment [99]. Another study of treatment with L-phe in combination with topical 10% L-phe gel, 0.025% clobetasol, and a sunlight/UVA lamp found a 75% improvement in 68.5% of patients, with the greatest amount of repigmentation present on the face [100]. L-phe has been found to be safe with few side effects [98–100].

Other studies have explored the use of natural extracts and vitamins in the treatment of vitiligo. *Ginkgo biloba* is a Chinese herb that has been used to treat a wide range of conditions, such as anxiety, dementia, and cardiovascular disease [101]. Its use in the management of vitiligo has been explored in some clinical trials. In a prospective study, 12 patients treated with 60 mg of *Gingko biloba* twice daily were followed for 12 weeks. They were found to have improvements in the mean total VASI score, with the trunk and legs having the greatest response [102]. Several vitamins and minerals, such as folic acid, vitamin B12, vitamin C, and zinc, have been used in addition to sunlight or UV exposure in the management of vitiligo. In one study, nine patients with active vitiligo were given a vitamin cocktail of vitamin C 500 mg, vitamin B12 1000 m/μg, and folic acid 5 mg twice daily along with broadband UVB two to three times/week. Progressive depigmentation was halted in all of the patients, and repigmentation was observed within 8 weeks of treatment [103]. Despite the promising results of that study, another randomized trial of 27 patients sectioned into NB-UVB only and NB-UVB + vitamin B12 and folic acid groups found that repigmentation rates did not significantly differ between the two groups [104].

These studies offer promising results of the utility of alternative medicine treatments to augment conventional therapy, particularly phototherapy. There is an opportunity for further research on a larger scale to determine the safety and efficacy of these treatments in the management of vitiligo.

25.6.2 Long-Term and Longitudinal Studies

Vitiligo disease progression can be unpredictable, with relapses common, and treatment can be challenging. Long-term studies can help to understand the natural history of this disease and guide disease management. Focal vitiligo is characterized by patches in a small area that are not in the typical segmental distribution. [105] The possibility of progression to segmental and nonsegmental vitiligo is not yet fully understood, and it is unclear if focal vitiligo may be a precursor to more extensive forms of disease. One study followed patients with focal vitiligo for a mean time of 7 years and found that 23% of patients progressed to nonsegmental vitiligo, 77% remained with focal vitiligo, and none of the patients progressed to the segmental subtype [105]. There were no specific demographic or clinical markers identified that predicted the spread of depigmented lesions. This poses an opportunity for further research into the natural history of vitiligo disease subtypes.

In a prospective cohort study from China, patients were followed for 12 months to evaluate if clinical signs such as the Koebner phenomenon, the trichrome sign, and confetti-like depigmentation can predict disease progression. Patients with these clinical signs were observed as having longer lengths of disease progression and more active disease compared to patients without. [106] Further studies of biomarkers and clinical signs can provide more understanding of those who are at risk for disease progression and therefore impact treatment decisions. Given that vitiligo lesions can change greatly over time, further longitudinal studies are warranted to observe what factors impact lesion progression and persistence.

25.6.3 Collaborative Global Research

Vitiligo affects people worldwide, with treatments varying by geographical region [107]. International collaboration of researchers, patients, and healthcare providers can promote understanding of the disease by sharing insight into the treatment and natural history of vitiligo. The VALIANT survey study assessed healthcare provider (HCP) and patient perspectives on vitiligo management and included participants from 17 countries [107]. Although HCPs and patients reported similar treatment goals, over two third of patients reported feeling as if their vitiligo could not be treated. [107] This highlights the need for the development of clinical recommendations that can guide treatment for practitioners worldwide to provide better care for patients with vitiligo. This study also highlighted a diagnostic delay in vitiligo, with patients receiving a formal diagnosis of vitiligo 2.4 years after the first appearance of lesions. [107] Delayed diagnosis can worsen a patient's prognosis, as early intervention can help arrest the spread of depigmenting lesions. Future studies can aim to develop standardized clinical guidelines that can aid practitioners worldwide in the diagnosis of vitiligo.

The VITAL study aims to determine a standardized set of outcomes for vitiligo trials. It consists of a large group of international stakeholders, including patients, vitiligo experts, and researchers, and is currently ongoing. [108] International efforts to be on one accord with outcomes and measures can facilitate more efficient dissemination of research findings.

An international vitiligo task force developed a consensus statement on topical, systemic, and procedural interventions for vitiligo [109]. Due to the chronic nature of the condition and the need for long-term treatments, it is helpful to establish clinical guidelines that practitioners can follow to successfully manage the disease [109]. Vitiligo is a disease with a great psychosocial impact on patients; therefore, it is helpful to include patients in the development of tools to monitor disease progression and treatment response. In 2017, three workshops were held with patients to determine the assessment of clinical response and to define successful repigmentation [110]. They concluded that a standardized repigmentation scale should be used across clinical trials to better understand treatment response [110]. The aforementioned efforts of vitiligo experts worldwide have helped promote a global understanding of vitiligo's natural history, management, and diagnosis. Continued international collaboration will be crucial to developing more insight into this complex disease.

25.7 Conclusion

Vitiligo research and treatment are undergoing transformative advancements, as highlighted in this chapter. Technological innovations allow us to better understand the disease at the molecular level. As we learn more about vitiligo pathogenesis—particularly through insights into its genetic foundations, immune system dynamics, and environmental influences—the path toward personalized medicine becomes increasingly attainable. Revolutionary diagnostic techniques, such as novel biomarkers and advanced imaging, are transforming early detection and disease monitoring, while innovative therapeutic strategies, including targeted immunotherapies and nanotechnology-based treatments, aim to improve treatment outcomes. These advancements enable more precise and effective therapeutic strategies, including identifying distinct disease subtypes that may respond to personalized approaches.

Equally important is the commitment to addressing the psychosocial challenges faced by vitiligo patients. Comprehensive care extends beyond physical treatment to include mental health support and patient advocacy. Efforts to raise awareness, reduce stigma, and promote inclusivity will play a critical role in improving the quality of life for those living with vitiligo. By prioritizing both cutting-edge molecular research and comprehensive psychosocial support, we ensure that the future of vitiligo treatment addresses the full spectrum of patient needs.

References

1. Ezzedine K, Eleftheriadou V, Whitton M, van Geel N. Vitiligo. Lancet. 2015;386:74–84. https://doi.org/10.1016/S0140-6736(14)60763-7.
2. Ezzedine K, et al. Vitiligo patient population and disease burden in France: VIOLIN study results from the CONSTANCES cohort. J Eur Acad Dermatol Venereol. 2023;37:2249–58. https://doi.org/10.1111/jdv.19447.
3. Mastacouris N, Strunk A, Garg A. Incidence and prevalence of diagnosed vitiligo according to race and ethnicity, age, and sex in the US. JAMA Dermatol. 2023;159:986–90. https://doi.org/10.1001/jamadermatol.2023.2162.
4. Gandhi K, et al. Prevalence of vitiligo among adults in the United States. JAMA Dermatol. 2022;158:43–50. https://doi.org/10.1001/jamadermatol.2021.4724.
5. Spritz RA, Santorico SA. The genetic basis of vitiligo. J Invest Dermatol. 2021;141:265–73. https://doi.org/10.1016/j.jid.2020.06.004.
6. Hayran Y, Özge Ergen G, Özmen F. The relationship between non-segmental vitiligo, HLA genotype and oxidative stress. Int J Clin Pract. 2021;75:e14024. https://doi.org/10.1111/ijcp.14024.
7. Bergqvist C, Ezzedine K. Vitiligo: a focus on pathogenesis and its therapeutic implications. J Dermatol. 2021;48:252–70. https://doi.org/10.1111/1346-8138.15743.
8. Marchioro HZ, et al. Update on the pathogenesis of vitiligo. An Bras Dermatol. 2022;97:478–90. https://doi.org/10.1016/j.abd.2021.09.008.
9. Farag AGA, Badr EAE, Ibrahim AF. Circadian clock gene expression and polymorphism in non-segmental vitiligo. Mol Biol Rep. 2024;51:142. https://doi.org/10.1007/s11033-023-09109-6.
10. Sabir A, et al. Oxidative stress among subjects with metabolic syndrome in Sokoto, North. Western Nigeria. Niger J Clin Pract. 2016;19:128–32.
11. Yang S, et al. Roles of blood metabolites in mediating the relationship between vitiligo and autoimmune diseases: evidence from a Mendelian randomization study. Int Immunopharmacol. 2024;133:112132. https://doi.org/10.1016/j.intimp.2024.112132.

12. Cantón I, et al. A single-nucleotide polymorphism in the gene encoding lymphoid protein tyrosine phosphatase (PTPN22) confers susceptibility to generalised vitiligo. Genes Immun. 2005;6:584–7. https://doi.org/10.1038/sj.gene.6364243.
13. Chivukula N, et al. ViCEKb: vitiligo-linked chemical exposome knowledgebase. Sci Total Environ. 2024;913:169711. https://doi.org/10.1016/j.scitotenv.2023.169711.
14. Gill L, et al. Comorbid autoimmune diseases in patients with vitiligo: a cross-sectional study. J Am Acad Dermatol. 2016;74:295–302. https://doi.org/10.1016/j.jaad.2015.08.063.
15. Wei G, et al. Role of HMGB1 in vitiligo: current perceptions and future perspectives. Clin Cosmet Investig Dermatol. 2022;15:2177–86. https://doi.org/10.2147/ccid.S381432.
16. Zhang J, et al. Extracellular HMGB1 exacerbates autoimmune progression and recurrence of type 1 diabetes by impairing regulatory T cell stability. Diabetologia. 2020;63:987–1001. https://doi.org/10.1007/s00125-020-05105-8.
17. Klarquist J, et al. Reduced skin homing by functional Treg in vitiligo. Pigment Cell Melanoma Res. 2010;23:276–86. https://doi.org/10.1111/j.1755-148X.2010.00688.x.
18. Song H, et al. Association of stress-related disorders with subsequent autoimmune disease. JAMA. 2018;319:2388–400. https://doi.org/10.1001/jama.2018.7028.
19. Stamu-O'Brien C, Kroumpouzos G. The role of lipids in vitiligo and schizophrenia. Clin Dermatol. 2023;41:89–94. https://doi.org/10.1016/j.clindermatol.2023.03.007.
20. Baird L, Yamamoto M. The molecular mechanisms regulating the KEAP1-NRF2 pathway. Mol Cell Biol. 2020;40:e00099-20. https://doi.org/10.1128/mcb.00099-20.
21. Xiong J, Yang J, Yan K, Guo J. Ginsenoside Rk1 protects human melanocytes from H(2) O(2)-induced oxidative injury via regulation of the PI3K/AKT/Nrf2/HO-1 pathway. Mol Med Rep. 2021;24:821. https://doi.org/10.3892/mmr.2021.12462.
22. Chen J, Li S, Li C. Mechanisms of melanocyte death in vitiligo. Med Res Rev. 2021;41:1138–66. https://doi.org/10.1002/med.21754.
23. Richmond JM, et al. Antibody blockade of IL-15 signaling has the potential to durably reverse vitiligo. Sci Transl Med. 2018;10:eaam7710. https://doi.org/10.1126/scitranslmed.aam7710.
24. Pan Y, et al. Survival of tissue-resident memory T cells requires exogenous lipid uptake and metabolism. Nature. 2017;543:252–6. https://doi.org/10.1038/nature21379.
25. Pan Y, Kupper TS. Metabolic reprogramming and longevity of tissue-resident memory T cells. Front Immunol. 2018;9:1347. https://doi.org/10.3389/fimmu.2018.01347.
26. Yu H, et al. Exosomes: the emerging mechanisms and potential clinical applications in dermatology. Int J Biol Sci. 2024;20:1778–95. https://doi.org/10.7150/ijbs.92897.
27. Shi Z, et al. The role of dermal fibroblasts in autoimmune skin diseases. Front Immunol. 2024;15:1379490. https://doi.org/10.3389/fimmu.2024.1379490.
28. Martins C, et al. Vitiligo skin T cells are prone to produce type 1 and type 2 cytokines to induce melanocyte dysfunction and epidermal inflammatory response through Jak signaling. J Invest Dermatol. 2022;142:1194–1205.e1197. https://doi.org/10.1016/j.jid.2021.09.015.
29. Jin R, Zhou M, Lin F, Xu W, Xu A. Pathogenic Th2 cytokine profile skewing by IFN-γ-responding vitiligo fibroblasts via CCL2/CCL8. Cells. 2023;12:217. https://doi.org/10.3390/cells12020217.
30. Peng L, et al. Mechanisms of action of Lycium barbarum polysaccharide in protecting against vitiligo mice through modulation of the STAT3-Hsp70-CXCL9/CXCL10 pathway. Pharm Biol. 2023;61:281–7. https://doi.org/10.1080/13880209.2022.2163406.
31. Speeckaert R, Bulat V, Speeckaert MM, van Geel N. The impact of antioxidants on vitiligo and melasma: a scoping review and meta-analysis. Antioxidants (Basel). 2023;12:2082. https://doi.org/10.3390/antiox12122082.
32. Michetti F, et al. The S100B protein: a multifaceted pathogenic factor more than a biomarker. Int J Mol Sci. 2023;24:9605. https://doi.org/10.3390/ijms24119605.
33. Passeron T, et al. 624—Vitiligo biomarker CXCL10 correlates with clinical response in the phase 2 randomized, double-blind, vehicle-controlled TRuE-V mechanism of action study. Br J Dermatol. 2024;191:ljae266.008. https://doi.org/10.1093/bjd/ljae266.008.

34. Yang Q, et al. Vitiligo skin biomarkers associated with favorable therapeutic response. Front Immunol. 2021;12:613031. https://doi.org/10.3389/fimmu.2021.613031.
35. Speeckaert R, van Geel N. Vitiligo: an update on pathophysiology and treatment options. Am J Clin Dermatol. 2017;18:733–44. https://doi.org/10.1007/s40257-017-0298-5.
36. Mosenson JA, Eby JM, Hernandez C, Le Poole IC. A central role for inducible heat-shock protein 70 in autoimmune vitiligo. Exp Dermatol. 2013;22:566–9. https://doi.org/10.1111/exd.12183.
37. Wang HF, et al. A new assessment method of vitiligo by combination of dermoscopy and reflectance confocal microscopy. Clin Cosmet Investig Dermatol. 2023;16:3615–23. https://doi.org/10.2147/ccid.S432169.
38. Lu L-Y, et al. Feasibility of high-cellular-resolution full-field, artificial-intelligence-assisted, real-time optical coherence tomography in the evaluation of vitiligo: a prospective longitudinal follow-up study. Bioengineering. 2024;11:196.
39. Zhong F, et al. Optimizing vitiligo diagnosis with ResNet and Swin transformer deep learning models: a study on performance and interpretability. Sci Rep. 2024;14:9127. https://doi.org/10.1038/s41598-024-59436-2.
40. Guo L, et al. A deep learning-based hybrid artificial intelligence model for the detection and severity assessment of vitiligo lesions. Ann Transl Med. 2022;10:590. https://doi.org/10.21037/atm-22-1738.
41. Hillmer D, et al. Evaluation of facial vitiligo severity with a mixed clinical and artificial intelligence approach. J Invest Dermatol. 2024;144:351–357.e354. https://doi.org/10.1016/j.jid.2023.07.014.
42. Su X, et al. Efficacy and tolerability of oral upadacitinib monotherapy in patients with recalcitrant vitiligo. J Am Acad Dermatol. 2023;89:1257–9. https://doi.org/10.1016/j.jaad.2023.07.1016.
43. Pan T, Mu Y, Shi X, Chen L. Concurrent vitiligo and atopic dermatitis successfully treated with upadacitinib: a case report. J Dermatolog Treat. 2023;34:2200873. https://doi.org/10.1080/09546634.2023.2200873.
44. Magdaleno-Tapial J, et al. Upadacitinib and its role in the treatment of vitiligo: a new possible therapeutic perspective. JAAD Case Rep. 2024;46:57–8. https://doi.org/10.1016/j.jdcr.2024.01.033.
45. Liu LY, Strassner JP, Refat MA, Harris JE, King BA. Repigmentation in vitiligo using the Janus kinase inhibitor tofacitinib may require concomitant light exposure. J Am Acad Dermatol. 2017;77:675–682 e671. https://doi.org/10.1016/j.jaad.2017.05.043.
46. Aickara DJ, Patel S, Rosen J, Alonso-Llamazares J. Significant improvement of vitiligo with oral tofacitinib treatment. Int J Dermatol. 2023;62:e358–60. https://doi.org/10.1111/ijd.16323.
47. Mumford BP, Gibson A, Chong AH. Repigmentation of vitiligo with oral baricitinib. Australas J Dermatol. 2020;61:374–6. https://doi.org/10.1111/ajd.13348.
48. Seneschal J, Guyon M, Merhi R, Andreu N, Cazenave S, Ezzedine K, Mazereeuw-Hautier J, Passeron T. Efficacy and safety of the combination of oral Baricitinib and NB-UVB for the treatment of active vitiligo: results from a randomized, double-blind, phase 2 proof of concept study. JEADV. 2023.
49. Domaszewska-Szostek A, Polak A, Słupecka-Ziemilska M, Krzyżanowska M, Puzianowska-Kuźnicka M. Current status of cell-based therapies for vitiligo. Int J Mol Sci. 2023;24:3357. https://doi.org/10.3390/ijms24043357.
50. Yousif J, Ceresnie MS, Hamzavi IH, Mohammad TF. Practical guidelines for the treatment of vitiligo with the melanocyte-keratinocyte transplantation procedure. Arch Dermatol Res. 2023;316:10. https://doi.org/10.1007/s00403-023-02761-9.
51. Huggins RH, et al. Melanocyte-keratinocyte transplantation procedure in the treatment of vitiligo: the experience of an academic medical center in the United States. J Am Acad Dermatol. 2012;66:785–93. https://doi.org/10.1016/j.jaad.2011.05.002.

52. Bellei B, Papaccio F, Picardo M. Regenerative medicine-based treatment for vitiligo: an overview. Biomedicine. 2022;10:2744. https://doi.org/10.3390/biomedicines10112744.
53. Alanazi RF, et al. Multilineage differentiating stress enduring (muse) cells: a new era of stem cell-based therapy. Cells. 2023;12:1676. https://doi.org/10.3390/cells12131676.
54. Mercuri SR, Vollono L, Paolino G. The usefulness of platelet-rich plasma (PRP) for the treatment of vitiligo: state of the art and review. Drug Des Devel Ther. 2020;14:1749–55. https://doi.org/10.2147/dddt.S239912.
55. Qadir A, Ullah S, Jahan S, Ali A, Khan N. Drug delivery of natural products through nano-carriers for effective vitiligo therapy: a compendia review. J Cosmet Dermatol. 2022;21:5386–404. https://doi.org/10.1111/jocd.15158.
56. Bishnoi A, Parsad D. Phototherapy for vitiligo: a narrative review on the clinical and molecular aspects, and recent literature. Photodermatol Photoimmunol Photomed. 2024;40:e12968. https://doi.org/10.1111/phpp.12968.
57. Li C, et al. Comparison of various excimer laser (EL) combination therapies for vitiligo: a systematic review and network meta-analysis. J Dermatolog Treat. 2024;35:2302064. https://doi.org/10.1080/09546634.2024.2302064.
58. Kato H, et al. Excimer laser for the treatment of incomplete rerepigmentation 1 year after cultured epidermal autograft use for carbon dioxide laser-ablated lesions in patients with stable vitiligo. JAAD Case Rep. 2024;47:80–3. https://doi.org/10.1016/j.jdcr.2024.02.033.
59. Seong SH, Oh SH. Up-and-coming drugs for the treatment of vitiligo. Ann Dermatol. 2024;36:197–208. https://doi.org/10.5021/ad.24.038.
60. Sharma D, et al. Analysis of patient experiences regarding JAK inhibitors for atopic dermatitis, psoriasis, alopecia areata, and vitiligo. Arch Dermatol Res. 2024;316:630. https://doi.org/10.1007/s00403-024-03325-1.
61. Searle T, Al-Niaimi F, Ali FR. Polypodium leucotomos as an adjunct to the treatment of vitiligo. J Am Acad Dermatol. 2022;86:e65. https://doi.org/10.1016/j.jaad.2021.05.073.
62. Ezzedine K, et al. Efficacy and safety of oral ritlecitinib for the treatment of active nonsegmental vitiligo: a randomized phase 2b clinical trial. J Am Acad Dermatol. 2023;88:395–403. https://doi.org/10.1016/j.jaad.2022.11.005.
63. Passeron T, et al. Once-daily upadacitinib versus placebo in adults with extensive nonsegmental vitiligo: a phase 2, multicentre, randomised, double-blind, placebo-controlled, dose-ranging study. EClinicalMedicine. 2024;73:102655. https://doi.org/10.1016/j.eclinm.2024.102655.
64. Fontas E, Montaudié H, Passeron T. Oral gliadin-protected superoxide dismutase in addition to phototherapy for treating non-segmental vitiligo: a 24-week prospective randomized placebo-controlled study. J Eur Acad Dermatol Venereol. 2021;35:1725–9. https://doi.org/10.1111/jdv.17331.
65. Pala V, Ribero S, Quaglino P, Mastorino L. Updates on potential therapeutic approaches for vitiligo: Janus kinase inhibitors and biologics. J Clin Med. 2023;12:7486. https://doi.org/10.3390/jcm12237486.
66. Polańska A, et al. Afamelanotide in protoporphyria and other skin diseases: a review. Postepy Dermatol Alergol. 2024;41:149–54. https://doi.org/10.5114/ada.2024.138818.
67. Inoue S, Suzuki T, Sano S, Katayama I. JAK inhibitors for the treatment of vitiligo. J Dermatol Sci. 2024;113:86–92. https://doi.org/10.1016/j.jdermsci.2023.12.008.
68. Dong J, et al. Baricitinib is effective in treating progressing vitiligo in vivo and in vitro. Dose Response. 2022;20:15593258221105370. https://doi.org/10.1177/15593258221105370.
69. Gharib K, Ibrahim A, El Sharkawi Y, Elmegrab N, Attia M. Methotrexate gel either alone or combined with narrow band ultraviolet B or excimer light for the treatment of vitiligo. J Clin Aesthet Dermatol. 2023;16:32–6.
70. Kitchen H, et al. Meaningful changes in what matters to individuals with vitiligo: content validity and meaningful change thresholds of the vitiligo area scoring index (VASI). Dermatol Ther (Heidelb). 2022;12:1623–37. https://doi.org/10.1007/s13555-022-00752-8.

71. Mahama AN, Haller CN, Ahmed AM. Psychosocial considerations in the management of vitiligo. Clin Dermatol. 2023;41:82–8. https://doi.org/10.1016/j.clindermatol.2023.02.008.
72. van Geel N, et al. Worldwide expert recommendations for the diagnosis and management of vitiligo: position statement from the International Vitiligo Task Force Part 1: towards a new management algorithm. J Eur Acad Dermatol Venereol. 2023;37:2173–84. https://doi.org/10.1111/jdv.19451.
73. Bhandarkar SS, Kundu RV. Quality-of-life issues in vitiligo. Dermatol Clin. 2012;30:255–68, viii. https://doi.org/10.1016/j.det.2011.11.013.
74. Shourick J, et al. Development of a shared decision-making tool in vitiligo: an international study. Br J Dermatol. 2021;185:787–96. https://doi.org/10.1111/bjd.20137.
75. Ezzedine K, et al. Psychosocial effects of vitiligo: a systematic literature review. Am J Clin Dermatol. 2021;22:757–74. https://doi.org/10.1007/s40257-021-00631-6.
76. Tan A, Schuster LM, Robbins MA, Holavanahalli R, Pandya AG. Evaluation of the psychosocial impact of a Social Interaction Skills Training (SIST) workshop for patients with vitiligo: a pilot study. J Am Acad Dermatol. 2020;83:645–7. https://doi.org/10.1016/j.jaad.2019.11.037.
77. Bibeau K, et al. Mental health and psychosocial quality-of-life burden among patients with vitiligo: findings from the global VALIANT study. JAMA Dermatol. 2023;159:1124–8. https://doi.org/10.1001/jamadermatol.2023.2787.
78. Ucuz I, et al. Quality of life, emotion dysregulation, attention deficit and psychiatric comorbidity in children and adolescents with vitiligo. Clin Exp Dermatol. 2021;46:510–5. https://doi.org/10.1111/ced.14196.
79. Fakih A, et al. Stigma in vitiligo: associated factors and severity strata of the Patient Unique Stigmatization Holistic tool in Dermatology (PUSH-D) score. Br J Dermatol. 2024;190:712–7. https://doi.org/10.1093/bjd/ljae020.
80. Linthorst Homan MW, et al. Impact of childhood vitiligo on adult life. Br J Dermatol. 2008;159:915–20. https://doi.org/10.1111/j.1365-2133.2008.08788.x.
81. Vitfriends. Vitfriends. http://www.vitfriends.org/ (2024).
82. International, V. S. Vitiligo Support International. http://vitiligosupport.org (November 27, 2023).
83. VitiligoStrong. V-Strong Vitiligo Support Community. (2024).
84. Foundation, V. R. Vitiligo Research Foundation. vrfoundation.org (2024).
85. Foundation, G. G. V. *GVFC—Global Vitiligo Foundation*, https://globalvitiligofoundation.org/gvfc/ (2024).
86. UMass Chan Medical School. Speaking of vitiligo! Blog—Vitiligo Clinic & Research Center UMass; 2014.
87. MyVitiligoTeam. Vitiligo Support Online | Vitiligo Social Network. (2024).
88. Maamri A, Badri T. Sexual disorders in patients with vitiligo. Tunis Med. 2021;99:504–5.
89. Representation of skin of color in social media discussions on melasma, keloids, and vitiligo. J Drugs Dermatol. 2024;23:510–4. https://doi.org/10.36849/jdd.7716
90. Subramanyam C, et al. Visibility of board-certified dermatologists on TikTok. JMIR Dermatol. 2024;7:e46085. https://doi.org/10.2196/46085.
91. Park JH, Christman MP, Linos E, Rieder EA. Dermatology on Instagram: an analysis of hashtags. J Drugs Dermatol. 2018;17:482–4.
92. Campbell J, Williams K, Woolery-Lloyd H. DermTok: how TikTok is changing the landscape of dermatology patient education. J Drugs Dermatol. 2023;22:302–4. https://doi.org/10.36849/jdd.6676.
93. Paller AS, et al. Stigmatization and mental health impact of chronic pediatric skin disorders. JAMA Dermatol. 2024;160:621–30. https://doi.org/10.1001/jamadermatol.2024.0594.
94. Majeed T, et al. Anti-stigma interventions in low-income and middle-income countries: a systematic review. EClinicalMedicine. 2024;72:102612. https://doi.org/10.1016/j.eclinm.2024.102612.

95. Kluger N. The Michael Jackson and Winnie Harlow effect: impact on vitiligo awareness on the internet. J Clin Aesthet Dermatol. 2019;12:12–3.
96. Murshidi R, et al. Public knowledge and attitude towards vitiligo: a cross-sectional survey in Jordan. Int J Environ Res Public Health. 2023;20 https://doi.org/10.3390/ijerph20126183.
97. Poondru S, Yang LJ, Kundu RV. Use of complementary and alternative medicine in vitiligo: a cross-sectional survey. Arch Dermatol Res. 2024;316:126. https://doi.org/10.1007/s00403-024-02872-x.
98. Schallreuter KU, et al. Decreased phenylalanine uptake and turnover in patients with vitiligo. Mol Genet Metab. 2005;86(Suppl 1):S27–33. https://doi.org/10.1016/j.ymgme.2005.07.023.
99. Siddiqui AH, et al. L-phenylalanine and UVA irradiation in the treatment of vitiligo. Dermatology. 1994;188:215–8. https://doi.org/10.1159/000247142.
100. Camacho F, Mazuecos J. Oral and topical L-phenylalanine, clobetasol propionate, and UVA/sunlight--a new study for the treatment of vitiligo. J Drugs Dermatol. 2002;1:127–31.
101. Cohen BE, Elbuluk N, Mu EW, Orlow SJ. Alternative systemic treatments for vitiligo: a review. Am J Clin Dermatol. 2015;16:463–74. https://doi.org/10.1007/s40257-015-0153-5.
102. Szczurko O, Shear N, Taddio A, Boon H. Ginkgo biloba for the treatment of vitilgo vulgaris: an open label pilot clinical trial. BMC Complement Altern Med. 2011;11:21. https://doi.org/10.1186/1472-6882-11-21.
103. Don P, Iuga A, Dacko A, Hardick K. Treatment of vitiligo with broadband ultraviolet B and vitamins. Int J Dermatol. 2006;45:63–5. https://doi.org/10.1111/j.1365-4632.2005.02447.x.
104. Tjioe M, Gerritsen MJ, Juhlin L, van de Kerkhof PC. Treatment of vitiligo vulgaris with narrow band UVB (311 nm) for one year and the effect of addition of folic acid and vitamin B12. Acta Derm Venereol. 2002;82:369–72. https://doi.org/10.1080/000155502320624113.
105. Lommerts JE, Schilder Y, de Rie MA, Wolkerstorfer A, Bekkenk MW. Focal vitiligo: long-term follow-up of 52 cases. J Eur Acad Dermatol Venereol. 2016;30:1550–4. https://doi.org/10.1111/jdv.13663.
106. Zhang L, et al. Association of Clinical Markers with Disease Progression in patients with vitiligo from China. JAMA Dermatol. 2020;156:288–95. https://doi.org/10.1001/jamadermatol.2019.4483.
107. Hamzavi IH, et al. Exploring the natural and treatment history of vitiligo: perceptions of patients and healthcare professionals from the global VALIANT study. Br J Dermatol. 2023;189:569–77. https://doi.org/10.1093/bjd/ljad245.
108. van Geel N, et al. Vitiligo International Task force for an Agreed List of core data (VITAL): study protocol of a vitiligo core outcome set (COS) and contextual factors for clinical trials, registries, and clinical practice. Trials. 2022;23:591. https://doi.org/10.1186/s13063-022-06497-1.
109. Seneschal J, et al. Worldwide expert recommendations for the diagnosis and management of vitiligo: position statement from the international Vitiligo Task Force-Part 2: specific treatment recommendations. J Eur Acad Dermatol Venereol. 2023;37:2185–95. https://doi.org/10.1111/jdv.19450.
110. Eleftheriadou V, et al. International Initiative for Outcomes (INFO) for vitiligo: workshops with patients with vitiligo on repigmentation. Br J Dermatol. 2019;180:574–9. https://doi.org/10.1111/bjd.17013.

MIX
Papier aus verantwortungsvollen Quellen
Paper from responsible sources
FSC® C105338

If you have any concerns about our products,
you can contact us on
ProductSafety@springernature.com

In case Publisher is established outside the EU,
the EU authorized representative is:
Springer Nature Customer Service Center GmbH
Europaplatz 3, 69115 Heidelberg, Germany

Printed by Libri Plureos GmbH
in Hamburg, Germany